I purchased Dee's first book in a local health food store, and thought, "Well, I'll give it a try." I never expected it to change my life, but it did. I have been "eating healthy" per Dee's recipes and suggestions for the past two months. I have lost 12 pounds and feel much better than I have in a long time. I have more energy, and at 53, I feel as though I have the energy I had years ago. I also find I don't need to sleep as much as I used to. "Real food" tastes so good now. I no longer buy processed foods or anything with processed flours/sugars, and do not crave those things. The only sweets I crave are fruit......and occasional small bites of dark (organic) chocolate. I also make my own salad dressings (per Dee's recipes), and they are so good I no longer buy store brands. I can't say enough about this new way of eating, and new way of life. I am so grateful that Dee has shared her knowledge and experience through this book. Blessings to you, Dee, from a thankful customer in Arizona.
   —*Nonni Johnson, Phoenix, AZ*

A wonderful guest…an important topic (nutrition). We are being pelted with diets and views as to what to do. Dee McCaffrey has done it and that message carries with those looking to lose weight.
   —*Mike Bellamy, Radio Show Host*
   WKLB – DeKalb, Illinois

Within three days of following Plan-D, I noticed I had less arthritis pain. Within four months, I lost 65 pounds. It has been over two years now and my weight loss has remained steady at a wonderful 125 pounds! My skin is better, my hair is shinier and I no longer take allergy medication. I rave about this plan to my family and friends!
   —*Colleen Politi, Peoria, AZ*

I purchased Dee's first book after hearing several of Dee's podcasts through her website. I have gleaned so much information about nutrients in food and how harmful sugar and processed food is to our bodies. I started Dee's food plan a month ago not only because I am overweight but because my right hip and back hurt so much I had trouble sleeping. In order to climb stairs, I need to take them one at a time. Today my pain level is down probably 80% and I have lost 12 pounds. Following the food plan isn't hard, it just takes preplanning and a desire. The recipes are very tasty. Dee writes well and shares her life experience having lost 100 pounds 17 years ago. I like the fact that Dee is a chemist and nutritionist. She really knows her stuff.
   —*C.M. Cameron, San Jose, CA*

I did not know what feeling good was until I started following Dee's plan. I have been able to naturally lower my blood pressure and get off all prescribed blood pressure medications. Within three months, I not only lost 15 pounds, I found that I had more energy than I had in years. Now three years later, I have kept off 20 pounds and at 63 years of age, I still have the energy to work 16 to 18-hour days.
   — *Ted Alber, Tempe, AZ*

Dee's program taught me what "healthy" really means and why it is so important for us. I wake up every morning – excited to prepare my healthy meals and this enthusiasm is carried through the entire day! My husband gets excited just watching me be excited about our new way of eating and he enjoys every meal. We feel more energetic and I can't say how good it makes me feel being pregnant and knowing I am giving my baby the best chance in life to be healthy…Thank you, Dee for your commitment and may you touch many more lives.

— *Vanessa Kirk, Vancouver, B.C., Canada*

Dee is an inspiration to anyone who's trying to lose weight. I'm telling everyone I can about her.

— *Mary LeVan, Hammond, IN*

I lost 13 pounds in 12 weeks. I would highly recommend Plan-D to anyone who has tried fad diets that don't work and wants to make a healthy lifestyle change.

— *Marie Samaniego, Tempe, AZ*

Dee is awesome! Everyone ought to be listening to what she has to say about how to eat healthy and lose weight.

— *Cheryl Nuhn, San Diego, CA*

Dee is a living example of permanent weight loss and a warehouse of knowledge on which foods to eat and which to avoid. Her message cannot be missed.

— *Rossi Mako, Houston, TX*

Dee McCaffrey is a fantastic diet counselor. I have learned so much on how to eat healthier and I feel so much better. My cholesterol dropped from 250 down to 185 without any medications! People think they can learn all this on their own, but it would take years of reading and research to learn what Dee presents in the pages of Plan-D.

— *Barbara Randel, Scottsdale, AZ*

I need to tell the world of the inspiration you have been for me. Thank you, Dee!

— *Judy Matthews, Quincy, Ill*

Dee McCaffrey was the first person to offer me nutritional advice that made sense. Within eight weeks of following Plan-D, I went from 215 pounds down to 180 pounds, dropped two pant sizes and never felt deprived!

— *John Bogumill, Tempe, AZ*

I have wasted countless hours and thousands of dollars on weight loss courses or programs advocating prepared and packaged foods! They don't work in the long run and it's like turning your body over to food chemists. Dee McCaffrey *is* a chemist and her plan shows you how to get the chemicals *out* of your diet while enjoying healthful, tasty food.

— *Larry Koslow, Scottsdale, AZ*

I found Dee's program to be over-whelmingly life changing. No other health program has been so fundamental in its approach and so eye opening. It made me aware of the importance of nutritional education. Dee McCaffrey presents all the information in an interesting, informed and easy to understand format. I highly recommend Plan-D!
— *Janice Palermo, Phoenix, AZ*

Before starting on this program, I "craved" sweets of all kinds. After the first 2 weeks of being on Dee's program, I have not had any desserts of any kind and have absolutely no desire for them. In the first 3 weeks, I have lost 13 pounds and feel better than ever.
— *Phil Marsh, Scottsdale, AZ*

Taking Dee's program marked a change in my life. I finally got the TRUTH about how to eat healthy and lose weight. I used to feel helpless, but now I am empowered with this information. I also feel more energy than I ever have before.
— *Katheryn Anderson, Scottsdale, AZ*

Since starting Plan-D, I am down to 160 pounds from 205 pounds. I just wanted to say thank you so much and let you know that to me a 45 pound weight loss has changed my life so much. I dropped my cholesterol 60 points the all-natural way and have managed to come off all medication, including sleep meds. Life is good. It took me a while to wrap myself around all your knowledge, but I've put a lot of it to good use. Thanks again.
— *Teresa Moore, Scottsdale, AZ*

Dee McCaffrey and her program have changed my life. I have been sick for years with diabetes, high blood pressure, high cholesterol, etc. and the food style Dee promotes has led to less medication and controlled health problems.
— *Diana Dooley, Scottsdale, AZ*

The information you presented was excellent and presented in an easy to understand format. The reading material provided was comprehensive...I have lost 14 pounds since starting your program. I "feel" better and plan to continue.
— *Katie Martin, Mesa, AZ*

This is the most informative class in nutrition that I have ever taken. Dee explained everything so well. An eye-opener – may put many doctors out of work.
— *Ruth G., Scottsdale, AZ*

What an inspirational class! It taught my family and me how easy and tasteful it is to eat healthy. The best information I have ever received.
— *D.K., Scottsdale, AZ*

Dee's class helped me maintain a healthy weight gain in my third pregnancy. I felt healthier and stronger than I have in a long time. It is a lifestyle I will be able to follow for the rest of my life. And I feel great about leading my children to a healthier lifestyle. I would recommend this plan to anyone!

    — *Martha F., Scottsdale, AZ*

Taking Dee's class and learning her program has been one of the best things I have done for myself.

    — *Marjorie H., Scottsdale, AZ*

I am amazed and thrilled with the knowledge and health benefits I have received by taking this program. I have lost 22 pounds, feel amazing, have my husband eating the same way and feel this knowledge has changed me forever! God bless Dee and her desire to share her educated knowledge with others. Truly life changing. Please do more TV ... how about Oprah?

    — *B.D., Phoenix, AZ*

PLAN·D™

THE AMAZING ANTI-DIET™
That Will Change Your Life Forever

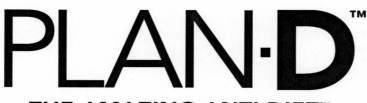

PLAN·D™

THE AMAZING ANTI-DIET™
That Will Change Your Life Forever

DEE MCCAFFREY, CDC

CENTER
FOR PROCESSED-FREE
LIVING
PUBLISHING

PLAN-D by Dee McCaffrey
Published by Center for Processed-Free Living
P.O. Box 27564
Tempe, Arizona 85285
www.processedfreeliving.org

Cover Designer: Jennifer Rose
Cover Photograph: Paul Markow

For those who share my experience.....
and for those who, after reading this book, may never have to.

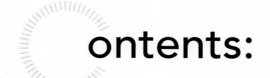ontents:

Preface

Plan-D is the anti-diet. When I tell people that I repeatedly failed at dieting for the majority of my life, but eventually claimed victory over my lifelong battle with obesity, the first question I am asked is "What did you do?" Most expect me to name a popular weight loss program or surgery, but the answer is deeply personal and intrinsically richer than expected. By disposing of my diet mentality and reaching beyond the conventional approaches to nutrition, I uncovered the true answer to weight loss and optimal health. I learned that true health doesn't come from a diet, a supplement, or a surgery. By simply eating foods in the form that our bodies are designed to eat them, thereby eliminating processed foods from my life; I released 100 pounds and have kept them off for nearly seventeen years.

Since then I have been guiding people of all ages and walks of life in their own quest for permanent weight loss and long-term health. As a chemist, nutrition educator and diet counselor, I am on a personal mission to transform the way our nation approaches food, health, eating, and weight loss. By taking a holistic approach to address the root cause of ill health—my own and subsequently the health of others—I developed a *way of eating for life*—not a diet—called *Plan-D*.

One evening in the fall of 2004, I was conducting a nutrition lecture at a local grocery store. Afterward, a middle-aged woman from the audience approached me and exclaimed, "That was amazing! You need to put all of that information into a book." It was the first time in her life she had ever heard that whole natural sugar cane contains an abundance of vitamins and minerals that actually *nourish* the human body if consumed in its whole natural state. She was astounded to learn that the most abundant mineral in the natural sugar cane is calcium—and it is that very calcium which is required by the human body to properly digest sugar. No doctor had ever told her that improper digestion of sugar leads to a number of common diseases. By listening to the lecture, she made the connection that her osteoporosis—a degenerative disease stemming from calcium-deficient bones—was most likely due to the fact that her flour and sugar-laden diet was leaching the calcium from her bones, rather than from a lack of calcium in her diet. Uncomfortably overweight, she was enlightened to the wisdom of our not-so-distant ancestors—that eating foods in their closest to natural form is the true path to sustained weight loss, and in fact the remedy for almost any "dis-ease."

In response to this woman's initial request, and with the support and encouragement of my partner and husband Michael, I wrote my first book—a cookbook titled *Dee's Mighty Cookbook: Tasty Cuisine for Flourless and Sugarless Living.* The premise for the cookbook was twofold: to educate readers on the health effects of eating refined white sugar and flour and to provide them with easy to follow recipes as a practical way to transition to a sugar-free and flour-free lifestyle.

In addition to the tasty and easy to prepare recipes, the book contained two chapters outlining what the astounded woman had heard in my lecture. "What's So Bad About Sugar and Flour?" detailed the reasons why white flour and white sugar are at the top of my list of *substances* that should never be ingested by the human body. "The Six Most Important Foods For Good Health and Weight Loss" assisted readers in finding suitable replacements for white flour and sugar in their diets. The chapter explained to readers the value of including these most essential foods into their lifestyle. A third chapter related my own personal struggle with food and weight, and how I was able to transform from an obese junk-food junkie into a slim, trim nutrition savvy expert. On the back cover of the book I invited readers to connect with me via e-mail to share their experiences with the recipes and improvements in their health.

Despite my own commitment to this lifestyle, I released the book with a bit of trepidation as to whether the American public was ready to embrace the idea that refined white sugar and flour really are the bane of weight loss and good health. However, my doubts were immediately allayed when suddenly people from all over the country and all walks of life sent me their success stories after following the simple guidelines outlined in the cookbook. To date, our self-published cookbook has sold over 7,000 copies.

Shortly after the release of the cookbook, I developed an eight-week weight loss course called *Health From the Heart* designed to educate people on how to implement the principles of flourless and sugarless living. The content of the eight-week class was the inception for *Plan-D.* The course included my then unnamed eating plan, with recipes and menu guidelines. Each week I explained the science behind the individual components of the plan, and also gave a cooking lesson featuring recipes from my cookbook so that students could see how easy it is to prepare healthy food and taste for themselves the delicious cuisine. Participants in the classes raved over the food, not to mention the success of their weight loss by following the plan.

At the same time, a natural food market chain picked up the cookbook and still to this day regularly features my lectures in their stores throughout the Southwest. Positive reviews appeared on Amazon.com, on-line cookbook review websites, and diet blogs. Feature stories in national magazines such as *Quick and Simple Magazine,* and *Obesity Help Magazine* catapulted my simple cookbook into the national spotlight. I landed regular cooking segments on local network channels, featuring favorite recipes from the cookbook. As a sought after nutrition and weight loss expert, *Woman's World Magazine* featured my advice in several of their articles on healthy food products and cooking.

Due to the sheer number of e-mails I received, I could not keep up with them all, so Michael established a message board on our website for people to post questions and get answers in a broad forum. We also created a podcast show called "Diet Science", which allowed me to expand on many of the topics from the book. We offered scientific nutritional information on current health related topics in a fun and informative format as a way to educate the public. The "Diet Science" Weekly podcast became so popular that it was nominated by Podcaster News as the best podcast in the Health and Fitness category for its straight talk nutritional information. The e-mails and message board postings from Diet Science listeners and followers of the cookbook gave me the opportunity to personally connect with individuals all over the world. As a result, I have been blessed with many new friends and followers.

As I heard from people around the globe, one thing became clear: they were hungry for the truth about food and they wanted and needed more. Many wanted more in-depth information about what is and isn't safe to eat. Some craved more science, while others just wanted new recipes and advice on new food products. Many asked for specific portion guidelines, and how much of each type of food to eat each day. They wanted daily and weekly menu plans, gluten-free ideas, and nutritional analyses of the recipes. They wanted to know which vitamins and supplements to take, what type of water to drink, where to find healthy food products, how to stock a healthy pantry, and what to do when you go out to eat. In other words, they wanted *Plan-D*.

All of this unexpected attention, however, did more than just spotlight the concept of flourless and sugarless cooking. It was the beginning of a growing movement that has since been coined "Processed-Free Living." Processed-Free Living is an individual's enlightened and staunch desire to avoid, as much as possible, the more than 3,000 synthetic chemicals that are added to the foods most Americans eat each day. These chemicals have shaped the landscape of America's food supply and include flavor enhancers, stabilizers, preservatives, colorings, hormones, antibiotics, artificial sweeteners, trans-fats and pesticides, just to name a few!

It is astounding that, in the name of science, we as a nation blindly and tragically denounced many of our traditional real foods as unhealthy, and replaced them with synthetically made chemicals. Out of fear of rising cholesterol levels and heart disease, we swapped real eggs for Eggbeaters and real butter for margarine. At the same time we added significantly more white sugar and white flour to our diets. Most recently we traded white sugar for an even more processed sweetener called high fructose corn syrup (HFCS). Studies show that metabolism of HFCS elevates triglyceride levels and promotes a serious health condition called fatty liver. Traditional wisdom and sheer intuition would tell us that not only does it not make sense to replace real food with chemicals; it simply cannot be sustained.

In an interview printed in the January/February 2007 issue of *Experience Life*

Magazine, wellness and weight loss expert Mark Hyman, MD points out:

> Healthy eating is about respecting how our bodies are designed. There are some foods our bodies naturally thrive on, and others that tend to make us sick and fat. At core, we're all designed to eat real food. By that, I mean foods without labels that haven't been highly processed, that aren't foreign to our DNA—essentially, whole foods that derive as directly as possible from the natural world.

> The foods most of us thrive on include unprocessed fruits and vegetables; beans and legumes; nuts and seeds; and lean, free-range, wild or pasture-raised animal proteins, including eggs and wild fish like sardines and salmon. These are the foods our bodies are designed to optimally function on and that support both good health and proper body composition.

Making the decision to eat processed-free foods can sometimes seem confusing and daunting. If you've ever wondered whether Newman's O's are really better for you than Oreos, you're not alone. Recognizing the need to provide affordable nutrition education to both young and old, in 2007 Michael and I established a non-profit organization called *The Center For Processed-Free Living*. The Center for Processed-Free Living is committed to providing education, support services, and an environment that supports living without processed foods—thereby helping to eliminate childhood and adult obesity. Its mission is to offer a sustainable, healthy lifestyle based on accurate scientific data where people of all ages can discover the personal power to improve health, lose weight and keep it off. Proceeds from the sale of this book and related products go toward the programs offered by The Center.

Plan-D is the culmination of the work we have been doing over the past several years, which includes the testimonials and success stories of people who have experienced weight loss and improved health by following its tenets. Our mailing list numbers in the thousands, and I know you will feel encouraged to begin *Plan-D* by reading some of the inspiring stories that people who are just like you have sent me.

The first part of the book introduces/reintroduces you to me. I will tell you my own personal health and weight loss journey—the struggle and eventual triumph—and will delve into the specifics of how I overcame my love affair with fast foods, donuts, and chocolate. I will also tell you what I have learned over the years since then about how the chemicals in those foods were probably more responsible for my weight problem than I ever realized.

I will recap the dangers of flour and sugar with a more in-depth explanation of the delicate balance between what we eat and how it ultimately affects our health. You will learn of two amazing nutritional studies that formed the basis for *Plan-D*, as I draw heavily upon my science background to illustrate and emphasize the importance of eating foods in their most closest to natural form.

Then we move on to the components of *Plan-D*. You'll learn the importance of reading ingredients lists, and discover the names of hidden food ingredients in so-called healthy foods that actually make you sick and fat. The world of fats and oils will be demystified, and you'll understand why low fat diets can be dangerous. I'll explain why the National Academy of Sciences has declared that there is *no safe amount* of trans-fat, and that if there is one thing you do to improve your health, it is to eliminate this devastating artificial oil from your life. The importance of eating organic foods is outlined, and I will explain how you can easily eat organic foods while remaining within your food budget.

Next, the specifics of *Plan-D* are outlined in detail. As most of the students in my classes have heard me emphasize, "The amount of vegetables you eat is directly proportional to the amount of weight you will lose and the amount of health you will gain." *Plan-D* emphasizes fresh vegetables and fruits, beneficial fats and oils, whole grains, lean protein sources, and of course water! You'll also discover that exercise, rest, relaxation, a positive attitude, and journaling are essential components of *Plan-D*.

You will find all of the information you have been asking for: weekly menus with portion guidelines and helpful cooking tips (like the best way to steam vegetables without losing nutrients) and I have included fifty new *Dee*-licious recipes. You'll also discover that eating processed-free is doable in restaurants if you're choosy and ask the right questions, and that traveling and staying in other's homes is easier than you think. I have also included a glossary and a list of resources where you can find more information about some of the studies, ideas, and products mentioned in this book.

There has been a wealth of questions posted on my message board over the years concerning *Plan-D* and other nutrition and health concerns. My research into the answers has been intriguing and enlightening, therefore the final part of the book is a compilation of the "best of" those questions and my honest answers. It is my intention to provide you with the straight truth about the food supply, and how to take nutritional responsibility for your own health.

It is important to point out that the word *diet* comes from the Greek word *dieta*, which means "discipline" or "way of living." The Latin root of the word means "a day's journey." I encourage you to approach adopting *Plan-D* as a process to be taken one day at a time. The key is to make real changes—changes you can live with successfully on a long-term basis—in the way you approach food, fitness, and the challenges and opportunities of living.

Each of the individual stories that you read in this book illustrate how each person's experience with *Plan-D* is unique. I've taken the liberty of modifying one of my favorite passages from the book *If the Buddha Came to Dinner* by Halé Sofia Schatz to encourage you along your own path to health:

> I invite you on a journey of inner growth through feeding yourself with great intention, care, and love. A true journey can't be made in a day, a week, or even eight weeks. Likewise, *Plan-D* isn't a quick fix-it diet program; it's a slow, steady, lifetime process. On this journey, there are a few rules—such as making the commitment to care for yourself on many levels—but there is no "getting it right." A Buddhist monk once told his

students: "There is no good meditation; there is no bad meditation; there is just meditation." So if you fall back into old unhealthy food patterns one day, then gently bring yourself back to center the next day, or even with the next bite. No big deal. Because your experience with *Plan-D* is *your* process, it will be uniquely your own.

Finally, while my own journey has been personal and unique, at the very core I am just like you. I have been there—100 pounds overweight, unhealthy and in the depths of hopelessness. If I can change, so can you.

My intention now is to use my experience to create a space for change; to educate and enlighten you on the value of proper nutrition, and to guide you in your transition to processed-free living. Welcome to *Plan-D*. Welcome home.

—*Dee McCaffrey*

Acknowledgments

Writing this book has been my dream for at least ten years. As I am certain most books do, it started as a completely different concept, which has evolved and come together over the years into a significant and special endeavor. At times it felt like an arduous chore, and I often wondered if I could actually ever finish it. In my head, I knew exactly what I wanted to say, but getting it out of me and onto the page proved to be more challenging than I ever realized. To make matters more difficult, the world of nutrition is so vast and ever changing, it took great restraint and discernment to stay focused on my original topics. In the end, a familiar quote has proven true—*God does not call the qualified, He qualifies the called.* This book is exactly what it is supposed to be—a message of health that I have been called and entrusted to carry.

Just as I did not lose 100 pounds on my own, there have been many people who have supported my dream and helped me write this book. First, this book and all its related enterprises would not be possible without the enormous support, creativity, dedication and unconditional love of my husband and partner Michael. You are my greatest teacher, my biggest fan, and the man of my life. I am forever grateful for your unwavering belief in me—it has kept me going when I didn't believe in myself.

The following people round out my literary gratitude list:

- Bob Cash, for taking precious time out of your busy life to meticulously proof and edit my words. I am privileged to have your literary expertise and honored by your belief in me. Your exquisite skills brought this book to life and fashioned me into a stellar writer. Any author would be grateful to be privy to your extraordinary talent and knowledge.

- Mary James, the unsung soldier for Plan-D. Thank you for the dozens of hours spent researching topics, re-writing articles, organizing my notes, creating charts and appendices, interviewing testimonials, and for your selfless dedication to the work. Your friendship, feedback, and admiration mean more to me than you will ever know.
- Bronwyn Marmo, for your guidance and assistance with securing endorsements, for coaching me through my fears so that I could see my worthiness and credibility for writing this book. Your shining example has been the glowing light at the end of my two-year long dark tunnel. Thank you for trudging this road before me, for willingly sharing your knowledge of the book biz, and for your clear demonstration of courage, integrity, and commitment.
- Jerry Bolfrass, whose culinary expertise, enthusiasm and charisma infused our test kitchen with high energy and fierce love for cooking. Thank you for your contributions in making the Plan-D recipes exciting and tasty. I value and treasure your loyalty and friendship.
- Martee Mann, who meticulously and carefully worked up the nutritional analyses on my recipes and for enthusiastically preparing many of them in our test kitchen. Your love for healthy cooking is inspirational.
- My mother and truest friend Carol, who instilled humble greatness in me through your own steady example, and who taught me that with God all things are possible. I am grateful that while I was growing up you shared and demonstrated the wisdom contained in the Edgar Cayce readings; as an adult it proved to be an invaluable lesson. A mother's love is like no other, and yours has carried me through the best and toughest of times. Thank you for always believing in me.
- My sister Rene, who is my closest friend and most treasured gift. Thank you for never hesitating to tout your horn about my plan to your friends and colleagues. I am deeply grateful for your caring and supportive nature.
- My brother Derek, whose decision to become a vegetarian continues to impress and inspire me. Distance and time have not kept me from noticing how much you love and support me.
- My father John and his wife Sophia, whose love and support were instrumental on my journey from obesity to health. You are forever and always in my heart.
- My husband's endearing family, his brother John and wife Brenda McCaffrey, and his mother Winnie McCaffrey, who have provided enormous support for this project in numerous significant ways. Words cannot express our deep appreciation and gratitude for your thoughtfulness and love—it makes us weak in the knees and bring tears to our eyes just thinking about it.
- Rossi Mako, who before I ever wrote my first book, affirmatively declared that I would publish three books before I reach the age of fifty. Your unbelievable friendship, support, encouragement, wisdom, and unconditional love set me on the path toward manifesting that reality. Thank you for walking alongside me through the peaks and valleys of my life and for holding me accountable to what I know I am capable of.

- Francene Adcock, who lovingly teaches me what it means to be courageous, honest, willing, and true to my dreams. Your friendship is a gift to my spirit. It is a joy to have you by my side in laughter, tears, and service. I am truly blessed to have you in my life.
- Jeanne MacLaughlin, who cast a new light on the meaning of integrity. Thank you for reminding me of who I am and what I am here for. Your invaluable coaching during the final lap of writing helped steer this book to completion.
- Lorrie Henry, who reminded me that my experience is the only credential I need.
- My support network, which continues to help me with my food and life choices. I would not be where I am today had it not been for the selfless service of those who trudged this road before me and beside me.
- My faithful supporters, followers, podcast listeners, message board members, clients and students, whose e-mails, contributions, recipes and testimonials have inspired me to complete this project. Thank you for the specialness you have brought to my life. I wish you all the best of health.

My deepest gratitude goes to the Great Creator, the deity I call God, who lifted me from the depths of despair and reawakened me to life. Your compassionate love empowered me to transform an otherwise shameful and demoralizing life experience into a purpose driven medium for helping others, and myself, stay on a path of health and healing. May I do your will always.

Introduction

What moves [individuals] of genius, or rather what inspires their work, is not new ideas, but their obsession with the idea that what has already been said is still not enough.
   —Eugene Delacroix

Plan-D is designed to enable your body to function at its optimal level. This is not a new concept, however health is still a mystery to most people. While there is a wealth of information available to us, we have only just begun to make a dent in our collective awareness about the healing properties of whole foods.

In my world, healthy eating is commonplace, and the information contained in this book is old news to me. It has all been written before by many others, perhaps more eloquently than I will present it here, however I wish to cast new light on an age old wisdom—*eating foods in their closest to natural form is the true path to sustained weight loss, and in fact the remedy for almost any health problem.*

One of the first things my nutrition students learn is that foods made with refined white sugar and white flour are the bane of weight loss and good health. Then they learn of all the other substances in the typical American diet that also compromise our body's ability to sustain health. In the past 50-100 years, our food supply has changed—*dramatically.* We have gone from growing, harvesting, and preparing our own food with our own hands, to mass-producing concoctions that are made in food laboratories. Refined sugar, white flour, artificial sweeteners, trans-fats, chemical preservatives, flavor enhancers, and stabilizers have replaced the real foods that our not-so-distant ancestors ate. We've become so far removed from foods in their natural state, that we now call them "health foods, " a sad admission that we've compromised our health for the sake of convenience. This brings up a disturbing question: If food in its natural state is considered health food, what does that make the rest of the food most people eat—*disease-food*?

Apparently so. The state of human health the world over is worse than ever before seen in human history. American fast-food chains have traversed the oceans into the most remote and developing countries, and as a result, obesity has become an international scourge. In America, we have been conditioned to believe that severe degeneration of our bodies is a natural consequence of aging. The number of seniors suffering from diseases of "old age" such as arthritis, osteoporosis, macular degeneration, hearing loss, and Alzheimer's, is staggering. While our modern technology has greatly extended our human life span, the quality of that life in our golden years has significantly declined. Too many of our elders spend their remaining years in assisted living facilities being cared for by people who don't really care for them.

The "old age" diseases are no longer reserved for the elderly. The baby boomers (people born between 1946 and 1954) and my generation, known as "Generation Jones" (people born between 1955 and 1964) have them too, in addition to cornering the market on widespread obesity. Simply being overweight isn't necessarily what's killing these generations—it's the diabetes, cancers and heart disease linked to being overweight that claim their lives before they reach old age.

Generation X is suffering too. Most of them have been led to believe they are victims of disease traits passed down in their genes. They are the first generation of young people to suffer in alarming numbers from chronic degenerative and autoimmune diseases such as multiple sclerosis, lupus, chronic fatigue syndrome, Chron's disease, celiac disease and other inflammatory bowel diseases, Type 1 and Type 2 diabetes, and even Parkinson's disease. In addition, the rates of infertility are staggering, causing more Gen-Xers to seek fertility specialists.[1]

Our youngest generation is suffering the most. In 2001, U.S. Surgeon General David Satcher asserted that our nation's youngsters may be the first generation who *will not outlive their parents*. The reasons for his assertion are on the rise. According to a 2006 report published by the International Journal of Pediatric Obesity, nearly half of all children in North and South America will be overweight or obese by the year 2010.[2]

The consequences of childhood obesity are sobering. Type 2 diabetes, previously called "adult onset diabetes" due to the fact that it used to be diagnosed only in adults in their 40's, is now being diagnosed at an alarming rate in children as young as 10 and 12. Additionally, according to new research presented at the 2008 American Heart Association's annual scientific sessions in New Orleans, 13-year old obese adolescents had damaged arteries more representative of a 45-year old.[3] These horrendous statistics are probably owing to the fact that sugary sodas are being given to children as young as seven months, French fries are the dominant vegetable for toddlers, and processed mac 'n cheese, with its ubiquitous dose of monosodium glutamate, seems to be the national "kid-food."

Why is this happening to us, and what can we do to change it? We are a fat and sick people because we eat foods that are taken out of their natural form, because we tax our livers with toxic food additives, because we don't understand how our digestive system works, and we know nothing of our true nutritional requirements. I wrote this book because I believe in the intelligent nature of our bodies and the intelligent nature of our most powerful medicine—food. We can change our health by understanding that our bodies can't sustain us if we pollute them, and more importantly they will push us to an early grave if we rob them of the vital life forces designed to keep us alive and thriving.

AN AMAZING MACHINE

The human body is an amazing machine. Given time and the right ingredients, it has an inherent ability to heal itself. When you break a bone, a doctor will set it and put it in a cast, but the doctor doesn't *heal* the bone. Nature does. There is a healing force in our world that mends bones and works behind the scenes to restore order. This invisible force is the basis for long-term health and healing. The same healing force that mends bones can also reverse illness and restore ideal body weight.

So it is with *Plan-D*. Improved health and safe weight loss occur naturally by following its tenets. A broken bone may be easier to repair than a degenerative health condition because broken bones are usually caused by a sudden trauma. The healing of arthritis, diabetes and obesity, on the other hand are not so simple. Chronic health conditions take many years to develop and are primarily attributed to poor dietary habits. A broken bone may still heal even if you eat junk food every day (although the healing may take much longer), but to reverse the effects of chronic health conditions, the underlying factors must be addressed and changed.

WHAT IS NATURAL?

The nutshell of *Plan-D* is this: *Eat foods in their closest to natural form as possible.* In order to do this, one must first understand what natural is. But even when the idea of eating natural foods is accepted, a larger problem remains; few modern people understand what following a natural diet really means, or even what constitutes a natural food. Are Newman's O's cookies really natural? What about soy milk and soy products? Are the newfangled trans-fat-free margarines with added omega-3 oils really the best substitute for real organic butter—a time honored staple food of many traditional diets? Are vitamin supplements even natural? *Plan-D* addresses these questions from the standpoint of the biological laws governing human nutrition and health.

America is in a severe health crisis, and people are in a desperate search for the truth about food, health, and healing. But even with a growing natural food industry committed to improving the quality of the food supply, there is still an immense amount of misleading information about what is and is not healthy to eat. A visit last year to Natural Products Expo West, the world's largest natural, organic and healthy products trade show, left me sadly disillusioned about the natural food industry. The majority of the food products showcased were glorified snack foods that contained one or more forms of unhealthy sugar, flour, or oil. Very few of the vendors were committed to empowering consumers to take charge of their health.

Plan-D provides ways for you to participate in the care of your own health. The underlying themes of *Plan-D* are nourishment, mindfulness, awareness, and taking nutritional responsibility. It is not a quick-fix food program. There are no pre-packaged meals to buy, no powdered drinks or energy bars to replace real meals, no weigh-ins (although you *are* encouraged to weigh yourself), and no counting calories. You will learn how to eat for long-term health. The focus is on nutrient density, variety, taste, and enjoyment—not calories, fat grams or glycemic index. In fact, you may to need to re-wire your brain and let go of the diet mentality as I did in order to clear some space for new concepts and scientific truths about food, fat, and healing.

If you do not need to lose weight, but are interested in improving your health through nutrition, you are in for a treat. You'll learn how to feed yourself and your family with high-quality nutritious food while building an arsenal of nutritional knowledge that will sustain you for the rest of your life.

PLAN-D

Plan A was a diet that failed. So was Plan B. Plan C was the low-carb craze that raised awareness about the effects of eating refined carbohydrates, but it did very little in teaching us anything about true health. Many of the low-carb foods are loaded with synthetic sweeteners, preservatives and flavor enhancers. Nearly every client that walks through my door for nutrition counseling has tried Plans A, B, and C. Their best efforts on these plans left them sick, fat, and exhausted.

Plan-D sets you on a path of lifelong learning about nutrition, the healing effects of whole foods, and a spiritual approach to food and to life. You will choose among a wide variety of healthy foods and eat them in proper portions to achieve proper body chemistry. Proper body chemistry is essential for maintaining weight, for assimilating nutrients, eliminating waste, and warding off disease. Daily exercise is moderate and designed to assist in balancing your body chemistry. You will better understand food and appreciate it as an instrument of personal healing. Nourishing yourself according to the principles of Plan-D becomes a wise, mature, and loving act of awareness cultivated through a "one day at a time" approach.

PROCESSED-FREE LIVING

"Processed-Free Living" is the nomenclature we have coined to describe the philosophy of *Plan-D*. Others have described it as *holistic nutrition* or *clean eating*. The nutshell of processed-free living is this: *Eat foods in their closest to natural form as possible*—avoid processed and refined foods, artificial sweeteners, and chemical preservatives, and you will reap the benefits of a healthy and happy body.

When I say "closest to natural form as possible," I mean eating a piece of fruit instead of a fruit roll-up, or a baked potato instead of French fries. It also means staying away from the junk that typically makes up the Standard American Diet (S.A.D). Edward Bauman, Ph.D., executive director of Bauman College for Holistic Nutrition and Culinary Arts, calls these types of foods *health banditos*. In his article *Eating For Health: A New System, Not Another Diet*, he writes:

> The usual suspects, also known as *health banditos*, are the stimulants, sugars, pastries, pastas, processed cheeses, artificial sweeteners, and margarine found in white-flour-laden, over-processed, frozen, microwaved meals served in restaurants or grabbed on the run. Such foods are formulated

in laboratories to over-stimulate our taste receptors so that we are no longer satisfied by the crunch of a carrot, the refreshingly sweet juice of a fresh mango, or the zing of fresh garlic. While it's easy to overeat nutrient-poor, sugary, salty, greasy snack foods, you can enjoy naturally satisfying, nutrient-rich vegetables, grains, seeds, legumes, and lean proteins in abundance.[4]

A person who eats processed-free generally adopts the following practices:

- Eliminates white sugar and white flour
- Eliminates artificial sweeteners
- Eliminates trans-fats and foods fried in unhealthy oils
- Eats a variety of whole grains
- Minimizes consumption of dairy products, with the exception of a daily serving of yogurt
- Minimizes exposure to pesticides
- Always eats breakfast and never skips meals
- Reads food ingredient lists and avoids as many chemical additives as possible
- Eats an abundance of vegetables and fruits
- Incorporates legumes, nuts, and seeds into their daily meals and snacks
- Cooks healthy meals
- Packs healthy meals and snacks
- Makes healthy choices when dining out
- Drinks an adequate amount of water
- Eliminates alcoholic beverages (or significantly limits it)
- Stays within healthy portion guidelines, but does not obsess about calories
- Has a healthy relationship with food and approaches it with reverence
- Surrounds themselves with a social community supportive to healthy eating

This list may seem like a tall order, but those who have been willing to give processed-free living an honest try, have found the improvements in their health astounding and remarkable. Our bodies need whole foods, as close as possible to the way nature provides them, in order to function well. Lucky for us, most of nature's foods are readily available, and this book will teach you how to enjoy nature's bounty in a way that is satisfying and delicious!

You may have to spend a little more time and money shopping for healthy foods, and a little more time in the kitchen preparing them, however it will be time well spent now to save yourself from having to spend more time and money later on doctor visits and medications. When you make the effort and adopt the "elements" of processed-free living, you may begin to rebuild your birthright of good health. Notice the words "elements of." Processed-free living is not to be approached with black and white thinking or a lofty goal for perfection. The willingness to strive for *progress*, not perfection, will bring about results simply by following the plan to the best of your ability.[5]

I encourage you to look at changing your eating as a *process* to be taken one day at a time. Changes are best achieved gradually, as an understanding of food and your own needs deepens. Trying to change everything all at once may create undue stress and a feeling of overwhelm. Yet without discipline and commitment, progress will be minimal.[6] You must be committed to sticking with the process, even if results are slow, and even if you stray from it temporarily.

If you have intuitively turned to nutrition as a means to better health, if you want to understand how and why foods affect us, and if you want to learn more about the place of food in the human story—then this book may become very important to you.[7] An understanding of food can lead to increased health and happiness, and has the potential to become a profound catalyst for spiritual growth, from experiencing a renewed sense of vitality and purpose in life to discovering your true vocation and making deeper connections in all of your relationships.[8]

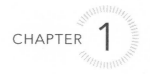

CHAPTER 1

From Obese Junk-Food Junkie to
Slim Trim Nutrition Savvy Expert:
SEVENTEEN YEARS OF SUSTAINED WEIGHT LOSS

My family history suggests I was a likely candidate for obesity and early death. My diabetic maternal grandmother weighed 300 pounds when she passed away. My fraternal grandmother, though not severely overweight, suffered a sudden fatal stroke at the age of fifty-two. Diabetes is rampant among relatives on my mother's side of the family, and all of the women on my father's side exhibit a strong tendency toward obesity in early adulthood. Current genetic theory would suggest the odds for escaping degenerative disease and maintaining a healthy body weight throughout my lifetime were stacked against me from my very first breath.

A child of the sixties, I was born in San Francisco, California in the summer of 1961 to twenty-one-year-old working class parents of both Irish and Mexican-American descent. Two years later my sister was born and six years after that our new baby brother arrived on Thanksgiving Day. My father worked as a service technician for the state utility company, while my mother held various clerical jobs to supplement our family income. Although we occasionally observed some of our cultural traditions when it came to food, we were not a typical Mexican-American family. We lived in mainly Caucasian neighborhoods, and for the most part we ate like every other American family during the 1960's—meat, potatoes, white bread, white rice, and canned vegetables. Although Popeye was among my favorite cartoon personalities, I was not able to stomach canned spinach with the vigor that he did. In fact, most vegetables made their way into my napkin to be stashed in the garbage can when my mother wasn't looking.

I openly admit that I am a recovered compulsive eater—a physical, emotional and spiritual condition characterized by a compulsion to eat when not hungry or frequent episodes of uncontrolled quantity eating, which may or may not lead to weight gain and obesity. My first recollection of compulsive eating is when I was five years old—I stole a Tootsie Pop from the corner store in our San Francisco neighborhood. Like most mothers, mine had an eagle eye for anything out of the ordinary, so before I was able to tally how many licks it takes to get to the center of a Tootsie Pop, she marched me down the street to apologize to the storekeeper for stealing his inventory. The memory of that confession marks a turning point in my story—at the age of five, I was already sneaking and stealing food, and hiding to eat it.

A HEALTHY ACTIVE CHILD

Toward the end of my kindergarten year in 1966, my parents bought their first brand new tract home in San Jose, California—a suburb fifty miles south of San Francisco in an area now famously known as Silicon Valley. As a child growing up in suburbia, I was very active and remained a normal healthy weight up until the age of nine. I loved riding my bike and climbing the trees in the walnut orchards that surrounded our neighborhood. As a child I had a great appreciation for physical activity and being outdoors, and I was known for climbing anything that presented a challenge.

Aside from climbing trees, I climbed up onto the roof of our house, the slides and jungle gyms at the playground, and numerous hills at the parks my mother would frequently take us to. The wooded creek bed running behind our neighborhood provided me with many hours of solitary walks when I would lose myself in daydreams and songs. This large capacity for solitude has remained with me my entire life. At times it has worked against me, but more often than not it has brought me peace in the darkest of times.

FOOD BECOMES COMFORT

Compulsive eating usually starts in early childhood when eating patterns are formed, or as the result of a significant emotional or physical trauma. In either circumstance, most people who become compulsive eaters are people who never learned the proper way to deal with stressful situations and instead use food as a coping mechanism. My parents had a stormy marriage, and after two separations followed by reconciliation, they divorced when I was eleven years old. During the separation years leading up to the divorce, I began to gain weight.

Around the age of nine I lost my desire for outdoor activity and became more of a bookworm. Instead of playing outside with my friends after school, I preferred to be alone and kept most of my feelings to myself. I began eating more food than I needed as a way to avoid feeling conflict, to comfort my fears, and to suppress anger at a situation over which I had no control. I remember sneaking slices of bread and hiding in my room to eat them. My sister and I hid chunks of salami in our kitchen cupboard and snuck bites when mom wasn't looking. I stole change from my mother's purse and secretly bought candy when we went to the grocery store. At family celebrations and holidays I gorged on all the goodies without inhibition. Eating made me forget about the emptiness I felt when my father left, and unconsciously food became my principal source of happiness.

LOGS WITH KNEECAPS

As my weight crept up, I became self-conscious about my body, especially my legs.

As early as fifth grade, I refused to wear dresses to school because I didn't want the boys to make fun of my fat legs. In junior high, one of my friends described my legs as "logs with kneecaps", a phrase that took permanent residence in my memory. On another occasion, a peer who hadn't seen me for a while remarked that when he first caught glimpse of me, I looked like a small whale. These and similar comments by others cut into my soul like icy daggers of insensitivity at a time when I myself had no idea why I was fat. Even my own mother, who I am convinced was only trying to motivate me, would often denigrate me for not being more active and for not choosing healthier foods.

In high school I tried to be more active, but despite playing on the tennis team (which I was good at and really wanted to do), I continued to gain weight. And although I loved singing in my high school choir and acting in community musical theater productions, I didn't have many friends and I never felt like I truly fit in anywhere. Those were especially painful years, as I became more aware of what I was missing out on because I was fat. Secretly, I longed to be popular—but I was quiet, shy and ashamed of my weight, so I related more to food and books instead of my peers. I compensated for being overweight by excelling in my classes, telling myself that I didn't need friends. Food was my best and most reliable friend. I could always count on food to make me feel better, but I was never happy about being fat.

WHEN LIFE GETS TOUGH, THE TOUGH GET GRATEFUL

My parents' divorce had a profound effect on our family as well as on my own psyche. I harbored an intense amount of anger and resentment at both of my parents, particularly my father, and because I wasn't capable of expressing my feelings verbally, they unconsciously showed up as overeating and weight gain. My mother did her best to provide a stable home and balanced meals, but at every opportunity, I overate.

Everything was different after the divorce. My sister and I had to take on many of the household tasks my dad used to do, such as yard work and taking out the trash. Without my dad's income, our family economics sharply declined. Like many single parents, my mom often worked two or three jobs to make ends meet, which meant she wasn't home some evenings. Because of this, I learned to cook at an early age. Thankfully, this was before microwave ovens came on the scene, so I actually learned how to cook rice on the stovetop and bake chicken in the oven.

My mother raised three children on a very meager amount of money, so much of the food we ate was from the discount grocery store, and on a few desolate occasions we ate from donated food boxes. Like most families, we did our big grocery shopping monthly—stocking up on the packaged and frozen foods that would last a month or more. The typical items we brought home were boxed pizza mixes (the kind that came with a can of pizza sauce and the just-add-water dough mix), boxed mac and cheese mix, spaghetti and other pasta, white rice, hamburger, chicken, eggs, milk, potatoes, canned vegetables, packets of taco seasoning and spaghetti sauce seasoning, white flour, white sugar, white bread, white flour tortillas, lunchmeats like bologna (and Italian salami as an occasional treat), hot dogs, pancake mix, biscuit mix, artificially flavored pancake syrup, Kool-Aid mix that required adding a whole cup of sugar per half-gallon (back then it was only ten cents a packet), Crisco shortening, margarine (because it was cheaper than butter), vegetable oil, and various frozen items like pot pies and tater tots.

To her credit, mom drew the line at most snack foods and overtly unhealthy stuff. She did not regularly buy chips, sodas, sugary cereals, candy bars, cookies, cakes, Twinkies, Ding-Dongs or any other treats. Those were saved for special occasions or when we had a little extra money. Our staple snack was popcorn, which mom herself popped in a large pot on the stovetop. We used the fresh peaches from the trees in our backyard to make pies and jams, and we baked our own cookies and cakes from scratch, using good old white sugar and white flour. As was the norm back then, we only occasionally ate fast foods.

Because she grew up in a large and very poor family, my mother really knows how to stretch a dollar, especially when it comes to food. Although the food we ate wasn't necessarily always the healthiest, it saved us from starvation. There were many material things we went without, but my mother taught us the meaning of gratitude. Often times she did not know where her next dollar would come from, but she clearly demonstrated a deep trust that we would always be taken care of.

NATURAL FOODS NOT FOR ME

During my adolescent and teen years, I witnessed my newly divorced mother go through a series of emotional and spiritual changes. While she wasn't exactly a hippie, (she was just a tad older than that generation), she definitely was not your typical suburban June Cleaver or modern day soccer mom. But there were certainly plenty of leftover hippies around during the mid 1970's, and my mom befriended some of them. During this time, she took an interest in "natural foods." She jumped on the counter cultural bandwagon and tried to overhaul our processed foods diet.

We started shopping at the "health food store" where the clerk's name was "Sunshine" and most of the food was fresh or in bulk bins. Unlike today, the health food store prices were actually *less expensive* than the processed foods in the mainstream grocery stores. For obvious reasons, this held great appeal to my mother. There were hardly any packaged foods, and back then there were no frozen foods in the health food store. Needless to say, this did not go over too well with my siblings and I, whose taste buds by this time firmly favored hot dogs, hamburgers, spaghetti and Rice Crispies. Aside from a natural candy bar called "Gypsy Boots" made of dates, carob and shaved coconut, we didn't take too well to healthy foods like whole-wheat pizza crust, wheat germ, brown rice, sprouts, raw honey, and heaven forbid—raw vegetables (ugh!). The experiment failed miserably!

Mom gave in and we went back to eating the way we were accustomed to for the most part. We did make one permanent change that I remember—we switched to "brown bread" (bread with a smattering of whole wheat flour in it so that it wasn't completely white). We could tolerate the brown bread, but at any opportunity outside the home, I chose white bread. I now know that I was addicted to it, and that addiction continued to rage into my adult years.

HERBS AND PRAYERS

Blame it on the hippies, blame it on the times—whatever the catalyst, my mom changed after the divorce. Part of the experimentation with natural foods came from information she gleaned through her study of spirituality and the philosophies of a relatively unknown health giant named Edgar Cayce. I will elaborate on Cayce's work in chapter 3, but suffice it to say that his health and spiritual teachings influenced my mom's life in a deep and effectual way.

Mom began reading to us at bedtime from the Bible and taught us to pray, not for worldly things, but for peace and comfort in our lives. From the books she read about the health teachings of Edgar Cayce, she started using herbal remedies and foods as medicine for aches, pains, and colds. Being the eldest of my siblings, I took a great interest in the information my mother passed on to us. As a teenager, I did not have much use for such things. As an adult, however, the prayers and remedies my mother passed on to me became invaluable tools that were instrumental in helping me overcome my life's greatest challenge.

MORE STORMY YEARS

While my mother was developing her inner life, I was still very angry about the divorce. My dad quickly remarried and was absent most of the time, even though he lived in a nearby town. When I was sixteen, economic pressures forced my mother to sell our house (the only home I remembered since the age of five). We moved to an apartment on the other side of town, which required me to change high schools in the middle of my junior year. Shortly afterward, due to a series of unfortunate events, we were homeless. We lived in shelters for six months before my mom was able to get herself back on her feet and into our own place.

My compulsive eating behaviors progressed rapidly during that year and I became more withdrawn. I had a part-time after school job at a Dairy Queen, which provided me with a steady supply of sweet treats and greasy foods, as well as my own pocket money, which I used to buy more junk food. After changing high schools, my enthusiasm for academics diminished, and I started skipping classes. Although I had dabbled in cigarette smoking since junior high, it was during my senior year that I started to smoke on a regular basis.

Despite my foray into quasi juvenile delinquency, I graduated from high school with National Honor Society standing. Although my parents had always encouraged me, and it was my sincere intention to attend college after high school, there was no money or guidance to get me there. While my grades were high enough to garner me acceptance to the Pharmacy schools at both Oregon State University and Kent State University, I clearly was not destined to follow that path. Instead, I got a job and moved out on my own, and it was then that my eating and weight soared. By the time I turned eighteen I was officially obese. By age 19 my weight had climbed to 180 pounds.

CUNNING AND BAFFLING

As mentioned before, compulsive eating usually starts very subtly, when a child turns to food whenever they are upset. From the age of five, I was upset *all the time*.

Over the years, I learned that food did in fact soothe my angry and upset feelings—it in fact buried them—to the point that I no longer recognized them. Unfortunately, the destructive pattern continued, as I never learned to trust that uncomfortable feelings eventually pass and that I could be capable of soothing myself without food. As a teenager, even though my mother had taught me to pray and worked to instill good dietary habits in me, my emotional pain was too great and I was distracted by our domestic upheaval.

Compulsive eating has only recently come to be taken seriously and straightforwardly as a chronic illness in our culture. Prejudice and stigma against the overweight and obese remain very strong. Overweight people are often stereotyped as lazy, gluttonous, and lacking in willpower or self-control. Consequently, their pain is overlooked, not just by other people, but also by themselves. They often feel guilty for overeating, and inadequate to others for their lack of self-control when it comes to food. But compulsive eating and addiction to certain foods (as I will explain in later chapters), is not a condition to be controlled by willpower. In fact, many compulsive eaters have a tremendous amount of willpower pertaining to other aspects of their lives.

In the following chart I have listed some of the signs of compulsive eating that I exhibited from an early age up into my adult years. My work with others has clearly demonstrated that many people show some of these same signs. It is my hope that if you see yourself or someone you love in this profile, you will take courage that your sanity around food can be restored as mine has.

COMPULSIVE EATING PROFILE

Eat when not hungry.	I always ate when I wasn't hungry. Unless I was dieting, I never knew what hungry felt like.
Go on eating binges for no apparent reason.	Who needs a reason? I ate for celebration, grief, comfort, companionship, entertainment, and just because it was there.
Feel guilt, remorse and shame after eating too much.	My entire existence was shame based. I was embarrassed of my weight and didn't feel like I deserved to be on the planet.
Give too much time and thought to food.	The first thing I thought about when I woke up every morning was about what I was going to eat that day. All day I thought about when I was going to get the food I wanted.
Plan secret binges ahead of time.	Friday and Saturday nights were usually my big binge times, and yes I often planned what I was going to stock up on for the weekend
Look forward with pleasure and anticipation to the time when you can eat alone.	Oh yeah baby, in fact I wanted to be alone quite often so that I could eat whatever I wanted and not feel embarrassed or judged by others.

Eat sensibly before others and make up for it when alone.	When I was around skinny friends or those who were not as enthusiastic about eating as I was, I usually restrained myself and ate sensible. In fact, one of my friends once told me that she was baffled at my obesity because she never saw me eating anything. Of course she didn't! I was too embarrassed to let her see me scarfing down French fries, tacos and donuts.
Repeatedly fail at dieting.	Every time I lost weight, the pounds came back— and brought friends.
Weight affects the way you live your life.	I never felt that I was fully participating in my life because I let my weight hold me back from being my true self. This ties in to what I mentioned earlier about being so embarrassed about my weight that I didn't feel I deserved to be on the planet.
Resent others telling you to "use a little willpower" to stop eating so much and lose weight.	People who don't have the compulsion will never understand that compulsive eating has nothing to do with willpower. If I was able to control my eating and lose weight with willpower, I would have been able to do it long ago. In order to truly recover sanity with food and eating, the physical addiction to certain foods must be removed.
Crave to eat at a definite time, day or night, other than mealtime.	Mostly I liked to eat at night, but I could overeat at any time of the day. Some people go all day without eating anything and then eat large amounts of food in the evening and late at night.
Despite evidence to the contrary, continue to assert that you can diet "on your own" whenever you wish.	It took a lot of motivation and determination to get me to go on a diet, but I always felt that I could do it on my own when I was ready. Problem was, I didn't want to give up eating all my favorite foods, so I wasn't really ready to change.
Eat to escape from worries or trouble.[1]	This was how my compulsive eating began, but I was never really conscious of it. It took a lot of self-honesty and personal "soul searching" to truly understand why I was eating myself to death.

Because I was too young to remember its inception, I had no idea why I loved to eat so much or why I had such a strange reaction to certain types of foods. I had done it all my life and didn't know any other way. Some foods I could comfortably eat a single portion of (like green beans), while other foods I had strong cravings for and felt compelled to eat another serving… and then another… and another. Sugary foods like donuts, pastries, cookies, candy bars, and mint chocolate chip ice cream were the foods I loved the most. Also, I couldn't resist crunchy salty snacks like corn chips, potato chips, and popcorn. My meals were high in starch, sugar and fat. Bread, pizza, sandwiches, spaghetti, macaroni & cheese, and Dr. Pepper were staples throughout my 20's. Nary a vegetable or a piece of fruit passed my lips. Peanut m&m's were my favorite. I could inhale a whole one-pound bag in one evening.

EARLY SIGNS OF POOR HEALTH

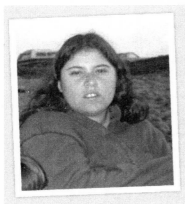

Summer 1984
What should have been a cool day at the beach was clouded by the unhappiness in my life. At age 23, I weighed over 200 pounds.

When I was eighteen, I began to experience sharp abdominal pain. It was affecting my ability to breathe, so one evening I went to the emergency room. After several tests I was diagnosed with gall bladder disease. The doctor told me that I had a large gallstone and that I would have to undergo surgery to have it removed. *What?* I was only 18! How could I have a gallstone? I thought only old fat ladies got gallstones.

Turns out young fat ladies get them too. Gallstones are clusters of solid material that form in the gallbladder. They are made mostly of cholesterol and can cause abdominal pain, especially after consuming fatty foods. During this time, I worked at Burger King and was consuming deep fried breaded chicken sandwiches and French fries on a fairly regular basis. On top of that, my morning fare was donuts or toast with gobs of margarine and my nightly snacking consisted of potato chips. Plenty of fatty foods to go around!

The doctor told me that people who are overweight have a higher risk for developing gallbladder disease, as they may have an enlarged gallbladder, which may not work properly. The idea that he was telling me this was quite ironic I thought, as the doctor's own girth was clearly outside a healthy normal range. Nevertheless, I consented to having the gallstone removed, along with my entire gallbladder. I now have a long scar etched across my mid-drift as a forever reminder of the innocent ignorance of my young years. Had I known then what I know today about the important role of the gallbladder, I would never have let them take it from me.

My instructions for diet upon release from the hospital after surgery were "do not eat fatty foods." That's it. Nothing further. So I went home and white-knuckled my way through about two weeks of no French fries or potato chips. That was the extent of my abstinence from fatty foods.

For the rest of my adult life up until I truly changed my diet, I suffered occasionally from pain while sleeping (it seemed to occur from being in a supine position) that can only be described as tightness in my mid-back region and difficulty breathing. The pain would wake me up and the only remedy would be for me to get out of the supine position and walk around or sit up until it subsided. This pain never occurred during the day—only while I was sleeping. Although the doctors could never find anything wrong with me, today I am convinced it was because I was eating too many fatty and processed foods.

THE BEGINNING OF A SERIES OF FAILED ATTEMPTS

When you compulsively overeat, you usually try every way you can think of to stop. I attempted to take control of my eating by becoming a chronic dieter. My first attempt to lose weight came at the age of nineteen—the beginning of a series of failed attempts. My story is typical—I never lost enough to reach a healthy goal weight, and I always gained back more than I lost.

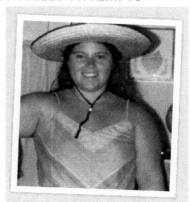

Summer 1986
Down to a svelte 170 pounds, I had just lost 30 pounds on a diet. I quickly gained the weight back.

I tried everything from Herbalife, Weight Watchers and Nutri-System to Slim Fast shakes, Richard Simmons' plans, and crazy diets I made up myself. While strict dieting may bring about temporary weight loss (which it did for me a few times), in the long run it doesn't do anything to remedy the emotional reasons for the compulsive eating. Moreover, my type of dieting was so limited and depriving that it set me up for big binges that set me back for long periods of time before attempting another diet.

Most of my attempts to lose weight never even materialized. They were *attempts* at attempts—never lasting longer than a fleeting thought or an hour of exercise. I never stayed the same weight from one month to the next. I was either losing weight or gaining weight, but I was never happy. I was in agony from overeating and I was in agony from trying not to eat.

By my late 20's I finally gave up trying to diet and my weight hovered steadily over 200 pounds. By the way, I'm 4'10" with a petite body frame—that's literally *twice* the normal weight for someone my size!

FINALLY IN COLLEGE

It was always my dream (and my parents' dream for me) to attend college. At age 21 I enrolled in general education courses at the community college while working full time in various unskilled jobs to support myself. I declared my major in pre-pharmacy with the intention of eventually transferring to a four-year university to get my bachelor's degree.

Although this may sound like advice from the outer reaches of new-age thinking, my mother had my astrology chart done when I was a teenager and it indicated that I would one day become a healer or develop a treatment for many people. We were limited in our ability to interpret that information, so we decided I should become a pharmacist, which would allow me to work with "drugs" that "cure" people.

The universe has a roundabout way of steering us in the right direction when we make choices that are not exactly in alignment with our destiny. During my introductory chemistry class, I fell in love with the science. Up until that point I never had much interest in science, in fact that was one of the only classes I flunked in high school (because I was absent, or skipped rather, most of the time). But in college, the world of chemistry fascinated me. I received an A+, and for the first time in a long time, I had confidence in myself. I changed my major to chemistry and closed the door on the idea of becoming a pharmacist.

Because I had to support myself, I couldn't attend college full time. I took a class here, a class there, and completed some of my general education, but my life started derailing me and I stopped classes altogether for a while. My eating was out of control; I was fat and unfulfilled.

At age 26, I experienced what I believe to be one of a series of turning points that set my entire life in a new direction. While working as a data entry clerk for an insurance company, one of my dear friends and co-workers asked me, "Dee, you are so smart. Why aren't you in college?" After spilling my litany of reasons, she encouraged me to bypass finishing out my general education at community college and apply straight to a four-year university. This I did, and was finally on my way to getting a bachelor's degree, but more importantly I was on my way to becoming my true self.

COLLEGE YEARS HARD FOR ME

I was thrilled to be in college full time, but I was also working full-time. Carrying a heavy load of chemistry, calculus and physics courses in addition to history, English and electives was stressful. An invitation to a fraternity party during my first semester led to a budding romantic relationship. My primary method for managing the stress and pulling all-night study sessions was to eat anything and everything I wanted. And all I wanted was to eat junk food. Super Big Gulps of Dr. Pepper, pizza, ramen noodles, sandwiches and candy bars sustained me during my first years of school.

During the second year, I decided to quit the insurance company for a paid summer research internship in the chemistry department. Although it was a huge pay cut and a real risk for me, I wanted the experience of working in a laboratory (instead of just taking classes in one!). The research job expanded my world, and I began to see future possibilities for my career. Looming largely in my life though, was my obesity. It kept me from truly feeling comfortable in my own skin, and denied me true happiness.

A REAL CHEMISTRY JOB

Life went on. College continued. My budding romance turned into an engagement and then marriage. We were both still in school and working. I was fatter than ever. After the summer internship ended I landed a part time job working for an environmental testing laboratory. This was a real chemistry job! My job duties entailed performing chemical tests on water and soil samples using sophisticated analytical instrumentation. The tests were established by the Environmental Protection Agency to detect a specific list of environmental pollutants. These pollutants included pesticides, herbicides, industrial solvents, chemicals used at water treatment plants, fossil fuel emissions like gasoline and diesel, and others. I learned the federal regulations governing the use and disposal of these chemicals, and the maximum government-allowed residual and exposure levels for humans. This job inspired me to once again change my college major to Environmental Studies with a chemistry emphasis. Although it meant staying in school for two additional years, I was excited at the prospect of becoming an environmental chemist.

OUT OF CONTROL AND MY LIFE IS A MESS

Despite my loving husband and my great job at the lab, I was still a compulsive eater. As much as I wanted to lose weight, I couldn't stop eating. I was obsessed with food. It was the first thing I thought of when I woke up in the morning. I snacked all day long and overate at nearly every meal. When I wasn't eating or thinking about eating, I was sleeping, which I did quite often. I slept through the

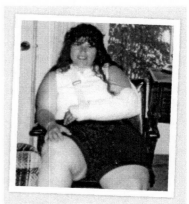

July 1990
Here I am in all my glory, just after my honeymoon at age 29. My weight had climbed to over 210 pounds, and I was still gaining.

day and ate through the night. Looking back, I was probably depressed. But just as I thought my compulsive eating was from a mere love of food, I thought sleeping was just a mere love of sleep.

Because I was so ashamed of my weight and my eating, I ate sensibly around other people and then made up for it later. I confined most of my eating to the hours when I was alone. That way I could eat to my heart's content without the fear of being judged. A typical binge consisted of eating beyond the point of being full, so stuffed that I could barely move. Afterward, like a sickeningly drunk alcoholic, I would pass out on the couch from the toxic overload. The next day I vowed that I would never again eat so much, only to find myself making the same vow days or even hours later. I lied to myself and to other people about what and how much I was eating. I stole food and I stole money to buy food. I loved food. It was my best friend. I could not imagine my life without it.

As much as I was struggling with food and weight, it should have been obvious that I had problems. I certainly felt exposed, because I wore 100 pounds of problems on my body for the whole world to see. I couldn't hide them from myself or anyone else.

The irony was that I did hide my problems. On the outside, it appeared that I had my life together. I was supporting myself through college with a job in my desired field. My husband, who loved me and adored me, was wonderfully supportive. Everyone I knew admired me for my strength, determination, and tenacity.

On the inside, I harbored a load of resentment and I frequently complained about how unfair life had treated me. I still resented my parents' divorce and continued to blame them for my struggles as an adult. Mainly, I blamed my father for everything that went wrong in my life and everything I was unable to achieve. Because I was unable to take responsibility for my own life, it was *his fault* that I had to work so many hours and didn't have enough time to devote to my studies.

Because of this, my grades were failing. If he would just *give me* enough money to get through college, my life would be perfect. This insane line of thinking spiraled back into my childhood and had me believing that somehow it was my father's fault that I was fat and my life was so completely unmanageable.

Because I never ate in front of people, no one could understand why I was so overweight. The way I conducted my life paralleled my eating behaviors. I was bright and intelligent yet I missed classes and failed exams. I was a dedicated and hard worker, but frequently late for my shift. My life was a collection of unpaid bills, broken commitments and procrastination. I was unable to be honest with myself or anyone else about my failings, so I only told people of my successes.

I felt like such a fake. I lived my life in lies and it became more difficult with each passing day to keep up the facade. My fierce independence kept me from believing that anyone or anything could help me with my life and I never dared to ask for help. To avoid facing my life, I often stayed home, missed work and classes, unplugged the phone, and shut myself off from the world.

One day in February of 1992, overstuffed from a super-sized lunch, I ransacked the cupboards looking for something more to eat. I found some old, stale candy from the previous Halloween that I didn't even like. As I sat on my couch eating this disgusting candy, it occurred to me that something was seriously wrong with me. In a moment of clarity, I had a vision of myself as an old woman nearing the end of my days wishing for a life that could have been. I saw that for most of my life, I had been an observer standing on the sidelines watching my life go by and not participating in it.

For as long as I could remember, I had let my weight hold me back from being my true self and pursuing the things in life that I knew would make me happy. Shame dominated my entire being and I never felt I had a right to be on the planet. Everything I said, everything I did, and every decision I made was based on whether I believed a fat person was entitled to it. I didn't even feel worthy of my husband's love.

I was so afraid of people, yet inside I longed for intimacy and friendship. I was quiet and shy, and did not actively seek out people as friends because I felt that no one would like me because I was fat. My obesity stripped me of my self-esteem, talked me out of taking risks, imprisoned me in isolation, and robbed me of my identity. The fat kept me from believing in myself and diminished my spirit. I felt trapped by my weight and I was in a state of hopeless despair.

It was as if I was living two lives: in one respect I was on the brink of a great future, on the other I was spiraling out of control. To the outside world my life seemed normal, but inside I silently suffered from a God-shaped hole in my soul. Filled with guilt and shame about my weight, I was incapable of loving myself enough to effect a change. I was lost and completely out of touch with my feelings because I stuffed them down with food. And because I was unable to truly share myself with others, inside I was tortured by isolation and loneliness.

COGNITIVE DISSONANCE

After working at the lab for a few months, I became acutely aware of three things:

1) thousands of chemicals are dumped into our water, air, soil, and food every day, 2) some of the chemical names of compounds I was using in my lab were the same chemical names on the ingredient lists of the processed foods I was eating, and 3) each person has a responsibility to revere and care for our environment (our planet and our bodies).

I began to experience a phenomenon social psychologists call "cognitive dissonance." Cognitive dissonance is an uncomfortable feeling caused by holding two contradictory ideas simultaneously. The "ideas" or "cognitions" in question may include attitudes and beliefs, and also the awareness of one's behavior. The theory of cognitive dissonance proposes that people have a motivational drive to reduce dissonance by changing their attitudes, beliefs, and behaviors, or by justifying or rationalizing their attitudes, beliefs, and behaviors.[2]

My cognitive dissonance surfaced with a growing enthusiasm for cleaning up the environment and a deep disgust at the chemical waste in our world. Yet I could not even clean up my own world, my own environment—my body. I had not yet become disgusted with the "pollution" I was dumping into my body every time I drank a Dr. Pepper, ate a Big Mac and smoked a cigarette. But the drone of dissonance was getting louder.

BACKPACK EPIPHANY

A month after the stale Halloween candy episode, I was on a field trip with one of my college classes that involved hiking up a steep hill. The dissonance hadn't yet reached decibel levels, and for some reason I thought it would be easy to hike up a hill. Never mind the fact that I was a "pack-a-day" cigarette smoker and by this time I was at my top weight, which had climbed to somewhere over 210 pounds. It was more than a struggle to pull my fat body up that hill. By the time I reached the halfway point, everyone else had scaled past me and were already at the top enjoying the glorious view.

I stopped at the halfway point because my legs were hurting, my heart was pounding in my chest, and I could hardly breathe. Then I had what I consider to be *the* most humiliating experience of my life—the very attractive young hike leader had to come back down the hill to see if he could assist me in some way. As I stood there trying to regain composure, he reached his hand out to me and asked, "Can I take your backpack?" *As if the backpack was the problem.* A tsunami of humiliation washed over me when I realized how out of shape my body was and that I could not keep up with the class. As I inched my way up the hill, huffing and puffing, I felt their eyes on me, waiting for the slow fat girl to reach the top.

Slowly and painfully, I made it to the top. I walked over to join the rest of the class and when I got there, my foot slipped out from under me and I fell flat on my rear. Humiliation and embarrassment filled me, and I turned and looked away from the crowd. At the top of the hill, looking out over the beautiful San Francisco Bay, I felt like the lowest thing on earth. Suddenly, a wave of realization overcame me. Dissonance broke, and I came face to face with my reality. It stripped denial from me, and my life stood starkly in front of me, demanding my attention. The physical condition of my body was symbolic of how I had let everything in my life get out of control. *I had let this happen. It wasn't my father's fault. What am I going to do?*

Then, I heard a voice. I don't know whether it came from inside of me or outside of me, but the message was loud and clear: ***CHANGE YOUR LIFE OR DIE***.

Those words haunted and frightened me in a way I cannot describe. There were many times in my life when I feared I would die of my obesity at an early age. I had frequent chest pains, and even though the doctors told me my heart was fine, my family history always kept me suspect. Stiff hip joints and the nocturnal pain in my back were evidence that my body was degenerating, and when I allowed myself to notice, I knew that I was already spiritually and emotionally dead.

Over the next few days, each time I relived the hiking trip in my mind, I heard the voice coming from within: ***CHANGE YOUR LIFE OR DIE***. I attempted to squelch the fear by turning to the only method I had ever known to cope with fear—I *ate*. And I continued to eat until the day came when the desire to remain the same was more painful than the risk to grow.

That day was April 3, 1992. On that day the motivational drive to reduce dissonance shifted something inside of me. I had what can only be described as a profound inner change—what the psychologist Carl Jung called a "vital spiritual experience." The old attitudes, ideas and emotions of my compulsive eater self, which until then had been the guiding forces of my life, were willingly cast aside. In exchange, I gradually allowed myself to explore new ways of thinking and acting.

In essence, I made the decision to give up the struggle of my life. Instead of dieting, I started learning and living. I began to believe in myself and became committed to making my dream of losing my excess weight come true.

A STRONG DESIRE TO CHANGE

The desire to change one's eating behavior can be a terrifying prospect, especially if one is entrenched in the belief that food provides relief from pain. With all of my experience at dieting, I knew that another diet was not the answer to my obesity. Using a diet to control my overeating was akin to using a fly swatter to bring down a jet airplane—the intention was real, I just wasn't very successful!

Previous dieting attempts failed because they were rooted in a flawed diet mentality. Instead of actually *changing* the types of food I was eating, I just tried to eat *less of* the same foods that had historically made me fat. I ate *less* cookies, *less* cake, *less* French fries, *less* ice cream. The problem with that approach was that because I was addicted to those foods, I was never satisfied with less of them, and I eventually reverted to eating larger and larger quantities.

AND NOW FOR SOMETHING COMPLETELY DIFFERENT...

In order to lose weight and keep it off, I needed to change my whole approach to eating and adopt the change as a permanent way of life. As I embarked on this endeavor, I was fortunate to become affiliated with a weight loss support group where a small faction of its members were refraining from eating all forms of sugar and flour. This at first seemed difficult to do, but I saw success in those who had been living sugar and flour-free for many years. People who had struggled their entire lives with obesity, now lived in normal-sized bodies—some of them 150 to 200 pounds lighter—without desire or pangs of deprivation for the starchy sugar-laden foods we had all grown up eating. Seasoned members claimed that sugar and flour were addictive substances, which when eaten on a regular basis, caused cravings that led to overeating. More than that, many of them claimed that their migraine headaches, arthritis, and diabetes had vanished after giving up flour and sugar. With trepidation, I decided to give it a try. The first new action I took in my weight loss process was eliminating all forms of refined sugar and flour from my life. Thirty days later, I had dropped 20 pounds.

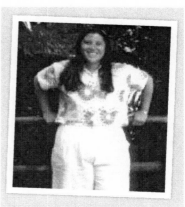

July 1992
Three and a half months after giving up flour and sugar, I had lost 48 pounds. At 162 pounds, I felt light and happy.

DIET MEANS "WAY OF LIFE"

Simultaneous to abstaining from flour and sugar, I began to educate myself about food. I spent countless hours reading nutrition books—educating myself on the most effective and balanced path to optimal health. I also spent lots of time in the kitchen creating healthier versions of my favorite comfort foods. Because of my work in the lab, I had become intimately familiar with the chemical names and toxic properties of the majority of common environmental pollutants, particularly those used in and on America's food supply. I made the connection that pesticides, preservatives, flavorings, colorings, and refined carbohydrates affect body chemistry in such a way that balanced health is difficult to sustain. It was this understanding that led to a deeper level of surrender—I began to read every food ingredient list with scrutiny in an effort to eliminate as many processed foods from my diet as possible. The result was a 100-pound weight loss and a lifestyle that I have sustained for 17 years and counting.

HERE'S HOW I DID IT:

From all of the reading and with the help of my organic chemistry background, I developed my own healthy eating plan and followed it like my life depended on it. I stopped eating all of the foods that had historically been problems for me. These included anything made with sugar and refined carbohydrates, fatty foods, processed foods, fried foods, alcohol, and caffeine. I started eating things I never liked before, such as fresh vegetables and fruits, unrefined whole grains, lean poultry and fish.

As I mentioned in the preface, the word diet comes from the Greek word *dieta*, which means "discipline" or "way of living." The Latin root of the word means "a day's journey." I adopted a healthy mindset of abstaining from processed foods for the current day only. The prospect of keeping it up for a lifetime was overwhelming, but I was confident that I could stick to my healthy plan for just one day.

For the first time in my life, I took nutritional responsibility and became accountable to myself by measuring my food at *every meal* and keeping a record of

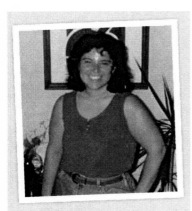

August 1992

It's amazing how quickly the weight came off after eliminating white flour and sugar. I had lost 61 pounds in 4 ½ months. I weighed 149 ½ pounds when this photo was taken.

everything I ate and how I was feeling. A food scale, measuring cups and measuring spoons became essential kitchen tools for helping me determine proper portion sizes. I never felt so much freedom around food before in my life. It seemed ironic, but once I introduced discipline into my food choices, I was free to enjoy food rather than being a slave to it. The structure and discipline helped me to put food in its proper perspective.

Having a set plan for eating is not much different from having a pre-planned driving route to get from point A to point B. The route keeps you from getting lost or distracted from your destination. Planning meals ahead of time allowed me to truly enjoy eating, knowing that I was getting closer to my goal—not distracted by my emotional fluctuations of the day. In essence, it taught me how to separate food from feelings. The eating plan became my anchor—the one constant in my ever-changing life.

Enlisting support played a crucial role in my ability to change my life. I continued to attend the weight loss support group because it helped me cultivate a belief in myself and connected me to others in a way that I didn't find in my other relationships. That fierce independence I was so proud of in my early life was actually my biggest downfall when it came to overcoming my food compulsion. The ability to ask for help, both from other people and through prayer, is a spiritual practice that continues to strengthen and deepen my commitment to balanced health.

HERBS AND PRAYERS REVISITED

Overcoming compulsive eating must happen on a soul level. My excess weight was but a *symptom* of a deeper problem. My life's greatest challenge was that I ate food as a way to fill many voids in my life, thus leading to an unhealthy relationship with food. No plan for healing that relationship was successful when it was based on diet alone.

When I was growing up, my mother taught me to pray for peace and comfort in my life. Somewhere along the way to becoming obese, I forgot that there was a healing power in the universe. But after my harrowing hiking experience, I reacquainted myself with the practice of praying. It began with a simple prayer, one that I have said every day since.

In the morning, I begin my day with a prayerful request: *"Please give me the courage, willingness, and strength to make wise and healthy food choices today."* To me, this prayer is a daily surrender, a "letting go" of my compulsive behavior with food. When I let go, I invite the universal healing power to guide me in my food and life choices. By letting go of my old eating behaviors and thinking patterns, I am able to increase my capacity for more meaningful and healthier ways of approaching food.

This mental and spiritual practice is quite different from dieting, because its goal is to heal the soul as well as the psyche. It is a daily ongoing process. For me, it brings a sense of wholeness—a wholeness that cannot be experienced without also learning the proper way to nourish my body.

As I began to deepen my spiritual connection, I was drawn to revisit the information my mother had taught me about Edgar Cayce, specifically the recommendations he gave for healthful eating. Avoiding white flour and sugar was confirmed by the Cayce teachings, in addition to including plenty of vegetables, fruits, small amounts of whole grains and lean proteins. He advised against eating pork, as it is an unclean animal, therefore I eliminated it from my plan. More importantly, the Edgar Cayce teachings emphasized the concept of purity in body, mind, and spirit. He taught that a healthier body allows us to be more fully developed emotionally and spiritually. These teachings shifted my thinking even further toward adopting a processed-free diet. As time has gone on, the task of sustaining my body, through proper nutrition, exercise, and other measures, has become a spiritual responsibility. It is a goal toward wholeness that allows me to fully experience my life in its totality.

A RETURN TO A CHILDHOOD LOVE

Not since childhood had I found any enjoyment in being outdoors, however my desire to be close to nature resurfaced and I returned to my childhood love of taking walks alone. In fact, walking became my mode of transportation on the road to healthy living. I started with slow and short walks, and quickly worked my way up to brisk, aerobic 60 minute walks. This is still a regular practice of mine. My preference is to walk alone because I use the time not only for exercise, but also for contemplative thinking. Walking helped to build and strengthen my body as well as to build and strengthen my relationship with myself. It gave me the nourishment and energy to change and reshape my life. As the days, weeks, and months passed, I watched my shadow on the ground get smaller and smaller, while my spirit inside grew larger and larger.

WRITING BECOMES A TOOL

Another discipline instrumental to my weight loss was the practice of writing and journaling. This enabled me to identify the emotions that were associated with my eating. I learned that the discomfort I felt when going on a diet—that sense of deprivation—was not about food and never had been. I had to write to find out what in my life was so painfully absent and what certain foods represented in my emotional life. For instance, one time after I binged on a big bag of popcorn, a good friend suggested that I write down everything I could remember about eating popcorn. It was through this exercise that I was able to identify my emotional attachment to popcorn.

When I was a little girl my mother used to make enough popcorn to fill a grocery bag when our family sat together to watch television. Mom was always happy, and when mom was happy, the mood in the room was loving and safe. At a

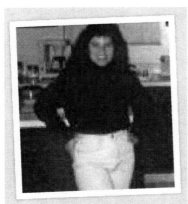

January 1993

After 9 ½ months of no sugar and flour, I had lost 92 pounds. Almost at my goal weight when this photo was taken, I weighed 118 pounds.

young age, I associated that big bag of popcorn with mom being happy and the family being close. Several years later after my mom and dad divorced, there was tremendous pain in the family.

During my troubled teen years, I only knew that eating popcorn gave me a good feeling, and I had subconsciously disassociated from the original emotional ties that had initiated those good feelings. The taste and smell of popcorn went straight to my heart, so whenever I was around it, I immediately wanted to eat it. When I dieted and didn't allow myself to eat popcorn, I felt *so* deprived. Eventually, and without fail, I would then binge on huge amounts of popcorn. In reality, I was looking to recapture the love and closeness from those days of old.

That was what was truly missing in my life, not popcorn. From then on, whenever I craved a particular food, I did this particular writing exercise to help break the emotional attachment. Over time, although slowly, I was able to free myself from these attachments. One by one, I worked hard to identify my weaknesses and erase the conditioning that trapped me for so long.

REALIZING MY DREAMS

It took me a little more than a year to lose the 100 pounds of excess weight. I went from a size 22 jeans to a size 4! In May 1993, two of my lifelong dreams were realized simultaneously. The first was that I finally reached my goal weight, 108 pounds. The second was that I finally earned my Bachelor of Science degree in environmental chemistry. I was the first female on my mother's side of the family to graduate from college, and the first ever on my father's side. Both of these dreams were such milestones, because I never believed that either one of them would come true. In November 1992, I quit smoking on the day before Thanksgiving. I haven't smoked a cigarette since, nor have I desired to.

The unwavering belief in myself, the commitment to a daily eating and exercise regimen, the release of those awful emotional attachments, and a deep sense of wholeness gave me confidence, self-esteem, and a freedom from shame and humiliation.

My life before losing weight was all about unfulfilled desires. I wanted to perform and dance and sing; I wanted to have a wealth of friends and acquaintances; I wanted a fulfilling profession; and most of all, I wanted to be comfortable just being in my skin.

Over the years, I have achieved all of those things and so much more. I have come into my own, reclaiming my true self that was buried so deeply for so many years. There have been many ups and downs in my life, and I have rarely succumbed to finding comfort, celebration, or relief in excess food.

It has been said that the definition of insanity is doing the same thing over and over again expecting to get a different result. Because I broke that cycle of insane eating and dieting, by changing my whole approach to food, my sanity has been restored. I am now *recovered* from compulsive eating, but this recovery is contingent upon the daily actions I take to nourish my body and my spirit. Even nearly 17 years later, it is still a conscious choice to eat healthy and exercise every day. I still write out my feelings and I continue to work on my personal growth.

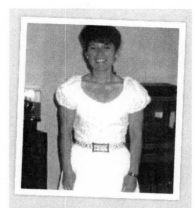

May 1993
My dreams have come true. Here I am on the day I graduated from college and one full year after staying away from flour and sugar. I lost 102 pounds and weighed 108 pounds. By staying away from flour and sugar and anything artificial, I have maintained this weight for over a decade.

A NEW CAREER PATH, A NEW LIFE

Because I was so successful with my own weight loss, others sought my advice for their own food and weight issues. As a result, I discovered a passion for helping others turn to nutrition as a means to better health, to help them understand how and why foods affect us, and to teach them how to prepare healthy food for themselves and their families.

In 2000, I decided to become formally trained in nutrition education and diet counseling at Bauman College (formerly The Institute for Educational Therapy), which included whole foods cooking classes and extensive study of nutritional therapies for achieving optimal health, including reversing chronic and terminal diseases. Bauman College specializes in training individuals for careers in holistic nutrition and culinary arts. The curriculum I studied focused on counseling clients in matters of diet and health, and on health-supportive cooking, which is based on preparing balanced meals using high-quality ingredients that are whole, natural (as opposed to man-made), unprocessed or minimally processed, fresh, in-season, and organic whenever possible. *(For a detailed description of what I learned at Bauman college, see Appendix C).*

My chemistry background was extremely valuable in helping me to understand not only the inherent chemical nature of food itself, but also the many aspects of how foods interact with the body to create health or disease.

Since receiving my nutrition certification in 2001, I have become a trailblazer in the world of nutrition education and whole foods cooking. I started my own practice, offering personalized nutrition counseling to help clients find the right nutritional balance for their health goals and lifestyle. Optimal nutrition for healthy weight loss is my specialty, although I have helped countless people improve other chronic health conditions. You will read some of their testimonials in Chapter 16.

Since I have a flair for cooking, I modified many of my old comfort food

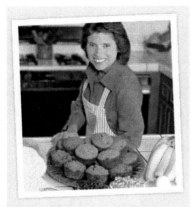

2004 - *Dee's Mighty Muffins™ were marketed.*

2006 - *Dee's Mighty Cookbook hit the store shelves.*

recipes into healthful gourmet fare. One of those recipes became my first product, *Dee's Mighty Muffins™*, flourless and sugarless oat bran muffins which now sell at natural food markets in Arizona, California and Texas.

To promote muffin sales, I began giving free nutrition seminars in local grocery stores and natural food markets. Soon thereafter, I wrote my first book, titled *Dee's Mighty Cookbook: Tasty Cuisine for Flourless and Sugarless Living.* Selling over 7,000 copies to date in the U.S., Canada and overseas, my self-published cookbook has become a sleeper sensation, helping thousands of people to change their approach to food, eating and weight loss.

In 2006 my husband and I founded *The Center for Processed-Free Living (affectionately called "The Center")*, a non-profit organization dedicated to eliminating childhood and adult obesity. The Center offers nutrition education and cooking classes specifically geared toward removing processed foods from the diet by teaching children and adults the health effects of processed foods and the healing properties of whole foods.

DISCOVERING MY TRUE LIFE PURPOSE

What started in my early years as a hollow desire to be thin has become so much more than I would have ever prayed for on that fateful day overlooking the San Francisco bay. Although I would never wish it on anyone else, I'm grateful for my experience as an overweight person. It has given me compassion for others, it's kept me mindful of where I could be again, and it's allowed me to more fully appreciate my life and my relationships with others.

I may not be dripping with degrees in medicine or nutrition, yet I hold a unique position of authority on sustained weight loss and improved health—I personally recovered from obesity and compulsive eating, gall bladder disease and ulcerative colitis without the use of drugs, diets, or weight loss surgery. Many have lovingly reminded me that although I do have academic credentials, *my experience is the only credential I need* for spreading the message of health.

Although degenerative disease may be too far advanced in some people for complete reversal, because of what I have learned and witnessed, I am convinced that every person can *greatly improve* their state of health. By following scientific and historically proven health principles and eliminating processed foods, an individual can embrace a way of eating that will lead to regeneration of the entire body, mind, soul, and spirit.[3]

A responsibility was instilled in me early in my weight loss process to extend my hand and heart to all who share my compulsion, and to those who are suffering from the effects of ill health. I have dedicated myself to serving others in this capacity, and live a gratified life from sharing my experience, strength, knowledge, and hope with others. Each day that I eat well, I am well, and I embody the principles of true health and healing, which attracts others who want what I've found.

The astrology chart my mother had done for me when I was a teenager was not so far off after all—in a roundabout way, I *am* a healer. My studies taught me a very important truth: *eating foods in their closest to natural form is our best medicine.* Incorporating the principles of *Plan-D* will help anyone who wants to avoid disease, lose weight and improve their health.

Many would say that my weight loss is the result of eliminating processed foods from my diet. That is true, however I believe that my weight loss is more the result of listening to the inner voice that called me to change my life, and my willingness to avail myself to the power and wisdom of that voice.

Some good friends have taught me to "seek the serenity to accept the things I cannot change, the courage to change the things I can, and the wisdom to know the difference." Such serenity and wisdom can bring a measure of happiness. But without the courage to change the things one can, a greater measure is missed. Processed-free living involves that greater measure.[4]

If you or someone you know identified with more than three of the signs of compulsive eating on page 6, please read the side box on page 22 for information about available help.

Finally, don't give up. If I can lose half my weight and keep it off for nearly 17 years, you can too. Read on, stay committed, and enjoy the beautiful life you have and the even more beautiful life that is yet to come.

ENLISTING SUPPORT

Changing the way you eat is a significant life change that is hardly ever successfully done alone, nor should it have to be. While it is true that we are each responsible for what goes into our mouths, we can surround ourselves with positive role models or people who share our same goals.

For some, being overweight can create a terrible sense of aloneness and isolation. Trying to lose weight on your own without being connected to others who share your same feelings and struggles may perpetuate those feelings. It can be a pretty lonely experience when you're the only one at the office birthday party who is not partaking in the cake. It is extremely valuable to have at least one person in your life that you can talk to, especially when you're feeling vulnerable or alone.

Support is crucial, because it helps us to cultivate a belief in ourselves and connects us to others in ways that we don't often find in other relationships. The ability to ask for help is a spiritual practice that strengthens us, rather than weakens us, in our moments of temptation. There's something magical that happens when two people who share a similar struggle work together to achieve a common goal.

Support has been essential in helping me maintain my 100-pound weight loss and healthy lifestyle for nearly 17 years. Remember, I was once a morbidly obese junk-food junkie who couldn't see past the next mouthful of m&m's. Once I decided to change my eating, I devoted countless hours to studying nutrition, attending lectures and classes, journaling my emotions, and counseling sessions to help change my thinking. But truth be told, the one thing that helped me more than any of those enlightening books and tools was the presence of a mutual support system in my life.

From the first day I gave up eating refined flour and sugar, I decided that I needed someone to help me stay committed to healthy eating. I can honestly say, since that day, I have never been without a supporting friend or mentor to help me with my food and life choices. Mutually, I support others in their health endeavors. We act as cheerleaders to each other, and don't allow each other to fall back into old habits. We lovingly hold each other accountable to what we say we will do, without judgment or scolding. And most importantly, we remind each other of our goals, even when we lose sight of them.

You will need your own support system to help you in your transition to processed-free living. Getting the support you need doesn't mean that you have to hire a life coach or join a weight loss group, although both of those would be excellent choices. You can enlist a family member, a good friend, a teacher, a co-worker, or anyone who will not let you give up on your goals. You can also join my on-line message board to get support from the growing community of Plan-D followers.

Log on to: www.plandee.org

If you identified with three or more of the signs in the Compulsive Eating Profile on page 6, you'll be doing yourself a great favor if you can experience an established support group with many members who have already achieved freedom from compulsive eating and maintenance of a healthy body weight. Overeaters Anonymous (OA) is recommended, as its philosophy is in alignment with the Plan-D principles. There are OA meetings in every part of the world, and in nearly every city in the United States. Many on-line and telephone meetings are also available. There are no dues or fees for membership, contributions to local groups is voluntary. To find a meeting in your area, log on to **www.oa.org** or call 505-891-2664.

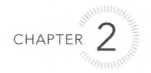

CHAPTER 2

Globesity and the Fatally Flawed Food Guide

My first recorded weight was five pounds, six ounces, which means that at birth I was a healthy normal weight for my age. Most of us enter the world this way, without a weight problem and without serious health concerns. Unfortunately, in today's world, the majority of us don't stay that way. As a species, we are currently facing a health crisis unlike anything seen in human history. According to the World Health Organization, 1.7 billion adults on the planet need to lose weight. Three hundred million of them qualify as obese, meaning that they weigh at least 50 pounds more than their ideal body weight. To put this into perspective, there are now more fat people in the world than there are gaunt, food-deprived hungry people, which numbers around 600 million.[1]

THE REAL GLOBAL TERROR

In the United States, 71 percent of adult men and 62 percent of adult women are overweight. Among those, 31 percent of the men and 33 percent of the women can be classified as obese.[2] A recent study conducted by Johns Hopkins Bloomberg School of Public Health published in the July 2008 online issue of *Obesity* suggests that if we continue the trend of the last three decades, 86 percent of Americans will be overweight or obese by the year 2030[3]. Analysis of the study data also revealed that, over time, heavy Americans become heavier. Whoa! If I had not altered my own personal trend, I am convinced that my already heavy American body would be much heavier by now.

Of more serious concern is the skyrocketing rate of overweight and obese children worldwide. A study published in the *International Journal of Pediatric Obesity* reports that the number of overweight children worldwide will increase significantly by the end of the decade. If present trends continue, *nearly half* of the children in North and South America will be overweight by the year 2010. However, the problem goes beyond American borders and has become a worldwide epidemic. Significant increases in the percentages of overweight children in the Middle East, Southeast Asia, Mexico, Chile, Brazil and Egypt are also expected.[4]

Neville Rigby, policy director of the International Obesity Task Force, is quoted as saying "It's [obesity] rapidly accelerating. We're even seeing obesity in adolescents in India now. It's universal. It has become a fully global epidemic—indeed, a pandemic." Certainly the United States leads the pack with its standard diet of sugary, greasy, high calorie, nutrient-deficient, chemically altered and preserved foods. However, a May 2004 Associated Press article lists several other places that are even worse:

- South Pacific islands like Tonga, Kosrae and Nauru, where traditional meals of reef fish and taro are replaced by cheap instant noodles and deep-fried turkey tails.
- Greece, birthplace of the Olympic Games, where the Mediterranean diet is as much a relic as the Parthenon.
- Oil-soaked Kuwait where Mercedes-driving mothers draped in black burqas feed French fries to their children while shopping for $375 giraffe-leather Italian loafers. [5]

If your mother was like mine, she guilted you into eating all the food on your plate by telling you that "children are starving in China"—referring to the Mao Zedong era when as many as 40 million people starved in the Great Leap Forward famine of 1958-1961. That statement doesn't hold true today. Ten percent of children living in Chinese cities are obese—a statistic that is increasing by 8 percent per year. Chinese cities represent the world's biggest growth market for restaurants that until recently were considered to be counterrevolutionary. Now a new KFC, Pizza Hut or Taco Bell opens almost every day.[6]

In Japan, obesity in nine-year-olds has tripled. Twenty percent of Australian adolescents and children are overweight or obese. "The prevalence of obesity in Europe has tripled in the past two decades; half of all adults and 20 percent of all children are overweight," according to an article by the Associated Press.[7]

This rapid and rampant spread of obesity to even the poorest of countries inspired the World Health Organization (WHO) to coin new verbiage for this rising global terror: *globesity*. Obesity is rapidly becoming one of the world's leading reasons why people die. Obese children are highly likely to become obese adults who will suffer earlier in life from heart disease, stroke and other ailments stemming from their weight. Dr. Phillip Thomas, a surgeon who works extensively with obese patients in England, said, "This is going to be the first generation that's going to have a lower life expectancy than their parents. It's like the plague is in town and no one is interested."[8] WHO decries obesity as a literal elephant in the room, one of today's most blatantly visible – yet most neglected – public health problems. If immediate action is not taken, millions will suffer from an array of serious health disorders.

SAD FOODS

Although obesity and its related illnesses have garnered the attention of the world's health experts, the number of normal weight people suffering from intestinal disorders, diabetes, hypertension, arthritis, osteoporosis, cancer, and heart disease—all diet related illnesses—is just as staggering. Our cheap plentiful food supply has created a blanket health crisis of epic proportions.

Dying of an inadequate diet in a land where there is a surplus of food is unheard of in the annals of history! People classically died of plagues, famines, and wars—not of a poor and imbalanced diet. Most of today's common health problems were rare as little as 100 years ago. Anthropologists and researchers agree by and large that our modern diseases *did not exist* in traditional cultures where people's diets consisted of high fiber foods such as fresh vegetables and fruits, legumes, whole grains, healthy fats, and lean protein sources. In the past century, our food supply has changed dramatically.

If you were to go into a grocery store at the beginning of the 1900's, you would find very little processed food. Back then, the shelves contained fresh produce, seeds and grains, along with a sparse amount of canned and boxed foods. The meat did not have hormones or sugar solutions injected into it, and there were no processed, fast, or convenience foods like the ones that make up the diets of Americans today.

The Standard American Diet of yesteryear was clearly healthier than what it is today. The current Standard American Diet, appropriately acronymed **SAD**, has many imbalances. First, it contains an excess of acid-forming foods, such as meat (proteins), fats, and sugar, which upset the delicate body chemistry required for optimal health. Second, it is lacking in raw plant foods, such as vegetables, fruits, nuts and seeds. Third, the food lacks nutrients, such as enzymes, fibers and antioxidants, due to the fact that the food is cooked and/or processed. Fourth, the foods are toxic due to the various additives, preservatives, pesticides, and hormones put into them to increase production or extend shelf life. It is no wonder we are a sick and fat nation.

The declining health of America has spurred several dietary freak-outs over which foods are harmful and which are helpful. Low fat diets failed to distinguish between beneficial oils and carcinogenic trans-fats. Atkins claimed that primitive man thrived on a high animal protein diet, not taking into account the fact that in primitive times humans had to hunt for days and expend tremendous amounts of energy to obtain their meat supply. They didn't have the luxury of eating meat three to five times each day while sitting for eight hours behind a desk. While low carbohydrate diets have raised our awareness of the dangers of eating too many bagels and donuts, as a nation we still haven't figured out how to eat.

FOOD SUPPLY DOES NOT SUPPORT HEALTHY EATING

Humans survived for two million years on earth without a printed guide for eating, but because we have strayed so far from our traditional diets, most of us need one. For a little more than 100 years, Americans have looked to the federal government to tell us what we're supposed to eat. But for all the time, research and resources spent over the last 100 years putting together food guides, most Americans don't follow them. We receive conflicting messages from nutritionists and the food industry. While our doctors and nutritionists urge us to eat limited amounts of snack foods, fast foods, and processed foods, take a walk down the aisles of any grocery store and you'll notice that the food supply does not support the guidance. Neither is healthy eating modeled in schools, the workplace, or at church. Grocery store shelves are filled with foods containing high fructose corn syrup, hydrogenated oils, artificial sweeteners, and preservatives. Ingredient lists are a mile long containing names of things most people can't even pronounce, let alone digest. The office "working lunch" usually consists of pizza or sub sandwiches, and the schools have been completely overtaken by the fast food industry. It is no wonder we are all so nutritionally confused.

Then, when we get too fat or too sick from our nutrient deficient diets, we look to our doctors and our government to take care of us. Not a bad ideal for a society that lives by the decisions of our elected lawmakers. Unfortunately, those decisions are often tainted.

WHO DECIDES WHAT YOU EAT?

Government intervention into the American diet began back in 1890 when the United States Department of Agriculture (USDA) began funding research to determine the correlation between agriculture and human nutrition. At that time, W.O. Atwater, the first director of the USDA's Office of Experiment Stations, reported that Americans were eating excessive amounts of "fat meats" and that dietary intake of such meats should be limited. When the USDA published its first national food guide in 1916, the advice from Atwater to reduce the amount of fat in the American diet was not included.

Thing haven't gotten any better since then, in fact they have gotten far worse. The USDA Food Pyramid is one of the most controversial guides to food and nutrition in the USDA's history, and has, in fact, changed is shape, style, and food group arrangement twice between 1980 and 2005. Moreover, what is most disturbing about the use of these food guides as the "true bible" for nutritional guidance for Americans is that, despite all of these government sanctioned food guides, we continue to be the fattest and sickest nation in the world.

My generation was raised on the USDA's *Food for Fitness—A Daily Food Guide*, published in 1956, which became widely known as The Basic Four, or the Four Food Groups. These four food groups consisted of Dairy, Meat, Fruits and Vegetables, and Breads and Cereals. The Basic Four was visually presented in schools as a circle divided into four equal quarters, indicating that each food group had an equal health value and that we should eat equal amounts from each group. By the 1980's, it was recognized that the method of eating equal amounts from each group was not nutritionally sound. In addition, the growing number of refined foods that fell into the bread and cereal group and the dairy group could be linked to a growing number of health problems.

In response to this nutritional disaster, the USDA hired a team of top-level nutritionists to develop a new food guide (now widely known as the Food Guide

Pyramid) to replace the "Basic Four" in the 1980's. Luise Light, MS, EdD, former USDA Director of Dietary Guidance and Nutrition Education Research, was leader of the team responsible for developing the original Food Guide Pyramid. Her article *A Fatally Flawed Food Guide*, describes the fatal flaws of a government bowing to industry interests. The following is an excerpt of her article:

Back in the early '80s, I was the leader of a group of top-level nutritionists with the USDA who developed the eating guide that became known as the Food Guide Pyramid. Carefully reviewing the research on nutrient recommendations, disease prevention, documented dietary shortfalls and major health problems of the population, we submitted the final version of our new Food Guide to the Secretary of Agriculture.

When our version of the Food Guide came back to us revised, we were shocked to find that it was vastly different from the one we had developed. As I later discovered, the wholesale changes made to the guide by the Office of the Secretary of Agriculture were calculated to win the acceptance of the food industry. For instance, the Ag Secretary's office altered wording to emphasize processed foods over fresh and whole foods, to downplay lean meats and low-fat dairy choices because the meat and milk lobbies believed it'd hurt sales of full-fat products; it also hugely increased the servings of wheat and other grains to make the wheat growers happy. The meat lobby got the final word on the color of the saturated fat/cholesterol guideline which was changed from red to purple because meat producers worried that using red to signify "bad" fat would be linked to red meat in consumers' minds.

Where we, the USDA nutritionists, called for a base of 5-9 servings of fresh fruits and vegetables a day, it was replaced with a paltry 2-3 servings (changed to 5-7 servings a couple of years later because an anti-cancer campaign by another government agency, the National Cancer Institute, forced the USDA to adopt the higher standard.) Our recommendation of 3-4 daily servings of whole-grain breads and cereals was changed to a whopping 6-11 servings forming the base of the pyramid as a concession to the processed wheat and corn industries. Moreover, my nutritionist group had placed baked goods made with white flour—including crackers, sweets and other low-nutrient foods laden with sugars and fats—at the peak of the pyramid, recommending that they be eaten sparingly. To our alarm, in the "revised" Food Guide, they were now made part of the Pyramid's base. And, in yet one more assault on dietary logic, changes were made to the wording of the dietary guidelines from "eat less" to "avoid too much," giving a nod to the processed-food industry interests by *not* limiting highly profitable "fun foods" (junk foods by any other name) that might affect the bottom line of food companies.

But even this neutralized wording of the revised Guidelines created a firestorm of angry responses from the food industry and their congressional allies who believed that the "farmers' department" (USDA) should *not* be telling the public to eat less of anything, including saturated fat and cholesterol, meat, eggs, and sugar.

"I vehemently protested that the changes, if followed, could lead to an epidemic of obesity and diabetes—and couldn't be justified on either health or nutritional grounds." To my amazement, I was a lone voice on this issue, as my colleagues appeared to accept the "policy-level" decision. Over my objections, the Food Guide Pyramid was finalized, although it only saw the light of day 12 years later in 1992. Yet it appears my warning has come to pass.

Here we are again, poised to be served up another helping of Dietary Guidelines in 2005, and a possible replacement for the failed Food Pyramid. This time, can we expect something less compromised and more reflective of what Americans need to achieve good health?

I think not. Ultimately, the food industry dictates the government's food advice, shaping the nutrition agenda delivered to the public. In fact, to the food industry, the purpose of food guides is to persuade consumers that *all* foods (especially those that *they're* selling) can fit into a healthful diet.[9]

NEW USDA FOOD PYRAMID STILL SUPPORTS PROCESSED FOODS

The 2005 Pyramid still contains information, which, as Luise Light, points out in her article, could be considered meaningless and deceptive. For example, it allows for consumption of refined carbohydrates (make half your grains whole is just another way of saying make half your grains refined), use of processed meats, and trans fats, as well as approval for "discretionary calories from added sugars and fats, once basic nutritional needs have been met." [10]

For example, the 2005 Food Guide Pyramid says you may have anywhere from 100 to 300 "discretionary calories" per day. These calories are the "extras" that can be used on luxuries like trans fats, added sugars, and alcohol, or on more food from any food group. According to the Food Guide Pyramid, you can use your discretionary calorie allowance to:

- Eat more foods from any food group that the food guide recommends.
- Eat higher calorie forms of foods—those that contain trans fats or added sugars. Examples are whole milk, cheese, sausage, biscuits, sweetened cereal, and sweetened yogurt.
- Add fats or sweeteners to foods. Examples are sauces, salad dressings, sugar, syrup, and butter.
- Eat or drink items that are mostly fats, caloric sweeteners, and/or alcohol, such as candy, soda, wine, and beer.[11]

A HEALTHIER FOOD PYRAMID

In his book, *Eat, Drink, and Be Healthy*, Walter C. Willett, M.D., addresses the USDA pyramid recommendations which he describes as "wishy-washy, scientifically unfounded advice on an absolutely vital topic—what to eat."[12] Dr. Willett is uniquely qualified to evaluate the USDA nutritional recommendations, as he is the chair of the nutrition department at the Harvard School of public health and one of America's foremost experts on nutrition. He was the pioneer researcher of the famous Nurse's Health Study, one of the longest running studies (several decades long involving over 238,000 dedicated nurse-participants) to investigate the factors that influence women's health. His extensive food and nutrition background has led to many published works, including the textbook *Nutritional Epidemiology* and over six hundred scientific articles. [13]

In, *Eat, Drink, and Be Healthy*, Dr. Willett calls the recommendations listed in the USDA food pyramid scientifically incorrect and states that "the USDA Pyramid hasn't really changed in spite of important advances in what we know about nutrition and health."[14] Instead, the USDA's Food Guide Pyramid recommendations provide misinformation that has contributed to obesity and other health issues faced by Americans.

As an alternative to the USDA pyramid, Dr. Willett created what he refers to as the Healthy Eating Pyramid. His nutritional recommendations are based on solid nutritional research, not the incomplete, inadequate, and politically influenced information used in the USDA pyramid. Dr. Willett's Healthy Eating Pyramid is a blueprint for solid nutrition, and involves seven healthy changes that will help control weight and promote good health. These are:

- Watch your weight and exercise daily
- Eat fewer bad fats and more good fats
- Eat fewer refined grains carbohydrates and more whole grains
- Choose healthy sources of protein
- Eat plenty of vegetables and fruits, but not potatoes
- Use alcohol in moderation
- Take a multivitamin. [15]

Plan-D provides a new and improved way of utilizing the food category components that comprise the typical American diet. Its tenets are based on scientific research and knowledge provided by experts like nutritionist Luise Light and Dr. Willett. In the following chapter, you will learn of three more nutrition experts whose work has shaped the foundation for Plan-D.

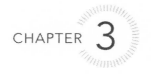

CHAPTER 3

Extraordinary Health:
A DOCTOR, A DENTIST AND A PSYCHIC

Our twenty-first century technological advancements allow us to process food so it will last for decades on a store shelf—yet our bodies are still "genetically wired" to function best on the foods favored by our ancestors.
—Jordan Rubin, The Maker's Diet

Now that we know we can't count on our government to steer us in the right nutritional direction, why don't we ask some real experts—our ancestors. In the development of Plan-D, I researched the role of food in the human story, and used the traditional diets of our not-so-distant ancestors as my guide.

To help me better understand the effect of food on human health, I studied the philosophies of three American nutritional giants. These American icons, Francis M. Pottenger, Jr., M.D., Weston Price, DDS, and Edgar Cayce, devoted their lives to investigating and disseminating information on the relationship between optimal health, nutrition, food choices, and the impact of food production techniques on America's food supply.

The work of Francis Pottenger and Weston Price spans over 100 years of study, observations, and research. Their work is maintained and expanded on today through the mission of the foundation named in their honor – The Price-Pottenger Nutrition Foundation. The foundation was founded in 1952, became a non-profit public education organization in 1954 and evolved over the years to be more commonly known as the Weston A. Price memorial foundation.[1]

The fascinating tale of their work shows a direct relationship between the rise in diseases and health problems in modern countries and the evolutionary trend toward a processed, refined, mass-produced food supply. Their research demonstrates the impact of poor nutrition on successive generations, which spans the globe and is as relevant today as it was when their studies were first conducted.

Edgar Cayce (1877-1945), known today as the "Father of Holistic Medicine," is the most documented psychic of the 20th century. For more than 40 years of his adult life, Cayce gave psychic "readings" to thousands of seekers while in an unconscious state. More than just a psychic, he had an amazing ability to diagnose illness and then "prescribe" holistic or other pathways of healing for sick people. He was not a medical doctor. Today he would be known as a medical intuitive, but his powers far exceeded any modern day seer.

In the Cayce readings, diet is featured prominently as both a preventative and a therapeutic measure.

Even back in the 1930's, Cayce warned about the dangers of eating processed foods. He advised against eating white flour and sugar, and recommended an abundance of fresh vegetables and fruits. Much of the contemporary "new" research about the preventative health properties of foods and herbs, were being espoused by Cayce in the early 1900's. The Edgar Cayce readings, of which there are over 14,000, are housed at the Association for Research and Enlightenment, the non-profit organization founded by Cayce in 1931 in Virginia Beach, Virginia.

In the remainder of this chapter, I will introduce you to these amazing men and their profound work. It is my intention to enlighten you as I was by the nutritional truths gleaned from their extensive studies and teachings.

DR. POTTENGER'S EARLY INTEREST IN NUTRITION

Dr. Francis M. Pottenger, Jr. was born in 1901 in Monrovia, California to Dr. and Mrs. Francis Pottenger, Sr. who founded the Pottenger Sanatorium for treatment of tuberculosis in 1903. Recognized internationally for its outstanding treatment of tuberculosis, good nutrition was one of the key components Dr. Pottenger, Sr. incorporated in the treatment provided at the sanatorium. So strong was his belief in the connection between nutrition and health that most of the food served to patients was grown on the premises. Dr. Pottenger, Sr. even worked with the U.S. Department of Agriculture to raise Holstein cows, which were the first to be accredited by the government as being free of tuberculosis. Over his lifetime Dr. Pottenger, Sr. wrote hundreds of articles and books on the treatment of chest disease, many of which were used in medical schools. [2]

As a member of this prominent family, Francis Pottenger, Jr. made his own mark early in his life with ingenious mechanical and electrical inventions. While only a teenager he created a system for his father's sanatorium that consisted of "tractor drawn, heated meal carts to deliver hot meals from the sanatorium kitchen to the outlying patient cottages." [3]

Despite Francis Pottenger, Jr.'s natural engineering skills, his father insisted that his son pursue a medical career. In abiding by his father's wishes, he attended and graduated in 1930 from the University of Cincinnati School of Medicine. From the start of his medical career, Dr. Pottenger, Jr. blended his mechanical and medical abilities with the invention of medical devices such as the Pottenger Suction system and Rubber Flask Connectors. Both devices were used for many years in the medical field until more modern pumps and equipment were developed.

While he was attending medical school, Dr. Pottenger developed a "hatred" for the way civilized man treated himself and his children. He wondered why people, so capable of advancing their technology, failed so miserably in promoting their biological health. He felt a driving need to know and understand how man could maintain good health and eliminate chronic illness. This missionary zeal led him to focus his medical career towards the field of nutrition. [4]

Dr. Pottenger's most famous and enduring project was a ten-year study from 1932 to 1942 to determine the effects of processed foods on the health of domestic cats. It is this study that contributed to proving that poor diets change DNA and create disease traits that affect future generations.

POTTENGER'S CAT STUDY

Dr. Pottenger's ten-year cat study was prompted by the high death rate among his laboratory cats undergoing operations to remove their adrenal glands. At that time, there were no chemical procedures to measure the strength of adrenal extract. So, manufacturers used cats. Cats die without their adrenal glands. So, the amount of extract the cats needed to keep them alive allowed the manufacturers to calibrate the strength of their product.[5]

In preparing his cats for surgery, Dr. Pottenger fed them what he believed was the optimum diet for cats. It consisted of "raw milk, cod liver oil and cooked meat scraps of liver, tripe, sweetbreads, brains, heart and muscle." [6] However, despite feeding his cats what he considered a healthy diet, many of these cats did not seem healthy; they exhibited nutritional deficiencies, and a high percentage of them did not survive the surgery.

Concerned with the cats' poor postoperative survival, Dr. Pottenger noticed the cats showed a decrease in their reproductive capacity and many of the kittens born in the laboratory had skeletal deformities and organ malfunctions.

By a quirk of fate, since the number of cats donated by his neighbors kept increasing, he couldn't handle the demand for cooked meat scraps. So, he ordered raw meat scraps from a local meat packing plant, including the viscera, muscle and bone. Always a scientist, Dr. Pottenger fed these raw meat scraps to a segregated group of cats so that he could observe any change. Within a few months, this group appeared healthier, their kittens more vigorous, and they had a higher survival rate after their operations.[7]

The contrast between the two sets of cats was so startling that it prompted Dr. Pottenger to conduct an experiment to verify these facts scientifically. Because pathological problems in cats eating cooked meats were similar to those in his patients, he believed a controlled-feeding experiment with animals would isolate variables of importance in human nutrition as well. This experiment is now famously known as the Pottenger Cat Study.

As explained in his book, *Pottenger's Cats*, he very carefully designed the study to research these questions:

Why did the cats eating raw meat survive surgery at higher rates than cats eating cooked meat?

Why did cats eating raw meat appear healthier and more vigorous?

Why did a diet consisting of cooked foods not provide adequate nutrients?

What was the relationship of these findings on human nutrition? [8]

His study encompassed four generations involving 900 cats. The cats were divided into five groups, each of which was fed different diets ranging from raw meat, raw milk, pasteurized milk, evaporated milk and condensed milk. Each cat's record was carefully documented with its own chart that tracked its history, weight, development, diet, and outcomes. Kittens born to the cats had their birth information, delivery details, and health issues carefully documented, and any stillborn kitten was immediately autopsied. Information collected included any birth defects, skeletal deformities, and calcium and phosphorus deficiencies. [9]

The experiments met the most rigorous scientific standards of their day. His outstanding credentials earned Dr. Pottenger the support of prominent physicians. Dr. Alvin Foord, professor of pathology at the University of Southern California and pathologist at the Huntington Memorial Hospital in Pasadena, co-supervised with Pottenger all pathological and chemical findings of the study.

As we proceed to look at the actual findings of The Pottenger Cat Study, you will be able to see for yourself how similarities in nutrition that impacted the health of his cats can be applied to the relationship between human health and nutrition.

FINDINGS OF THE POTTENGER CAT STUDY

All the groups were supplied the same basic minimal diet, but the major portion of their diets was varied. Two of the groups were fed whole foods (raw milk and raw meat - real foods for cats). The other three groups were given processed foods: pasteurized, evaporated and condensed milk. The findings of the five groups over four generations were carefully recorded. In addition, at the end of the 10-year study, recorded histories of 600 of the 900 cats were completed. The study was designed to demonstrate the health effects of eating raw foods versus eating cooked and processed foods over successive generations of cats.

The following table clearly summarizes the health effects on the four generations of cats studied.

GROUP	A	B	C	D	E
FOOD FED	**Raw meat**	**Raw milk**	**Pasteurized milk**	**Evaporated milk**	**Condensed milk**
1st Generation	Remained healthy	Remained healthy	Developed diseases and illnesses near end of life		
2nd Generation	Remained healthy	Remained healthy	Developed diseases and illnesses in middle of life		
3rd Generation	Remained healthy	Remained healthy	Developed diseases and illnesses in beginning of life; many died before six months of age		
4th Generation	Remained healthy	Remained healthy	No fourth generation was produced; either third generation parents were sterile, or fourth generation cats were miscarried before birth		
Source: Pottenger's Cats, a Study in Nutrition [10]					

All four generations of the raw meat and raw milk groups remained healthy throughout their normal lifespans. The three groups of cats receiving processed foods developed diseases and illnesses earlier in their life spans with each succeeding generation, to the point where they were no longer able to reproduce their species.

The results document that through each successive generation the levels of health *decreased,* and the rates of degenerative diseases *increased.* Here are the specifics of the impact of processed foods on each generation studied as described in Ronald Schmid's book *Traditional Foods Are Your Best Medicine*:

> The cats eating only raw food were disease-free and healthy, generation after generation after generation. They reproduced easily, and as each generation developed there was for each sex, striking uniformity in size and skeletal development. A broad face with wide dental arches and no crowding of teeth was the rule. Fur was uniform, with good sheen and little shedding. Inflammation and diseases of the gums were rare.
>
> These animals were resistant to infections, fleas, and other parasites. They were friendly, even-tempered, and well coordinated—when dropped from up to six feet or thrown, they always landed on all four feet. Miscarriages were rare, and litters averaged five kittens. Cause of death was generally old age, or occasionally fighting among males. Autopsies invariably revealed normal internal organs.
>
> The cats eating the cooked and processed foods had myriad health problems that grew with successive generations. Litter mates varied greatly in size and skeletal structure, particularly in dental and facial pattern. Often by the third generation, bones became so soft as to be actually rubbery. Vision problems, infections of internal organs and bones, arthritis, heart problems, underactivity of the thyroid gland, inflammation of the joints

and nervous system, skin lesions, allergies, intestinal parasites and vermin, and a host of other pathologies were common. Coordination was poor; when tossed a short distance, the cats had trouble landing on all four feet. Pneumonia and lung abscesses were the most usual causes of death in adults; pneumonia and diarrhea were the usual causes in kittens.

At autopsy, analysis of the bones of processed-food cats determined calcium and phosphorous content to second- and third-generation kittens to be one-third to one-half that of the raw-meat kittens.

Many processed-food kittens exhibited behavioral changes; females were irritable and aggressive, while males were often docile and unaggressive with little interest in females but keen interest in other males (an interest never seen in raw meat-fed males). Abnormal sexual activities also were seen between females in the processed food group. At autopsy, females often showed small ovaries with a congested uterus; males frequently showed testes that had failed to develop the ability to produce sperm.

The miscarriage rate among first generation processed food cats was about 25 percent, among the second generation about 70 percent. Many cats died in labor; deliveries were difficult; many kittens were born dead or too frail to nurse. The kittens born of processed food mothers, weighed an average nineteen grams less than those of raw-meat mothers.

No fourth generation of kittens was born to the processed food groups in the ten years of the study. In the third generation, the cats suffered from most of the degenerative diseases encountered in human medicine; the kittens always died before reaching six months of age, terminating the strain.[11]

Dr. Pottenger also studied and documented the effect of the mother cat's diet on her nursing kittens. He found that when normal, healthy kittens were born, their state of health was either maintained or reduced based on the diet fed to the mother cat. In other words, if the diet of the nursing cat was changed from the raw based components to the less healthy diet, she could not pass on adequate nutrients to the nursing kittens. This directly impacted the health of the kittens. For kittens born to deficient mother cats to whom the deficient diet consistently was given, the milk the kittens received was deficient in nutrients and that reinforced the deficiencies with which the kittens were born. However, if the deficient kittens were given feedings in which proper nutrients were provided during the nursing period, improvements to their general condition occurred. [12]

CORRELATIONS TO HUMAN HEALTH

These results clearly show that without a doubt, nutrition impacts health. It may not appear until later in life, or not until the next generation, but genetic weaknesses do develop over time. Those weaknesses develop when generation after generation continues to depend on diets that are devoid of correct nutrients. That impact can be lessened only when diets with proper nutrients are adopted! When healthy diets are eaten, illnesses and degenerative diseases can be improved. That point is clearly shown in both Dr. Pottenger's cat studies and the research conducted by Dr. Weston Price, as you will read shortly.

As for applying his results to human nutrition, Dr. Pottenger said, "While no attempt will be made to correlate the changes in the animals studied with malformations found in humans, the similarity is so obvious that parallel pictures will suggest themselves." [13]

The Pottenger Cat Study gives insight into why children today are getting degenerative diseases that used to only show up in humans at an age of 50 years or older. What's alarming about this study is that the levels of health get progressively worse with each generation, just as we are seeing with humans. It takes approximately 20 years to beget a generation of humans, so the same study would take over 80 years in people. Of course no such study is being done on humans, but it's easy to observe that there is a tremendous increase in heart disease, cancer, arthritis, and autoimmune diseases over the last eighty years.

Does this give you an understanding of and make you wonder why so many children are now developing cancer, diabetes, and other rare medical conditions that were once only found in adults? Could our processed SAD foods be the reason why Generation X is experiencing high rates of infertility? A fertility clinic was all but unheard of a mere 50 years ago.

Dr. Pottenger's study is not a gloom and doom story. He proved that diseases are *not* inherited; rather only the *tendency or potential* of a disease is passed on from parents to offspring. The disease tendency is transferred by way of the genetic code (DNA), and will only manifest as a disease unless there are factors that exploit that weakness (poor diet, for example).

Throughout the study he pulled some of the sick cats out their processed food groups and put them into the raw food groups. The results showed that within a short amount of time, the sick cats got well. And more than that, the disease tendencies no longer manifested in subsequent generations when those generations continued on the raw diet.

My understanding of the results of the Pottenger Cat Study is that we have the ability to improve our health simply by improving our diet. We can reverse disease traits that have been passed on to us if we take the necessary steps to correct nutritional deficiencies.

THE NUTRITIONAL WORK OF A PROMINENT DENTIST

Just as you may have never heard of Dr. Francis Pottenger, the name Weston Price probably eludes you as well. Although he was a Harvard trained dentist, Dr. Weston Price is most likely the greatest nutritionist who ever lived.

After receiving his degree in dentistry in 1893, Weston Price became a prominent, well-respected dentist, professor and researcher in his field. He taught to thousands at dental schools and wrote textbooks on dentistry that became standards at universities throughout the country.

During his years in private dental practice, Dr. Price began to notice that the children of his patients were developing dental problems that their parents had not experienced. Besides having more decay, in many children the teeth did not fit properly into the dental arch and were, as a result, crowded and crooked. Dr. Price suspected that changes in nutrition were responsible.[14]

These problems were not seen just ten or fifteen years earlier, which peaked his curiosity as to why it was it happening now. Dr. Price also noticed a strong correlation between dental health and physical health: a mouth full of cavities went hand in hand with a body either full of disease, or generalized weakness and susceptibility to disease. In Price's time, tuberculosis was the major infectious illness, known as the White Scourge. He noticed that children were increasingly affected, the ones with the lousy teeth.[15]

He also noticed that the condition of the teeth reflected overall health. Considering possible reasons, a revolutionary idea occurred to him: perhaps some deficiency in modern diets caused the problems.[16] Solid scientific evidence indicates that all three symptoms Dr. Price noticed in his young patients signal physical degeneration and an increased vulnerability to diseases such as heart attacks and cancer.[17]

Dr. Price knew that the observations of anthropologists had long documented the excellent teeth found in primitive cultures. Being rather well off financially, he and his wife Monica Price, R.N., decided to travel the world to study primitive societies. They were specifically looking for healthy peoples who had not been touched yet by civilization—at that time, such groups were still around, however many of them were just beginning to adopt modern diets.

Price's work is often criticized at this point for being biased. Critics claim that Price simply ignored native peoples that were not healthy; therefore, his data and conclusions about primitive diets are unfounded. These critics are missing the point and motivation for Dr. Price's work. Dr. Price was not interested in examining sick people because he'd seen enough of them in America. Dr. Price wanted to find HEALTHY people, find out what made them so, and see if there were any patterns among these people.[18]

DR. PRICE'S WORLDWIDE JOURNEY

As Ronald Schmid writes in his book, *Traditional Foods are Your Best Medicine*:

> Price visited and studied cultures where people who were following traditional ways and diets lived near kinsmen who were eating the foods of modern civilization. Throughout the world in the 1930's, groups in the early stages of modernization were using foods imported from western countries—sugar, white flour, canned foods, and vegetable oils. These people often lived close to fellow villagers and people of the same ancestry living in nearby villages who still ate entirely according to native ways.
>
> Price's time in history was unique. The cultures he observed were still truly indigenous, with groups of people living entirely on the local foods. Photographic emulsion was commonly available for the first time; he could easily record his observations. World travel too was readily available for the first time for anyone able to afford it. This combination of old and new enabled him to see and record a picture of a disappearing world.[19]

Dr. Price and his wife went just about everywhere in their journeys. They traveled to isolated villages in the Swiss Alps, to cold and blustery islands off the coast of Scotland, to the Andes Mountains in Peru, to several locations in Africa, to the Polynesian islands, to Australia and New Zealand, to the forests of northern Canada, and even to the Arctic Circle. In all, Price visited with fourteen groups of native peoples.

In every village they visited, Dr. Price conducted dental and physical exams, and documented all of his findings. He recorded the components of each group's daily diets, and even preserved samples of the various foods his research subjects ate, in order to later conduct chemical analysis of those foods. To further document his observations, Dr. Price and his wife took 18,000 photographs, many of which are contained in his book.[20]

Dr. Price's discoveries were remarkable. He found entire cultures with beautiful straight teeth—no children with misshapen dental arches and crowded teeth. Dr. Price interviewed an American medical doctor living among the Eskimos and northern Indians who reported that in thirty-five years of observation, he had never seen a single case of cancer among the natives subsisting on their traditional foods. When natives eating the white man's foods developed tuberculosis, this doctor eventually took to sending them back to their native villages and native foods; they then usually recovered. In every culture where the people were immune to dental and degenerative disease, biochemical analysis showed the diet to be rich in nutrients poorly supplied in modern diets.[21]

Dr. Price recorded his findings from his travels to all fourteen countries in his book *Nutritional and Physical Degeneration*, published in 1939. Many in his profession viewed his work as profound and significant. So too did many anthropologists; for years, the book was required reading for anthropology classes at Harvard. But because the book is long, tedious, and technical, it was never widely read by the general public.

What is clear from Dr. Price's studies is that there is a definite connection between consumption of traditional and natural food diets and the maintenance of good health. This connection is emphasized by studies of groups who followed their traditional diets, and lived near relatives who had adopted a more westernized diet. This gave Dr. Price the opportunity to *compare* the health of two related groups whose only difference was their diet. Dr. Price was even allowed to examine skeletal remains of ancient people in various groups he studied. In Peru alone, "he examined 1,276 successive skulls without finding one with the narrowed dental arches of modern people." [22]

Before discussing Dr. Price's specific findings, I want to clarify what the groups were eating when I refer to traditional foods versus the foods consumed on more modernized diets. The following table demonstrates the drastic differences between them.

Traditional Diet Foods	Modernized Diet Foods
All traditional diets studied were rich in *animal foods** containing *saturated fat* and *cholesterol* such as butter, eggs, fatty fish, wild game, and organ meats. The fats in these foods are rich in the fat-soluble vitamins A, D, E and K	Consumption of naturally raised meats and seafood declined while the increase of canned meats and seafood increased

Artificial vitamins were taken to make up for deficiencies |
Raw dairy products: milk, yogurt, butter, cheese	Pasteurized, homogenized milk and dairy products made from this milk
Tropical fruits; raw honey	Refined sugar or corn syrup
Legumes, sprouted grains, raw nuts and seeds soaked in water, naturally leavened breads	White flour products, roasted and salted nuts
Cold-pressed oils	Refined or hydrogenated vegetable oils
Naturally preserved, fermented vegetables, fruits, beverages, meats, and condiments	Canned Foods Additives and colorings
* Unlike the meats eaten today, the animals eaten in traditional diets were pasture raised (grass-fed) without hormones or antibiotics. **Source:** http://www.westonaprice.org/brochures/wapfbrochure.html [23]	

Diets would vary from country to country. For example, in the Loetschental Valley in the Swiss Alps, the villagers lived primarily on butter and cheese made from unpasteurized milk, rye bread, berries, and occasional beef when one of the older cattle were slaughtered. Very little vegetation grew due to the altitude, so whatever could be grown in the short summer months was pickled for use in winter months.[24]

Populations which lived near seas and oceans, such as Gaelic peoples of the Outer Hebrides, Eskimos and Maori of New Zealand all consumed large amounts of seafood including cod, shellfish, walrus, seal, shark, octopus, and sea worms, depending on what was common to their area. Additionally, while the Maori had a variety of plant foods and fruits, Eskimos only gathered nuts, berries and some grasses in short summer months and depended almost 100 percent on animal products. The Gaelic were limited to growing oats and used them as a major part of their diet.[25]

Diets of the tribes in Africa that were studied greatly varied. In the Sudan, diets consisted of fermented whole grains with fish, red meat, particularly liver, vegetables, and fruit. A number of other tribes throughout Africa were primarily agricultural and their diets consisted of corn, beans, sweet potatoes, bananas and millet, along with some fish and milk, while the Muhima tribe raised cattle and lived on meat, milk, blood, and wild plant foods.[26]

Some commonalities among all diets that Dr. Price noted were the daily use of fermented foods which ranged from cheeses, yogurt, grain drinks, fish, and seaweeds. Additionally, native diets were *rich in fats, particularly animal fats*; the use of saturated fats is necessary for the body to assimilate and utilize proteins. Finally, foods were natural, unpasteurized, pesticide-free, and unprocessed with no added sugar, white flour, preservatives, additives, or colorings. [27]

DR. PRICE'S FINDINGS

In every group he visited, Dr. Price did what he was best at—he counted cavities and physically examined teeth. Imagine his surprise to find, on average, less than 1 percent of tooth decay in all the peoples he visited! He also found that these people's teeth were perfectly straight and white, with high dental arches and well-formed facial features. And there was something more astonishing: none of the peoples Price examined practiced any sort of dental hygiene; not one of his subjects had ever flossed or used a toothbrush! However, kinsmen of groups studied who had left their isolated village and had spent time in modern cities eating modernized foods, experienced large amounts of dental diseases.[28]

The Loetschental Valley, nearly a mile above sea level in an isolated part of the Swiss Alps, had been for more than a dozen centuries the home of some two thousand people when the Price's first visited in 1931. At this time in Switzerland, tuberculosis took the lives of more people than any other disease. Astonishingly, no deaths had occurred from tuberculosis in the history of the Loetschental Valley, despite frequent exposure to the disease. Dr. Price noted this was evidence of a good diet and natural forces at work.[29]

In general, Price found, in contrast to what he saw in America, no incidence of the very diseases that plague modern people with our processed food diets: cancer, heart disease, diabetes, hemorrhoids, multiple sclerosis, Parkinson's, Alzheimer's, osteoporosis, chronic fatigue syndrome (it was called neurasthenia in Price's day), etc. But, groups who no longer only ate their traditional diets were highly susceptible to tuberculosis and other degenerative diseases.[30]

Dr. Price saved and preserved a variety of foods obtained from each country that he sent back to the United States for analysis of the vitamin and mineral content. The results showed that the traditional foods contained ten times the amount of fat-soluble vitamins (A, D, E, and K), and four times the calcium, minerals and water-soluble vitamins found in the Western diets of the 1930's.[31]

Dr. Price also noticed another quality about the healthy primitives he found: they were happy, hardy and strong, despite the sometimes difficult living conditions they had to endure. While depression was not a major problem in Price's day, it certainly is today: ask any psychiatrist. While certain natives sometimes fought with neighboring tribes, within their own groups, they were cheerful and optimistic and bounced back quickly from emotional setbacks. These people had no need for antidepressants.[32]

There are so many more stories and details about specific groups and foods Dr. Price studied than I can include in this chapter. But, what I can summarize for you from the highlights of Dr. Price's findings is that one's health—both physical and dental—is directly related to food choices. Poor nutrition leads to chronic and degenerative diseases, and contributes to the development of obesity.

The good news that Dr. Price's findings show, and that I have personally experienced, and have seen with my clients, is that when a person changes their poor food choices and adopts a processed-free lifestyle, good health follows.

THE PARALLELS BETWEEN THE WORK
OF DR. POTTENGER AND DR. PRICE

The health problems of the cats Dr. Pottenger studied provided parallels with the human societies that Dr. Price studied. Again, Schmid details the parallels:

> The cats developed the same diseases as humans eating refined foods. The cats eating processed foods also developed the same dental malformations that children of people eating modernized foods developed, including narrowing of dental arches with attendant crowding of teeth, underbites and overbites, and protruding and crooked teeth. The shape of the cat's skull and even the entire skeleton became abnormal in severe cases, with accompanying marked behavioral changes.
>
> Price observed these same physical and behavioral changes in both native and modern cultures eating refined foods. Humans don't have the same nutritional requirements as cats, but whatever else each needs, we have strong empirical evidence that both need a significant amount of certain high quality foods to reproduce and function efficiently.[33]

In the 1940's Dr. Pottenger recognized and acknowledged the importance of Dr. Price's work. Believing that Dr. Price's findings on the connection between diet, nutrition and health were a confirmation of his own studies, Dr. Pottenger "became chairman of a committee established for the purpose of disseminating Price's work through exhibits, lectures and printed materials." This committee later formed the Price-Pottenger Nutritional Foundation in 1952, later to be known as the Weston A. Price Foundation.)[34] I encourage you to visit the Foundation's website (see Appendix B) which is a storehouse of cutting edge articles and research on whole foods nutrition.

EDGAR CAYCE, THE FATHER OF HOLISTIC MEDICINE

During the same period that Dr. Pottenger and Dr. Price were conducting their nutritional studies, Edgar Cayce was helping thousands of people recover from physical ailments through natural treatments he prescribed while in a hypnotic state. Often the cures he prescribed focused on eating whole foods, herbs, and lifestyle changes, such as you might find with today's holistic medicine or naturopathy.

Edgar Cayce was born on a farm in Hopkinsville, Kentucky, in 1877, and his psychic abilities began to appear as early as his childhood. As an adult, his profession was as a photographer, but Cayce discovered that he had the ability to put himself into a sleep-like state by lying down on a couch, closing his eyes, and folding his hands over his stomach. In this state of relaxation and meditation, he had the amazing ability to see into a person's body, to detect the root cause of ill health, and to accurately prescribe a natural treatment. The information he gave to people concerning health and other topics came to be called "readings," and their insights offer practical help and advice to individuals even today.

The majority of Edgar Cayce's readings deal with holistic health and the treatment of illness, for which he is best known. He viewed the human body as a miracle of creation in its ability to heal itself when given the proper nourishment, exercise, and rest. As it was at the time Cayce was giving readings, still today, individuals from all walks of life and belief receive physical relief from illnesses or ailments through information given in the readings—some readings were given as far back as 100 years ago!

In an article written by Sydney Kirkpatrick, *Edgar Cayce's View of Health and Healing*, he describes Cayce's remarkable gift:

> When Edgar Cayce, fully awake, considered human anatomy, it was with the eye of a professional portrait photographer. In trance, however, when "the Source" spoke through the sleeping Cayce, he was the "psychic diagnostician," reporting on temperature, blood pressure, and other physical and anatomical details of a patient's body. Cayce could describe a patient's condition in such a cool, calm, and detached manner that observers were left with the impression that he was a physician describing to fellow colleagues an examination he was in the process of conducting, except for the fact that Cayce's patients didn't have to be in the same room or even in the same country as Cayce. He appeared to be able to see right into his patient's body, to examine each organ, blood vessel, and artery with microscopic precision, and then recommend treatments to restore or enhance a patient's health. Many of Cayce's recommended treatments, once dismissed as the fanciful products of an overactive imagination, are now considered state-of-the-art medical treatment and have earned Cayce the distinction of being called the father of holistic medicine.
>
> In the chaotic early years of Edgar Cayce's career as a psychic diagnostician (1911-1927) – before his trance readings were properly recorded and indexed, and when the patient's detailed medical records were not shared with Edgar - it was nearly impossible to view his contribution to medicine in a broader context. Unless a patient experienced immediate recovery Edgar and those around him had limited knowledge of the outcome of the treatments he recommended while in trance. Little or no effort was made to trace a patient's progress or to determine the effectiveness of the treatments recommended. Only files containing letters of thanks offered insights.
>
> This changed in 1928 when the Edgar Cayce hospital was founded in Virginia Beach, and Cayce would go on to give approximately 7,000 more medical readings before his death in 1945. With a dedicated conductor to put Cayce into trance, a stenographer to supervise and record trance sessions, and a team of board-certified physicians to study, chart, and interpret a patient's progress over a long period of time, it was possible to begin seeing the scope of Cayce's contributions and to gain a better understanding of the general principles of health he communicated in the readings. As medical

scholars would point out a generation later, together, Cayce's trance readings provided a primer on the emerging field of holistic medicine.

Although the information Cayce imparted was often in keeping with the practice of both homeopathic and allopathic medicine at the time, it became clear by the late 1920s that Cayce also drew information from the medical knowledge of ancient cultures, especially those in Egypt and Greece. And a fair percentage of Cayce's ideas were entirely new at the time the readings were given—sometimes given on the very same day the treatment or product was becoming available to the public. Some of Cayce's medical insights have since been confirmed by modern medical science, while others are yet to be validated.

The fact that many of the treatments Cayce recommended were in keeping with the standard medical approach to illness made it easier for doctors to follow his advice. As a general rule, these treatments varied only in the combination of medicine and therapies, but often involved more hard work on the part of both the doctor and patient than has become the norm in modern medicine. Invariably, however, the hard work paid off. In many instances, Cayce was clearly ahead of his time. For instance, he once recommended that an infant with digestive problems be kept on a strict diet of bananas, which in the 1920s was generally considered to be poisonous to infants. Now, the all-banana diet is standard medical treatment for celiac children.

The greatest surprises of Cayce's health readings were the apparent causes given for various illnesses and his warnings against eating processed foods. Just as mass-produced foods were beginning to appear, and decades before the whole-food movement became popular, Cayce was issuing warnings. He repeatedly stated that refined foods, sugars, red meat, and fried food were generally harmful to the body. He stated that pork was to be avoided, with the exception of a little crisp bacon at breakfast occasionally.

Cayce did not just warn patients away from certain foods, he encouraged the consumption of others. For instance, in keeping with what is now known about the importance of ingesting active food enzymes, he recommended eating one meal per day of primarily raw vegetables. He also consistently instructed patients to eat whole rather than refined grains, saying that refined products not only lacked nutrients the body needs, but that such foods, with all enzymes and other elements removed, are actually toxic to the human body. And although he didn't use the contemporary term *phyto-chemicals*—the nutritional element related to the color of foods—he often recommended foods of a certain color for particular ailments.

Cayce also spoke of the acid-alkaline balance in the body, which he said was affected by the foods we eat—an area of nutrition that was virtually unheard of in the 1920s, and has only recently become popular. Cayce's general diet guidelines recommended the consumption of twenty percent acid producing foods, such as meats, starches and sugars, and eighty percent alkaline producing foods, such as vegetables, fruits and dairy products. To a forty-eight-year-old woman, Cayce said: "The less physical exercise...the greater should be the alkaline reacting food taken. Energies or activities may burn acids, but those who lead the sedentary life can't go on sweets or too much starches."

He also recommended that vegetables from below the ground, such as carrots, beets, and potatoes, should constitute only twenty-five percent of one's diet of vegetables, while above the ground vegetables, such as lettuce, squash, and tomatoes, should account for the other seventy-five percent. He recommended that only ten percent of our diet be fats, another ten percent proteins, five percent refined starches and sugars and the other seventy-five percent complex carbohydrates such as vegetables, fruits and grains.

Long after Cayce's death, many of the seemingly radical guidelines he offered in the 1930s would be seen as having merit. But some of Cayce's recommendations still seem strange to this day. For instance, he stated in several readings that while tomatoes contain more nutrients than any other single food, when not vine-ripened, they are toxic to the human body. He also stated that carbonated drinks were to be almost always avoided, not just because of the sugar or artificial sweetener in them, but because they interfered with the interaction between the liver and the kidney. Other gems offered by Cayce included such statements as: apples should never be eaten raw, only baked or cooked, unless used for fasting purposes; only the peel of the white potato was of any real nutritional value; and coffee and tea become toxic when combined with milk or cream.

Poor elimination was cited as being at the root of a great number of illnesses, and references to it appeared in over half of Cayce's medical readings. Apart from taking in nourishment, human cells must also eliminate waste products and toxins to remain healthy.

Cayce suggested many different aids to elimination. One of the simplest was to drink a cup of hot water with a squeeze of lemon juice each morning upon rising and before eating, which apparently helped the body eliminate the toxins thrown off during sleep. Similarly, he recommended doing deep breathing exercises each morning to eliminate toxins pooled in the lungs from the shallow breathing characteristic of sleep. Dietary measures were also recommended to improve bowel activity, which included eating leafy vegetables and stewed fruit such as figs and raisins. He also suggested drinking as much as six to eight glasses of water a day.

An important aspect of sustaining good health, according to Cayce, was circulation. "The circulation...is the main attribute to the physical body, or that which keeps life in the whole system," he often said in trance, and references to circulation turned up in approximately sixty-percent of the readings. Highlighting the role that circulation plays in assimilation and elimination, he pointed out that "there is no condition existent in a body that the reflection of same may not be traced to the blood supply, for not only does the blood stream carry the rebuilding forces to the body, it also takes the used forces and eliminates same through their proper channels." In the same reading, Cayce made a startling prophetic remark: "The day may yet arrive when one may take a drop of blood and diagnose the condition of any physical body."

Cayce made reference not only to arterial circulation, but lymphatic circulation, which he considered to be just as important. The Source referred to the fluid in the lymphatic system as "white blood" or "lymph blood," and pointed out that unlike the arterial system which has both the heart and the muscle-lined wall of the arteries to move the blood along, the lymph system has no pump of its own, and it relies on other methods to move waste matter out of the body. One method Cayce recommended was massage. Although it was considered by many to be nothing more than idle pampering, Cayce saw massage as curative, particularly for the inactive.

The most natural way to sustain good overall circulation, both of the lymph and the blood, Cayce said, was exercise. As he pointed out in a reading for a forty-six-year-old woman, "Exercise is wonderful, and necessary—and little or few take as much as is needed, in a systematic manner." To another patient he said exercise "is not something merely to be gotten through or gotten rid of." Daily stretches, head and neck rolls and walks, preferably of twenty minutes, were all recommendations Cayce gave.[35]

The recommendations on proper diet given by Edgar Cayce have come to be known as The Cayce Diet. The recommendations basically make up the basis of modern day food combining rules and the pH balance diet. Much of the information we have today about digestive wellness, alkalinity, and food combining were recommended by Cayce long before such contemporaries as Harvey Diamond (*Fit for Life*), Elizabeth Lipsky (*Digestive Wellness*), Theodore Baroody (*Alkalize or Die*), and Robert Young (*The pH Miracle*) wrote their books.

As you will see, the elements of Plan-D closely follow the health recommendations of Edgar Cayce, and the findings of doctors Pottenger and Price.

Further details of Cayce's life and work are explored in the classic book, *There is a River* by Thomas Sugrue, and *Edgar Cayce: An American Prophet* by Sidney Kirkpatrick.

Thousands of people have improved their health by following the advice in the Cayce readings. You may find more information about his health remedies by visiting the websites listed in Appendix B.

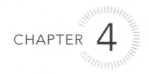

CHAPTER 4

The Perfection of Whole Foods

Healthful food has a spiritual value, for as we digest the life forces it contains, it becomes a part of us.
—Dee McCaffrey

As the studies of Dr. Pottenger and Dr. Price proved, and as the readings of Edgar Cayce suggest, our bodies are not designed to operate at optimum levels on junk food, fast food, sugar, flour, and convenience foods prepared in microwave ovens. There are biological laws that govern our bodies and our health, just as there are physical laws that govern our world. Those laws have been in place since the beginning of humankind. Just as the physical law of gravity cannot be changed, neither can the biological laws that dictate our health, whether or not we accept that they are in place. As much as we would like to be able to eat cookies, burgers and fries every day and still enjoy beautiful bodies, straight teeth and tons of energy, it just doesn't work that way.

Our bodies were specifically designed to function best on foods that have either not been changed from their original form, or only minimally changed (as in making butter and yogurt from milk, making bread from whole grains or cooking meats, fowl, and fish). Dr. Price's study of traditional societies eating their traditional diets revealed that the healthiest people in the world did not die from the diet- and lifestyle-related illnesses that kill most modern people before their time, mainly because they ate more healthfully and had more active lifestyles. Our not-so-distant ancestors ate foods such as wild game, fresh-caught fish from the sea or inland waterways, wild berries, nuts, and plant foods.[1] Some of them also ate dairy products made from the milk of cows or goats that fed on organic green grass (the optimal food for cows and goats).

So just what is it about whole natural foods that make them so optimal for our bodies? In order to understand this, we must first examine the inherent perfection of food. Studying food and nutrition has given me a great appreciation for its design and its designer. When we examine how food exists in nature, it is undeniable that our food was provided for us by an intelligent nature and does not occur by random chance.

IT IS A MYSTERY SCIENCE HAS NOT BEEN ABLE TO EXPLAIN

It is a mystery science has not been able to explain, but it is still true—every food that grows on the planet is uniquely and precisely designed for our bodies. There are no two foods that are exactly the same. Each food contains differing amounts and types of nutrients, that when eaten together, provide our bodies with complete and balanced nutrition. Additionally, the foods themselves contain specific combinations of vitamins, minerals, phytochemicals, fibers, and enzymes that work together, synergistically, to help our bodies digest those particular foods.

For example, the minerals required by our bodies to digest sugar are calcium, phosphorous, chromium, magnesium, cobalt, copper, zinc and manganese. Sugar cane in its natural form is rich in these vitamins and minerals. It also contains vitamins A, C, B1, B2, B6, niacin, iron, and pantothenic acid, which work synergistically

PHYTOCHEMICALS

Fruits, vegetables, grains, and legumes contain a group of health-promoting nutrients called *phytochemicals*. Phytochemicals are the biologically active substances in plants that are responsible for giving them color, flavor, and natural disease resistance. They are the magical mysterious healing substances that research has proven can prevent and reverse cancer and other diseases.

Nutrition researchers have identified thousands of phytochemicals, yet there are still many more that remain a mystery. It is estimated that there are **thousands** of different phytochemicals in a typical fruit or vegetable. To understand how phytochemicals protect the body against cancer, it is necessary to understand that the formation of cancer is a multistep process. Phytochemicals fight cancer by blocking one or more of the steps that lead to its formation.

For instance, cancer can begin when a carcinogenic (cancer causing) molecule—from the food you eat or the air you breathe—invades a cell. But if sulforaphane, a phytochemical found in broccoli, also reaches the cell, it activates a group of enzymes that whisk the carcinogen out of the cell before it can do any damage.

Other phytochemicals are known to prevent cancer in other ways. Flavonoids, found in citrus fruits and berries, keep cancer-causing hormones from latching on to cells in the first place. Genistein, found in soybeans, kills tumors by preventing the formation of the capillaries needed to nourish them. Indoles, found in cruciferous vegetables such as cabbage, Brussels sprouts, broccoli, and cauliflower, increase immune activity and make it easier for the body to excrete toxins. Sapopins, found in kidney beans, garbanzo beans, and lentils, may prevent cancer cells from multiplying. P-coumaric acid and chlorogenic acid, found in tomatoes, interfere with certain chemical unions that can create carcinogens. The list of protective substances goes on and on. Tomatoes alone are believed to contain an estimated 10,000 different phytochemicals!

with natural sugar cane's fiber and enzymes to *nourish the body*. Imagine, whole natural sugar cane actually nourishes our bodies! The natural fibers specific to the sugar cane help slow down the absorption of the sugars and prevent the sharp rise in blood sugar levels associated with eating sugar in an unnatural refined form. Similarly, other plant foods like fruits, carrots, and beets, also supply our bodies with the specific nutrients needed to properly digest their sugars.

Another example of the perfect design of food is found in seed-bearing plants. Dr. Rex Russell, M.D., explains, "A scientific examination of seeds indicates that they could not have developed by random chance." Seeds (which include grains, beans, and nuts) grow everywhere in the world, in any climate, and reproduce quickly. They have a long storage life: Kernels found in Egyptian tombs can still be sprouted after 4,000 years. Nutritionally—if they are not processed or refined—these intelligently designed seeds meet nearly all of our nutritional needs, since they are filled with vitamins, minerals, fibers and even protein.[2]

FRUITS AND VEGETABLES - THE GIVERS OF LIFE

Consider also the perfection of fruits and vegetables. The vast array of colors in fruits and vegetables owes to their high content of a special family of nutrients called

It is important to point out that each of the different phytochemicals protect our bodies in different ways, therefore we must eat a wide variety of plant foods in order to benefit from all the different functions. Cancer is reversed by the synergistic effect of all the different actions of the different phytochemicals—from whisking carcinogens out of cells, preventing hormones from latching on to cells, cutting off blood flow to tumors, and interfering with the creation of carcinogens. Meals that contain a variety of plant foods ensure an abundant supply of phytochemicals. On the other hand, if all we eat are a few of the same vegetables over and over, we may be missing out on some of the best cancer fighting agents.

By following Plan-D, it will be easy to get a healthy dose of phytochemicals at every meal. Almost every fruit, vegetable, grain, and legume tested has been found to contain these amazing substances. Moreover, unlike many vitamins, phytochemicals do not appear to be destroyed by cooking or other food manipulation. Genistein, the substance found in soybeans, for instance, is also found in fermented soybean products such as tofu and miso (fermented soy foods are the only soy foods recommended in Plan-D). Similarly, the phytochemical phenethyl isothiocyanate, found in cabbage, remains intact even when the cabbage is made into coleslaw or sauerkraut. It is also important to eat the edible peels and skins of fruits and vegetables such as apples, carrots, potatoes, cucumbers, and kiwis, as this is where many of the phytonutrients are contained.

I'd like to warn you against the use of isolated phytochemicals that a number of companies are now selling as concentrated supplements. These pills can never be a replacement for whole foods. Because several ***thousand*** phytochemicals are currently known to exist, and new ones are being discovered all the time, a supplement of one single phytochemical cannot possibly contain all of the cancer-fighters found in a shopping cart full of fruits and vegetables.[10]

phytochemicals. These important compounds give plant foods their colors, flavors, and disease-fighting abilities. The more intense the color of a fruit or vegetable, the greater the concentration of phytochemicals. Nutrition researchers today have only skimmed the surface in identifying these powerful compounds, which give plant foods their tremendous healing potential. Thousands of phytochemicals have been identified, yet there are still many more that remain a mystery. It is estimated that there are **thousands** of different phytochemicals in a typical fruit or vegetable.

The word "vegetable" comes from the Latin word *vegetare*, meaning "to enliven or animate." The name describes the very essence of the purpose of vegetables, which is to provide our bodies with life. Fruits also fulfill this purpose, however it is the vegetables that contain some of the most powerful life-giving qualities. It is these life-giving qualities that scientific studies have proven can prevent, as well as treat, many diseases, especially chronic degenerative diseases such as heart disease, cancer, diabetes, and arthritis. Our ancestors ate an abundance of vegetables; hence, until recently, cancer and other diseases were a rare or nonexistent occurrence in human history. Many Plan-D followers have experienced the healing effects of vegetables by including an abundance of them in their daily meals.

In many cases, fruits and vegetables provide the same, if not better, remedies for common ailments. For instance, doctors often prescribe taking an aspirin every day to prevent heart problems. But studies have shown that taking an aspirin every day actually increases the risk of other serious problems, such as hemorrhagic strokes. This is because the main ingredient in aspirin, salicylic acid, is chemically manufactured and does not work the same way in the body as naturally occurring salicylic acid. If doctors would prescribe fruits and vegetables instead, the harmful side effects of synthetic aspirin could be avoided.

Not only do fruits and vegetables contain salicylic acid, but they also help the body make more of its own natural salicylic acid. Studies have shown that people who do not take aspirin, but eat an abundance of vegetables and fruits, have the same levels of salicylic acid in their blood as patients taking low doses of aspirin but not eating an abundance of vegetables and fruits. Fruits and vegetables provide just the right amount salicylic acid to prevent both kinds of strokes—unnecessary clotting (which leads to heart attacks) and hemorrhagic strokes. Eating just three vegetable servings a day decreases the incidence of strokes and heart attacks by a significant amount.[3]

LIFE-FORCE ENERGY

In the introduction to this book I described a universal force that works behind the scenes to heal and bring life where it is needed. In ancient Chinese medicine this force, or energy, was named *chi* or *qui*. The Japanese term for it is *ki*. In India they call it *prana* and in Hawaii it is known as *manna*. African Bushmen call it *boiling energy*. In the West we refer to this timeless force as *Life Force Energy*. All cultures and traditions recognize that Life Force Energy needs to be able to flow freely and abundantly into our bodies in order for us to experience the full range of physical, emotional, and spiritual well being. So where does this Life Force Energy come from? It comes from our food!

Phytochemicals in plant foods absorb sunlight in the visible region of the electromagnetic spectrum causing them to be vibrantly colored. Green veggies owe their green color to a special phytochemical called chlorophyll. Chlorophyll is the green pigment of all green plants, including green foods such as leafy vegetables like lettuces, spinach and kale, broccoli, wheat grass, and the algae superfoods known as spirulina and chlorella. The colors in plants are a form of stored energy, which is housed in the plant's cells. When we eat colorful fruits and vegetables, we experience a noticeable difference in our energy levels. This is because the energy in the food is transferred to us as vital life force. Therefore, the more fresh and alive the food is, the more life force we receive. These foods have been called *bio-genic*, or life-generating foods.

In her book *Raw Food Life Force Energy*, Natalia Rose describes how food, like all matter, is vibrating energy:

> Everything that exists, be it natural or synthetic, has a vibration. The earth itself, the moon, trees, animals, even your dining room table, all have a specific vibration that not only affects their own being, but also the energy of those around them. Things that have a lot of Life Force Energy vibrate at a much more rapid rate than things that have very little Life Force Energy. For example, a plant vibrates at a much more rapid rate than a table. An apple vibrates at a much faster rate than a serving of fries. Human beings are designed to have a relatively high vibration.

> However, if we fill our high-vibration bodies with low Life Force Energy substances, our natural vibration will slow down, effectively distorting and slowing down our human energy pulse. Instead of progressing into healthier, more beautiful beings, we are digressing into inferior versions of ourselves. In this way, modern living, which includes the widespread consumption of low-vibration, low Life Force Energy foods and drinks, fails to honor our natural design as individuals and as a species.[4]

MEASURING OUR LIFE FORCE

Life Force Energy is a real, measurable force. Most of us can't see this life force with our naked eye, but it can be measured by Kirlian photography. This remarkable form of electrophotography captures the energy field around living things.

In 1988 a book was published called *The Dark Side of the Brain* by Harry Oldfield and Roger Coghill. Harry Oldfield is the world's leading researcher in Kirlian photography and electrotherapy, and Roger Coghill is a Cambridge Scientist. Their book contained many Kirlian photographs, most notably those which showed energy fields around both junk food and organic food such as oranges and cabbage. The oranges had a brilliant energy field in the shape of a corona, followed by another ring of what looked like lightning. The junk food had no such corona, hardly a trace of light. The energy field of half a head of fresh cabbage was bright while the other half, which had been cooked, was a pale shadow. Meusli (a live grain cereal) was full of energy while cornflakes showed none at all.[5]

Additionally, Oldfield and Coghill selected twelve average individuals who were eating an "everyday diet." After feeding these people a 24-hour "junk food" diet consisting of processed foods including the usual chemicals, preservatives, artificial ingredients and colorings, the initial Kirlian photography of the subjects showed a weak energy field. [6]

They continued the experiment by asking the same people to go on a whole foods diet for the next 24 hours—a balanced diet of natural foods to which no chemicals had been added. Coghill and Oldfield reported that a dramatic difference in the energy fields surrounding each subject appeared in the next set of Kirlian photographs. After the subjects ate balanced diets of just whole foods, the quality of their personal energy fields, as seen in their Kirlian photos, were brighter with a more sharp and vibrant glow. This proves how quickly high Life Force Energy foods can trigger healing. Many people have cured themselves of cancers and other terminal illnesses by consuming only raw high-Life Force Energy foods.

One of the reasons that processed foods rob us of our Life Force Energy is because they are extremely difficult (in some cases impossible) to break down and thus remain in our bodies, occupying previously clean, healthy cells. This is especially true of pesticides, additives, preservatives, and other artificial chemicals that our bodies were not designed to handle or break down.

A second reason is that the chemical reactions that take place as these substances struggle to move through our bloodstream and intestines make us grumpy, bloated, and exhausted. Eating processed foods chips away at our health, meal after meal, consistently removing our Life Force Energy, sneaking in dark lifelessness where light, beauty, and energy should be![7]

FOOD TECHNOLOGY NO
SUBSTITUTE FOR LIFE FORCE ENERGY

While technology has made great strides in extracting vitamins, minerals, and enzymes from foods and putting them into powders, capsules, and meal replacement bars, there is still something missing from those altered foods. The difference between a real live food and a pill is just that—life! We cannot extract life-force energy and put it into a pill. It is the life force that tastes so good and is so good for us!

Harvey Diamond, author of *Fit For Life*, is one of the most celebrated and successful health authors credited with helping shift people toward a healthier eating lifestyle. In the book *The Christ Diet*, author Charles J. Hunt III shares Harvey Diamond's explanation about the importance of eating natural foods:

> "Right now, technology exists that can create a grain of wheat in the laboratory. Every chemical component can be duplicated and made into a grain of wheat. But if it is put into the ground, it won't grow. Yet grains of wheat taken from tombs that are 4,000 years old will sprout if put into the ground. There is a very subtle ingredient missing in the synthesized wheat; life force!" [8]

Anything that dramatically alters the state of a food, such as canning, freezing, pesticides, chemical additives, and cooking, will affect the amount of Life Force

Energy contained in the food. This is why processed-free living is so important in maintaining a healthy body. When following Plan-D, you will learn to incorporate an abundance of raw fruits and vegetables into your meals so that you receive a high dose of Life Force Energy every day.

In the words of Michael Murray, N.D., "The human body, the vessel of your soul, is something to be cherished."[9] I agree. We must also cherish our food. It is a sacred and beautiful gift. Our designer cared for us and our nutritional needs by specifically designing and providing food in a perfect form. It was only when we forgot how perfect it is, and thought we could make it better, that we began to experience problems with our health.

Our society's desperate quest for a miracle cure or magic pill is tragically futile. There is simply nothing on the planet more perfect and good for us as the Life Force Energy in whole natural foods. Truly, when our life force is in balance, it is a powerful, magical healing force.

Get Your Own Dirt!

The following is a joke I tell to my nutrition classes to illustrate the idea of the perfection of whole foods. Our designer cared for us and our nutritional needs by specifically designing and providing food in a perfect form. Somewhere along the way we forgot how perfect it is, and thought we could make it better...

At the world summit of "Cloning and Other Miraculous Scientific Discoveries," a group of highly esteemed scientists decided that Man had come a long way in his technological abilities. It was unanimously agreed upon that Man would no longer need the services of God, the original creator and designer of all things vegetable, animal and mineral. In a deviation from their highly advanced methods, they followed the rudimentary process of drawing straws to decide which of the scientists would be the one to tell God they didn't need Him anymore.

The cocky scientist, who had picked the shortest straw, went to God and said, "God, I've been sent to tell you that you are no longer needed. We've made amazing scientific breakthroughs and are now to the point where we can clone people and animals, make our own food, replace failing hearts with artificial ones, and do many other miraculous things. So, you can just leave us be. We're perfectly fine without you."

God listened patiently and with great interest to everything the scientist had to say. When the scientist was finished talking, God said, "That is very interesting. You say you can make your own man?"

"Yes," replied the scientist. "And, not to be disrespectful, but we can do it better than you."

At this God became highly amused, and said, "Very well. I will leave you be if you can prove to me that you can make a man that is just as good as the one I make. I'd like to challenge you to a Man-making contest."

The scientist, grinning with great arrogance, said, "Fantastic, you're on!"

God added, "But there's one rule. We're going to make the man just like I did back in the old days."

The scientist, still arrogant, and now even cockier, said "Sure, no problem!" He was quite confident in his ability to make a man the old fashioned way, and went straight to work. He bent down and grabbed a handful of dirt.

Observing this, God was even more amused. He just looked at the scientist, and exclaimed, "Whoa! Whoa, whoa! Wait a minute! *Get your own dirt!*"

CHAPTER 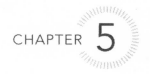 5

The Truth and Nothing But the Truth

ABOUT SUGAR AND FLOUR

Have you ever eaten a piece of broccoli and found that you just couldn't stop? Do you have urges for eggplant and find it hard to satisfy your craving unless you eat it? Do you wait hours in line for the perfect apple, or drive across town because you heard a new shop now carries the most scrumptious oranges? Most people would probably say "no" to all of the above. On the other hand, isn't it true that people *do* find that after eating one cookie or one chip, they just can't stop? When the Krispy Kreme donut shops first opened their doors in the city where I live, people were camping out the night before just to get their fix of the deep-fried sugary rings of white flour.

What is it that makes a person *crave* a food? The same thing that makes a person crave a cigarette, a drug, or alcohol—a chemical dependency. The initial reason for eliminating white flour and white sugar from my diet was the strong personal evidence that I was addicted to the stuff. In 1992 I read a groundbreaking book written by Kay Sheppard called *Food Addiction: The Body Knows*. Her book opened my eyes to the concept of addiction to certain foods, specifically refined carbohydrates. It was like a dark corner in my brain was suddenly flooded with light, and I finally understood why I was never successful with my diets.

The premise of Sheppard's book is that a large segment of the population is genetically predisposed toward addiction. They have inherited a peculiar brain chemistry, similar to that of an alcoholic, which causes them to react differently than other people when they ingest refined carbohydrates. For instance, while some people can sanely eat just one cookie or one piece of bread, those who are genetically predisposed to food addiction find that they have difficulty controlling their intake of these types of foods. Sheppard claims that *the body knows* which foods it is addicted to. When you eat broccoli, or any other whole food, there is no biochemical reaction that causes a physical craving for more and more broccoli. However, even when only small amounts of refined carbohydrates are consumed, knowingly or unknowingly, the addiction is triggered, and it becomes impossible to control cravings. Attempting to restrict consumption of refined carbohydrates, as in dieting, is usually short-lived, claims Sheppard, as the addiction eventually gets its way.

This made huge sense to me, considering my own food history, and I embraced the concept of food addiction readily. Kay Sheppard's book has helped thousands recover from compulsive eating and food addiction, and I encourage you to read it if you feel you fall into that category. However, I continued to research and explore beyond the food addiction model, because even the segment of non-food addicted people who eat refined carbohydrates are suffering in large numbers from diet related illnesses. Being a scientist and wanting to reach both populations, I needed a more compelling reason than just the concept of food addiction for convincing people to eliminate flour and sugar from their diets. Fortunately for me, many in the medical and research community now believe that excessive consumption of refined carbohydrates is a contributing factor in a wide variety of diseases and premature aging.[1]

THE TRUTH ABOUT SUGAR

According to Nancy Appleton, author of Lick the Sugar Habit, we are a nation of sugarholics, slaves to and victims of sugar. Nearly two hundred years ago, the average American consumed about 10 pounds of sugar per year. Today, we gobble and slurp down about 170 pounds of sugar per person per year. But, I don't eat any sugar, and I know a lot of other people who don't eat it either, so that means the numbers are a little skewed and many people are actually eating a lot more than that.

Seductive and sweet, sugar is more a drug than it is a food—a poison to our bodies. While quickly adding pounds of fat to our bodies, sugar slowly and deleteriously robs us of many important nutrients. The result is a myriad of health complications and degenerative illnesses such as diabetes, hypoglycemia, heart disease, gallstones, mineral deficiencies, osteoporosis, arthritis, cancer, and others. This chapter outlines some of the real truths about sugar, which may help you understand why it is so difficult to let go of, and the dangerous consequences of holding on to it.

Your Body Does Not Need Refined Sugar

Refined white sugar, as sweet and delicious as it may be, is a highly refined carbohydrate and can technically be classified as a pharmaceutical drug, due to its chemical, refined and addictive nature. There is absolutely no nutritional value in refined sugar. In fact, a person could live their entire life without consuming it.

Our bodies only need the equivalent of two teaspoons of blood sugar (glucose) at any one time in order to function properly. This small amount of glucose is easily obtained by digesting proteins, essential fats, and complex carbohydrates such as vegetables and whole grains. Compare the two teaspoons of sugar your body needs at any one time to the amount in the typical American diet. According to 1996 U.S. Food Supply Data, the average American consumes 32 teaspoons (128 grams) of sugar per day. One twelve ounce can of a soft drink contains 10 to 12 teaspoons of sugar.[2] Every extra teaspoon of refined sugar we eat works to throw our bodies out of balance and compromises our health.

Refined sugar, in one form or another, is found in almost all packaged foods. The most common form of refined sugar is high fructose corn syrup (more on that later). Sugar and high fructose corn syrup are lurking in many foods that you might not even consider sweet. For example, you might be surprised to learn that:

- Many meat packers feed sugar to animals prior to slaughter. This improves the flavor and color of cured meat.
- Sugar (in the form of corn syrup and dehydrated molasses) is often added to hamburgers sold in restaurants to reduce shrinkage.
- The breading on many prepared food contains sugar.
- Before salmon is canned, it is often glazed with a sugar solution.
- Some fast-food restaurants sell poultry that has been injected with a flavorful processed honey solution.
- Sugar is used in the processing of luncheon meats, bacon, and canned meats.
- Sugar is found in such unlikely items as bouillon cubes and dry-roasted nuts.
- Some iodized salt contains sugar (in the form of dextrose).
- Some brands of vanilla extract contain sugar or corn syrup.
- Seasoning mixes, such as taco seasoning, sauce mixes, and salad dressing mixes, often contain some form of sugar.
- Almost half the calories found in the average can of cranberry sauce come from sugar.[3]

Sugar is also found in many other foods such as crackers, tortillas, bagels, bread, canned beans, canned vegetables, frozen entrees, pickles, peanut butter, macaroni and cheese, spaghetti sauces, and breakfast cereals, including Cheerios. Sugar sweetens jams, jellies, pork and beans, mustard, relish, flavored yogurt, canned fruit, salad dressings, and nearly all fat-free foods, not to mention chocolate and the endless list of desserts that are loaded with sugar.

Human evolution has not yet caught up with the sugar industry. For many *thousands of years*, humans survived without eating refined sugar at all. Even the naturally occurring sugar in fruits was only eaten when the fruit was in season, maybe one or two months out of the year. The past two hundred years of sugar consumption is but a moment compared to thousands of years, and our bodies are just not equipped to metabolize such large amounts of sugar on a daily basis. Our bodies do their best to adjust, but they become overworked and exhausted, and eventually begin to degenerate, manifesting in a host of diseases.[4]

Sugar Is An Addictive Substance
With sugar in virtually every food, it's no wonder so many people are addicted to it. Some of you may not believe in the concept of sugar addiction, but consider this:

nearly all addictive substances are highly refined white crystals or powders. Refined white sugar comes in both forms—white crystals and white powder!

All addictive substances start as something natural, and are then refined into unnatural chemical forms of the starting substance. After all, heroin is nothing but a chemical. The juice of the poppy is refined into opium and then refined into morphine and finally to heroin. Sugar is nothing but a chemical, the legal heroin of the food family. The juice of the cane or beet is refined into molasses and then refined into brown sugar and finally to strange white crystals. This highly concentrated form of sugar *does not exist anywhere in nature*, not even in the original sugar cane or sugar beet plants themselves!

To understand what happens to sugar when it is refined, you must first understand what's in a natural sugar cane. If you walked into a field of natural sugar cane (growing in the sun) and cut off a piece to chew on, you would experience a yummy sweet, yet dark flavored treat. Eating this piece of natural sugar cane would actually nourish you, because natural sugar cane is brimming with vitamins, minerals, enzymes, fibers, and phytonutrients that help the body digest the naturally occurring sugar. The refinement of sugar removes all of these wonderful nutrient components, leaving a nutritionally empty substance.

Refined sugar is 99.4 to 99.7 percent pure calories—no vitamins, minerals, enzymes, fibers, or proteins, just simple carbohydrates.[5] This is where the term "empty calories" comes from—calories with no nutrition.

Sugar Depletes Calcium and Other Minerals From Your Body

Although most people don't understand their bodies' nutritional requirements, *the body knows* what it needs. For instance, the minerals required to digest sugar are calcium, phosphorous, chromium, magnesium, cobalt, copper, zinc and manganese. Sugar cane in its natural form is rich in these vitamins and minerals. It also contains vitamins A, C, B1, B2, B6, niacin, iron, and pantothenic acid, which work synergistically with natural sugar cane's fiber and enzymes to nourish the body. The natural fibers specific to the sugar cane help slow down the absorption of the sugars and prevent the sharp rise in blood sugar levels associated with refined sugar.

By contrast, refined sugar is devoid of the nutrients and built-in enzyme systems that exist in naturally sweet foods. So when you eat a cookie, your body freaks out. It knows that in order to properly digest the sugar, it needs these minerals and the corresponding enzymes. When these are not eaten along with the sugar, the body, being the amazing machine that it is, adapts by pulling stored nutrients from your bones, tissues and teeth, to be able to properly digest the cookie you just ate. This is called *leaching*—sugar robs calcium from your bones, tissues, and teeth in order to be digested.

Most of us are fed sugar from the time we are children. Imagine having calcium leached out of your bones and teeth on a daily basis over a period of years. You may end up with crooked teeth (like Dr. Price's young patients), a calcium deficiency in your mid-years, or perhaps even younger. Your doctor may prescribe a calcium supplement, but it won't do any good because as long as refined sugars are continually eaten, essential nutrients, including calcium, are unavailable to the body. The depletion of calcium leads to a whole host of health problems, including obesity.

Sugar Negates a Healthy Diet

In addition to keeping our bones and teeth strong and healthy, minerals are used to help us digest our food and to maintain proper body chemistry (alkalinity). Many people think that they can eat anything they want as long as they exercise and take their vitamin and mineral supplements daily. But eating sugar totally *negates the effects of an otherwise healthy diet*. Eating sugar changes your body chemistry in such a devastating way that many of those essential nutrients will be unavailable to your body. Vitamin supplements may actually become toxic to the body.[6]

Sugar Suppresses Your Immune Response

Your immune system is your body's only defense against foreign invaders such as viruses and bacteria. It is your white blood cells that have the ability to attack and destroy these invaders. Nearly all forms of sugar interfere with the ability of white blood cells to perform their job. In one study, when healthy volunteers consumed a large amount (100g) of refined sugar, their white blood cells' ability to destroy bacteria was impaired for at least 5 hours.

Ironically, sugar is in almost every over-the-counter cough syrup, cough drop and flu remedy designed to help us fight coughs and colds. Sugar is also in chicken soup, another remedy we take when our immune systems are already compromised!

Sugar is a Cancer Fuel

Dr. Otto Warburg, a Nobel Prize winning doctor, discovered that normal cells need oxygen, while cancer cells despise it. Dr. Warburg concluded that cancer metabolizes through a process of fermentation, which as any brewer or wine maker knows, requires sugar. Cancer cells require sugar in order to perpetuate their growth. When you eat sugar, you are actually feeding cancer cells. Additionally, if you don't eat enough life force energy foods loaded with cancer-fighting phytochemicals, it is almost certain that the stage is being set for cancer to develop in your body.

In order to stop cancer cells from growing, they need to be starved. Additionally, cancer cannot grow in the presence of an alkaline body chemistry. As I have discussed, sugar is one of the major contributors to upset body chemistry, creating an acidic rather than an alkaline environment in the body. A highly acidic body chemistry is the main cause of all diseases, especially cancer.

HIGH-FRUCTOSE CORN SYRUP: WHY IT'S EVEN WORSE THAN SUGAR

High fructose corn syrup (HFCS) is not the bottled stuff you buy at the grocery store to make pecan pies and caramel. And it isn't natural, as some advertisers might claim. High fructose corn syrup is a synthetic sweetener that is cheaper and easier to use than plain old sugar and has become a ubiquitous ingredient in nearly all processed foods. It is the sweetener of choice in everything from soft drinks, snack foods, and cookies to ice cream and yogurt. Like the sugar it has replaced, it also turns up in foods that you don't think of as sweet, like soups, breads, pizza dough, crackers, and salad dressings.

Over the last few years, HFCS has been labeled "the crack of sweeteners" due to its addictive qualities and its impact on the health of Americans. More than one scientific article has documented that since 1980, obesity and diabetes rates have climbed at a rate remarkably similar to that of HFCS consumption. Right around the time that manufacturers started replacing sugar in sodas with the more cheaply produced HFCS, there was a sharp rise in male and female obesity in the United States. From 1980 to 2000, the incidence of obesity doubled, after having remained relatively flat for the preceding 20 years. Concurrently, per capita consumption of HFCS increased by more than 1,000 percent from 1970 to 1990, exceeding the intake of any other food group tracked by the Department of Agriculture.[7]

Food Chemistry Creates Fake Sugar

The highly processed syrup is a far cry from the natural corn it's derived from. And it's not a product that you could whip up at home using a few ears of corn. It's a 15-step process using some pretty sophisticated laboratory equipment. It starts with corn kernels and takes place in a series of stainless steel vats and tubes in which a dozen different mechanical processes and chemical reactions occur—including several rounds of high-velocity spinning and the introduction of three different enzymes to incite molecular rearrangements.[8]

The enzymes turn most of the naturally occurring glucose molecules in corn into fructose, which makes the substance sweeter. This 90 percent fructose syrup mixture is then combined with regular corn syrup, which is 100 percent glucose molecules, to get the right percentage of fructose and glucose. The final product is a clear, goopy liquid that is roughly as sweet as sugar.[9]

The manufacturers of HFCS say that their product is natural because it is made from plain old corn and contains no synthetic materials or color or flavor additives. They must have forgotten about those unnatural molecular rearrangements that occur during the refinement process. HFCS *is artificial* because the resulting molecular rearrangement is not found anywhere in the natural corn.

Still, some companies still pitch their products as being "natural" even if they contain HFCS. Cadbury Schweppes promotes 7-Up, which is sweetened with HFCS, as "100 percent natural." Capri Sun fruit flavored drinks have also been promoted as all-natural, although they, too, are sweetened with HFCS.[10]

The Crux of the HFCS Problem

While food scientists can convince themselves that HFCS is natural, *the body knows* it is not. Many experts argue that there is no difference between sugar and HFCS and that the body handles them both in the same way. Other experts are gravely concerned. Richard Anderson, a scientist at the Federal Human Nutrition Research Center in Beltsville, Maryland, thinks it's a huge problem. He claims, "high fructose corn syrup is metabolized differently than other sugars, and it has a different effect on health. [It] upsets me when people say there's no difference… there's a big difference."[11]

The syrup contains about five percent more fructose than sugar does—an amount so insignificant that it should not produce any greater effect than eating white sugar—and certainly not a significant enough amount to cause the skyrocketing rates of obesity, say some experts. However, they're not taking into account the fact that the fructose in HFCS is molecularly altered, whereas the fructose in refined white sugar is not. It's that difference that is the crux of the problem.

When we eat refined white sugar, as bad as it may be for us, our body at least knows what it is and knows how to handle it. In normal sugar metabolism, the fructose is broken down in the digestive tract and processed in the cells. Once this occurs, the cells send a signal to the brain, which stimulates the pancreas to secrete a hormone called insulin. Insulin is then used by the body to convert the sugar into energy, and helps provide a sense of fullness. Any excess sugar that does not get converted to energy goes to the liver to be stored as fat. This is why, if you eat too much sugar, you get fat.

Because of its altered molecular structure, the body doesn't know what to do with HFCS. It does not get metabolized the same way that sugar does, in fact it doesn't really get metabolized at all. When we eat HFCS, the cells do not send a signal to the brain, therefore the pancreas does not release insulin. As a result, the sugar (fructose) does not get converted into energy, and goes directly to the liver to be stored as fat. This large glut of sugar turning to fat in the liver has been linked to fatty liver disease (a condition where the liver is literally choked by fat globules and cannot perform its normal detoxifying and fat burning functions), elevated levels of triglycerides and cholesterol; high triglycerides in the body are linked to heart disease and diabetes. HFCS also lowers chromium levels in the body, further increasing the risk of type 2 diabetes.

Since HFCS goes directly to the liver and never sends a signal to your pancreas to secrete insulin, you will never feel a sense of fullness, in which case you will more than likely eat more than you need to. Eating more results in weight gain. Aha! That's another reason I discovered as to why I was never able to stop eating sugary foods.

GETTING THE SUGAR OUT OF YOUR DIET

The only way to make sure you are not eating sugar is to read ingredient lists of any food that comes prepared or in a package. If you eat in restaurants, you should know that you are probably getting some form of sugar in your food, either in the seasonings, sauces, salad dressings, or the meat. Try to avoid sugar as much as possible to reduce your exposure. Because of the prevalence of sugar in the food supply, you probably won't be able to avoid it entirely without becoming a complete neurotic. However, you should make every effort to eliminate it as much as possible.

Ingredients must be listed in order of their predominance by weight in a food product. In other words, when reading an ingredient list you should know that the ingredient that weighs the most is listed first, and the ingredient that weighs the least is listed last. Some people subscribe to the idea that if a form of sugar is listed after the third ingredient, the sugar in that food product is not in a significant amount. This is a flawed method for avoiding sugar.

One of the most deceptive methods that food companies use to deal with a load of sugar in a food product is to use a variety of different sugars in lesser amounts, or to distribute sugars among many other ingredients, so that no one sugar appears in the top three. For example, a manufacturer may use a combination of sucrose, high-fructose corn syrup, corn syrup solids, brown sugar, dextrose and other sugar ingredients to make sure none of them are present in large enough quantities to attain a top position on the ingredient list. If the sugars were combined on the product's ingredient list, sugar might very well be the first (most predominant) ingredient on the list!

Check food ingredient labels for these forms of sugar:

Sugar	Corn Syrup	High Fructose Corn syrup
Brown sugar	Corn Syrup Solids	Fruit Juice Concentrates
Glucose	Molasses	Evaporated Cane Juice
Dextrose	Lactose	Barley malt
Fructose	Maltose	Maple syrup
Sucrose	Honey	Rice syrup
Corn Starch	Modified food starch	Rice syrup solids

One way to tell if a product has a lot of sugar in it is to look at the nutrition fact panel for the number of grams of sugar per serving. If a product has a high number of grams of sugar per serving, it's a sure bet that sugar has been added.

A nutrition fact panel will not distinguish between naturally occurring sugar and added sugar. For instance, one cup of plain yogurt has 15 grams of sugar listed, but those sugars are from the naturally occurring lactose in the milk. On the other hand, one cup of vanilla flavored yogurt has 28 grams of sugar, nearly twice the amount! That means that nearly half the sugars have been added to the yogurt. The only way you will know whether sugars have been added is to read the ingredient list to see if there are any sugars listed.

THE TRUTH ABOUT ARTIFICIAL SWEETENERS

By now you get the gist—anything artificial is not a part of Plan-D. As bad as sugar and high fructose corn syrup can be, the pink, blue, and yellow packets are even worse. When I was growing up, my mother, who was always watching her sugar intake, used tiny little white tablets of saccharin to sweeten her coffee. Saccharin, later marketed as Sweet-n-Low, was found to cause cancer in laboratory animals, and we thought that it would be banned from the sweetener landscape. However, it persists in the marketplace as a non-caloric alternative to sugar, but the cancer-causing warnings still appear on package labeling.

There has been much documentation on the ill-effects of artificial sweeteners—weight gain, disruption of sleep patterns, sexual dysfunction, increases in cancer, MS, Lupus, diabetes, and a list of epidemic degenerative diseases—but the companies who own their patents continue to deny any connection.

Dr. Janet Starr Hull has written extensively on the subject of artificial sweeteners.

She claims, "Artificial sweeteners are a mix of unnatural chemicals combined in a laboratory that the body can't process. Basically, these chemicals either accumulate in your vital organs (*causing severe damage later*), pollute your bloodstream (*causing severe damage later*), or form the basis for eventual mutations of your cells (*causing severe damage later*)."[12]

It's hard to say which of the other two commonly used artificial sweeteners, the blue packets and the yellow packets, is the worst. Since Aspartame, also known as Equal (the blue packet) has been in use longer, there are more documented problems from its use than from the use of the new kid on the block Sucralose, also known as Splenda (the yellow packet).

The Accidental Discovery of NutraSweet

A chemist working for the G.D. Searle Company accidentally discovered aspartame while he was testing for a drug to treat ulcers. He got some of the substance on his finger, and then *accidentally* touched his finger to his mouth. When the substance was found to be sweet tasting, the company realized that it could be more lucrative as a food additive than as a limited-market ulcer drug. As a chemist I can tell you that it is not good laboratory practice to put anything in your mouth while working with toxic chemicals, but that is exactly how aspartame came to be! Soon, nearly every commercially produced sugar-free food and drink was laced with it. Next, it became available for home and restaurant use in those little blue packets, labeled as Equal and Nutrasweet.

Early testing of aspartame was wrought with results showing that it was not safe to consume, yet it was still approved for food use by the FDA in 1982. Since then, seventy-five percent of complaints to the FDA about food reactions pertain to NutraSweet. The FDA once listed 92 different symptoms associated with the use of NutraSweet. Symptoms confirmed through controlled studies include headaches/migraines, weight gain, dizziness, confusion, memory loss, drowsiness, depression, irritability, anxiety attacks, tingling and numbness, convulsions, heart palpitations, shortness of breath, chest pain, nausea, diarrhea, aggravation of diabetes, menstrual problems, joint pain, decreased vision, eye pain, ear ringing, noise intolerance, hyperactivity in children, and excessive thirst.[13] In 1995, the FDA stopped reporting aspartame reactions.

What Exactly is Splenda?

With all of these problems and a growing public concern, the time was ripe for a new sweetener to come on the scene—Sucralose (Splenda). Splenda is the trade name for Sucralose, the newest man-made artificial sweetener. The manufacturer of Splenda markets the product as being "natural" because it comes from sugar (sucrose). They are only telling a partial truth.

Although the starting substance is sugar (sucrose), it undergoes a complex 5-step chemical process involving many caustic chemicals which selectively substitutes three atoms of chlorine for three hydrogen-oxygen groups on the sucrose molecule. This chemical reaction essentially forces chlorine atoms to form an unnatural bond with the sugar, resulting in a new molecule called Sucralose, marketed under the name Splenda.

Sucralose does not exist anywhere in nature. It is a patented compound, meaning no one else can make it or sell it. Whereas the starting substance (sucrose) belonged to the class of compounds called sugars, the three chlorine atoms attached to the Sucralose molecule put it into the class of compounds called "polychlorinated compounds." You may be familiar with some other polychlorinated compounds—they're called pesticides! Splenda shares many similar molecular characteristics to pesticides like DDT that can accumulate in the body's fat and tissues. It is impossible to predict the long-term consequences of ingesting this substance over many years.

Figure 5.1

Through a complex five-step chemical process, Sucralose is synthesized by adding several chlorine-containing compounds to the sugar molecule, resulting in the substitution of the hydroxyl (**OH**) groups with chlorine (**Cl**) atoms.

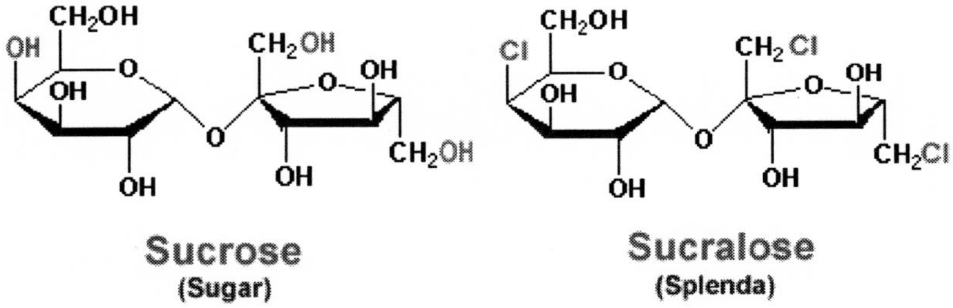

Sucrose
(Sugar)

Sucralose
(Splenda)

Image Source: http://www.feingold.org/Research/Splenda.html

In her book, *Splenda: Is It Safe Or Not?* Dr. Janet Starr Hull explains the dangers of Splenda:

Splenda contains chlorine, which is a carcinogen. The Splenda marketers insist it is chemically "bound" so it cannot be "released" in the body during digestion. I question that, and wonder if this artificial chemical can safely pass through the human body. Wait until you read what chlorine can do to the human body. You decide if you want to ingest this chemical.

Sucralose (Splenda) is a chlorocarbon – a chlorine-containing compound. The chlorocarbons have long been known for causing organ, genetic, and reproductive damage. It should be no surprise then, that testing of sucralose revealed organ, genetic, and reproductive damage. Research on lab rats showed up to forty percent shrinkage of the thymus gland, a gland that is the very foundation of our immune system. The contamination of water supplies by chlorocarbons is a serious problem in most European countries today, making many people very ill. Due to the chlorine content in Splenda, sucralose can cause inflammation and swelling of the liver and kidneys, in addition to calcification of the kidney, as shown in animal studies. If you experience kidney pain, cramping, or an irritated bladder after using sucralose, stop using it immediately.

Man-made chlorine (found in Splenda) is essentially bleach. There is natural chlorine in nature, but it is totally different from Splenda's laboratory invention. Manufactured chlorine is an extremely toxic biohazard, and I was shocked when I first learned chlorine is in Splenda.

So, feel like munching on a few sugar-free cookies made with sucralose about now? What are the guarantees that this poisonous chlorine chemical won't break down in your extremely efficient digestive system—a complex machine with seven organs all valiantly trying to break it down for absorption? After all, your body thinks that's why you ate it, right? So chances are, it can be digested and assimilated into your body to some degree. As with aspartame, after people get ill, will we hear another "oops!" from the industry and "I told you so" from independent scientists? Why take the chance?[14]

NATURAL SWEETENERS AND NATURALLY OCCURRING SUGARS

Many people have a false understanding about sugars in general. The popular notion is that sugar is sugar—whether it comes from white sugar, whole sugar cane, honey, or a piece of fruit—and that it all behaves in the body the same way. *This is not true.* The naturally occurring sugars in whole sugar cane, fruits, milk products, and even maple syrup and raw honey have an advantage over refined sugars in that they are balanced by a wide range of nutrients that aid in the utilization of the natural sugars contained within them.

As humans, we have a natural desire for the taste of sweet foods. There is nothing wrong with acknowledging that desire and satisfying it on occasion. However, when we do indulge our sweet tooth, we need to do it with sweet foods that will nourish us, rather than deplete us. Therefore, we want to keep in mind the nutrient value and the health benefits of the sweet foods we choose. Plan-D incorporates the *occasional* use of the following natural sweeteners:

Stevia – The sweetness of stevia comes from the leaves of a perennial herb that the Paraguayan natives call "sweet leaf." *It is not a sugar*—it is an herb that just happens to be sweet. Just 1 teaspoon of the liquid extract has the same sweetness as one cup of sugar. Stevia has been used as a traditional remedy for diabetes and gum disease among the indigenous people of Paraguay and other South American countries for over 1,500 recorded years (and for probably many thousands of more years prior to the records). Since stevia is not a sugar, its use does not affect blood sugar levels. In fact, scientific research shows stevia has the ability to actually heal the cells in the pancreas, thereby improving glucose tolerance in people with diabetes. According to the generations of people who have used stevia as part of their daily diet, stevia has also been proven to regulate blood sugar. Unlike any other sweetener, stevia has been reported to have anti-viral properties and may also lower blood pressure. Stevia is the only sweetener I recommend for daily use. For a more detailed discussion on the history and use of stevia, see chapter 11.

Raw Honey – Throughout history, honey has been regarded as "nature's gold"—a medicinal food capable of healing the body and soothing the spirit. Honey has a long history as a component of folk remedies for many ailments, including colds, coughs, and digestive difficulties. In East Indian Ayurvedic medicine, honey is used as a blood purifier, a decongestant, and a kidney tonic.

When I was a teenager my mother would give us chamomile tea with a teaspoon of honey in it when we had a cold or flu. She learned about the value of honey from the Edgar Cayce readings. The Cayce readings consistently point to honey as the preferred sweetener, particularly raw honey. Honey was recommended to individuals suffering from a variety of ailments, including anemia, arthritis, diabetes, toxemia, and psoriasis. According to Cayce, honey may also naturally suppress the desire for other sweets. An epileptic with an excessive craving for sweets was told: *"Once a day, early of morning, take a teaspoonful of honey (teaspoonful, not a tablespoonful), and there will not be the desire so much for other sweets."*[15] In another reading, a fifty-two year old woman suffering from insomnia was advised to take *"each evening before retiring, about a cupful of heated milk (organic milk, preferably), in which there would be stirred a level teaspoonful of pure honey."* The reading cautions: *"Do not boil the milk but just let it come to the heating point, and then stir in the honey."* In folk medicine around the world, the combination of warm milk and honey is well known for its soothing, relaxing effects.[16]

For those who believe that honey is just another type of sugar, it's nutritional profile may be surprising. Honey contains protein, the B vitamins thiamin, riboflavin, and niacin, vitamin C, calcium and iron. According to honeyologist Joe M. Parkhill, professor of agriculture and author of *The Wonderful World of Bee Pollen*, honey is the only food that provides all the substances necessary to sustain life, including water. Parkhill credits the enzymes in raw honey with activating a number of biochemical reactions within the body, notably those associated with digestion.[17]

Honey also has antibacterial properties. Bacteria cannot survive in raw honey, whereas refined sugar and refined honey creates an ideal breeding ground for harmful bacteria. A 1998 issue of the *Journal of Apicultural Research* also confirms that honey, in its raw form, is a rich source of antioxidants, which stop disease-causing free radicals in their tracks.[18]

Most of the honey found in supermarkets is not healthy. It is basically the refined white sugar version of honey, which makes it just as bad for us. When honey is heated (pasteurized) and processed, many of its natural enzymes and nutrients, are destroyed. Therefore, the best way to enjoy the benefits of honey is in its natural form: raw, unfiltered, and unpasteurized. You can find raw honey in natural food markets, specialty shops, and farmer's markets.

Store honey in a dry place. If it begins to crystallize, which is normal for raw unfiltered honey, you can place the jar in a pot of hot, not boiling, water until the crystals dissolve. Make sure the water is not too hot as you may risk destroying the valuable nutrients.

One final word about honey: most labels warn not to feed infants and toddlers honey because it can cause infant botulism, a rare and serious form of food poisoning which affects a baby's nervous system. This warning only applies to pasteurized honey, which does not have the same antibacterial properties as raw honey. Pasteurized honey is a known source of bacterial spores that cause infant botulism. As already mentioned earlier, bacteria cannot survive in raw honey.

Pure Maple Syrup – This is not Log Cabin or Aunt Jemima pancake syrup, which are artificially flavored processed foods. Pure maple syrup is derived from various maple trees by tapping the tree bark and allowing the sap to flow out freely. The sap is clear and almost tasteless and very low in sugar content when it is first tapped. It is then boiled to evaporate the water, which concentrates the sugar and creates the flavor and color profile of the syrup. The darker the color, the longer the syrup has boiled, shifting it further from its original state.

Pure maple syrup contains fewer calories and a higher concentration of minerals than honey, although it contains no protein or vitamins. Maple syrup is an excellent source of manganese and zinc. The trace mineral manganese is essential for helping antioxidants disarm free radicals in the cells. In addition to acting as an antioxidant, the zinc contained in maple syrup can decrease the progression of atherosclerosis. Zinc and manganese are both important for strengthening the immune system, as many types of immune cells in the body depend upon them.

Maple syrup has a wonderful rich flavor and is the secret ingredient in my famous wheat-free chocolate chip cookie recipe (see page 266). Enjoy maple syrup on oatmeal, mixed into yogurt, or mixed with some flaxseed oil to top your French toast or pancakes.

Raw Blue Agave Nectar – Agave (Ah-gah-vay) nectar, interchangeably called agave syrup, is obtained from a cactus plant called agave, which is similar to the aloe plant. The nectar is filtered and heated (raw agave nectar is heated only to 118 degrees F to avoid destroying enzymes) to create a syrup of a consistency slightly thinner than honey. Its sweetness is light and more intense than white sugar, so less is needed to get the same sweetness as sugar. Agave nectar contains nutrients, including iron and calcium that aid in the functioning of the gall bladder, helping to break up and dissolve dietary fats. Agave nectar also works against the blocking of arteries and veins due to high cholesterol levels.

Though blue agave plants are grown in most places of the southern and western United States, the Mexican Blue Agave Nectar remains the most popular of all, as the blue agaves from this country are more hearty and plentiful than anywhere else in the world. The primary reason for this is that the Mexican soil in the regions where agave is grown contains volcanic ash rich in nutrients.

Agave has the lowest glycemic index of all the natural sweeteners, owing to its unique form of fructose. Due to its slow absorption by the human body, agave nectar works as intelligent caloric food, since it is absorbed according to the body's needs. Because of its extremely low glycemic index, it will not over stimulate the production of insulin, making it a safe sweetener for people with diabetes. In fact, agave nectar has met the "food exchange requirements" by the American Diabetic

Association and American Dietetic Association for product labeling.

Agave is used as the sweetening ingredient in many of the Plan-D recipes.

Unsulphured Blackstrap Molasses – Blackstrap molasses is a dark thick viscous liquid that comes from processing raw sugar into its more refined form. While not a whole food, blackstrap molasses is a sweetener that is actually good for you. Unlike white sugar and corn syrup, which are stripped of all nutrients, blackstrap molasses contains significant amounts of health-promoting minerals found in the original whole sugar cane. One tablespoon of blackstrap molasses provides up to 20 percent of the daily value of calcium, magnesium, potassium, and iron. It also contains copper, manganese, selenium, chromium, B-vitamins, and protein. I recommend buying organic, unsulphured blackstrap molasses. It is made from mature sugar cane and does not require treatment with sulphur dioxide, a preservative, used during the extraction process of other types of molasses.

Brown Rice Syrup – Brown rice syrup is an amber colored syrup with a mild butterscotch-like flavor. Brown rice syrup is prepared by fermenting brown rice with special enzymes to disintegrate the natural starch content of the grain. Once fermentation is complete, the fermented liquid is strained off, and the rice is allowed to slowly cook until it reaches a smooth liquid consistency. The health benefits of brown rice syrup come from its main ingredient, the brown rice, which contains protein, bran, and fiber. The bran also contains the minerals magnesium, manganese, and zinc. The syrup therefore is rich in protein and fiber, which help to slow down the absorption of the natural sugars contained in the syrup. Brown rice syrup has a light flavor and is only half as sweet as sugar.

Rapadura™ (Organic Unrefined Whole Cane Sugar) - Rapadura™ is an unrefined organic whole cane sugar that can almost be considered a whole food. It is prepared by pressing the juice from the sugar cane stalk and then evaporating off the water. The remaining coarse, golden crystals retain a significant amount of the essential vitamins, minerals, and nutrients contained in the natural sugar cane. A 100-gram serving of Rapadura contains 110 milligrams of calcium, 1,000 milligrams of potassium, and 100 milligrams each of magnesium and phosphorous. It also contains 1,200 IU of Vitamin A, and trace amounts of the B vitamins. Refined white sugar contains none of these; therefore Rapadura is a much healthier alternative.

Rapadura granules are a dark brown color, round, porous and easily compressed, and can replace refined white sugar cup for cup in recipes. Some of the Plan-D recipes call for Rapadura. It can be purchased in natural food markets or online.

If you cannot find Rapadura, you can use its close cousin, Sucanat, which seems to be more widely available. Sucanat (**Su***gar* **Ca***ne* **Na***tural*) contains less of the nutrients contained in Rapadura, but significantly more than white sugar. A 100-gram serving of Sucanat contains 110 milligrams of calcium, 570 milligrams of potassium, 8.7 milligrams of magnesium, and 37 milligrams of phosphorous. It also contains trace amounts of the B vitamins, and less than 20 IU of vitamin A.

When it comes to natural sugars, you need to be aware of false claims.

"Evaporated cane juice" or "evaporated cane sugar" shows up on the ingredient lists of many "natural" and "healthy" cereals and snack foods. It is more refined than you would think, and doesn't contain nearly the amount of vitamins and minerals that Rapadura and Sucanat contain. Because of their low or nonexistent nutrient values, other "natural" sugars such as Florida Crystals, Turbinado, and "Sugar in the Raw" definitely *do not qualify* as healthy alternatives.

No Comparison to Pure Maple Syrup

Pure Maple Syrup can strengthen the immune system and aid antioxidant functions in the body. Its ingredient list, which contains only one, cannot be matched by artificial substitutes. Check out the ingredient list on a bottle of a leading brand of artificial pancake syrup, taken from the company's website:

Ingredients: Corn Syrup, High Fructose Corn Syrup, Water, Cellulose Gum, Caramel Color, Salt, Sodium Benzoate and Sorbic Acid (Preservatives), Artificial and Natural Flavors, Sodium Hexametaphosphate.

WE EAT THIS???

THE TRUTH ABOUT FLOUR

When I was eating compulsively, I must have eaten enough bread and pasta to feed a third world country. I loved bread! I remember when I was 12 years old my cousin and I ate a whole loaf of Wonder bread between the two of us. We just kept popping slices into the toaster, spreading them with butter, and chowing down. It was as if the bread melted in our mouths. We were so embarrassed that we had eaten the whole loaf, we walked down to the corner store and bought another loaf to replace the one we'd eaten. But when we got back home, we ended up eating half of that loaf also.

Pasta was another one of my downfalls. Any kind of noodle excited me. Ramen, mac-n-cheese, and spaghetti were my favorites. I often ate cold spaghetti for breakfast. In fact, sometimes, I would make a spaghetti sandwich, by putting a scoop of cold spaghetti onto a slice of white bread, folding it over, and eating it. It was like nirvana!

Today I know why I was able to eat so much bread and pasta in one sitting. Like sugar, white flour is so highly refined, that the body doesn't recognize it as food. White flour has very little nutrition in it (white sugar doesn't have *any* nutrition in it), therefore when we eat foods made from white flour, our bodies do not get nourished. White flour stimulates our hunger sensation, but it doesn't satisfy us. As a result, even though we're filling our bellies, the rest of our body isn't getting nourished, so we think we're still hungry and eat more.

ANATOMY OF A WHOLE GRAIN

Figure 5.2 Anatomy of a Whole Wheat Kernel

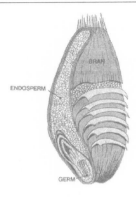

Image Source: http://wbc.agr.mt.gov/Consumers/diagram_kernel.com

White sugar originates from a whole natural sugar cane, brimming with vitamins, minerals, fibers, enzymes, and phytonutrients. White flour originates from a whole-wheat kernel, brimming with vitamins, minerals, fibers, enzymes, and phytonutrients. To understand how white flour is made, you must first understand the components of a whole-wheat kernel.

Figure 5.2 is a diagram of a whole-wheat kernel, although you can think of it as the anatomy of all whole grains, as they are all basically the same. Whole grains contain three main components: the bran, the germ, and the endosperm. The bran and the germ are part of the outer husk of the wheat kernel. They are two very important fibers that are required by our bodies for the proper digestion of wheat. They both contain B-complex vitamins and trace minerals. The wheat germ contains a small amount of oil, called wheat germ oil, which is also required by our bodies for the proper digestion of wheat. The germ also contains the embryo, or sprouting section of the grain (meaning it's the part of the grain that will form a new sprout if the kernel is placed in water or planted in the ground).

The endosperm, which is on the inside of the wheat kernel, contains most of the carbohydrates and proteins in the wheat kernel. I call it the starchy, spongy part of the wheat kernel. It also contains B-complex vitamins.

The Refinement of Wheat

To produce white flour, the outer husk of the wheat kernel is removed, thereby removing all of the bran and the germ, leaving only the endosperm (the starchy spongy part). This is unfortunate, because all of the fiber and nutrients contained in the bran and germ are also removed. The remaining endosperm is milled and bleached to remove its original brown color, and as a result, all of its nutrients and enzymes are destroyed.

We refine our wheat and other grains to give the resulting flour a longer shelf life, but it is so nutritionally void that even bugs won't eat it! Our government doesn't seem to care that refined sugar is void of nutrition, even though it is used to make thousands of foods. However, the USDA was concerned that refined white flour was also nutritionally empty, so they enacted a law, called the enrichment law, which requires the manufacturers of white flour to add back in some nutrients. This is where the term *"enriched flour"* comes from—a pitiful attempt to replace key nutrients that have been destroyed in the refinement process. Enriched flour is refined white flour that has had all of its nutrients stripped out of it, and only a sprinkling of synthetic vitamins have been added back to the flour—usually iron and the B-vitamins thiamine, niacin, and riboflavin.

But they don't and can't possibly enrich it enough. The original whole-wheat kernel contains over 100 vitamins, minerals, and phytochemicals, in addition to essential oils, fibers and enzymes, which act together, synergistically, to assist our bodies in digesting the wheat. Enriched flour becomes deadly to our bodies, because not only can we not digest it properly, it too robs us of vital stored nutrients. In fact, if you tried to live on white bread alone for 60 days, you would literally die, because there isn't enough nutrition in the flour to keep you alive for that long. And in fact, you get a double whammy effect. Like sugar, white flour leaches calcium and other minerals from your bones, tissues, and teeth, just to be able to digest it.

Unfortunately, the American diet is rife with products made from white flour and other refined grains. Examples include breads, crackers, pastries, baked goods, pastas, most commercial cereals, pizza dough, tortillas, fast foods, and snack foods of all types.

Excessive consumption of refined white flour has led to an epidemic of obesity and digestive illness in our country. The lack of fibers, and oil from the wheat germ, make it difficult to break down and utilize the proteins in the endosperm of the wheat kernel. One such protein, called gluten, has become one of the most feared food components of our time. Many people have a digestive disease called "gluten intolerance", or "celiac disease," which causes severe inflammation of the small intestine. Such people must avoid all grains containing gluten, including wheat, rye, barley, spelt, kamut, and oats. Could it be that our overexposure to this protein, without the accompanying fibers, oils, and other nutrients, has created a widespread food allergy and a change in DNA, such that this disease is now being passed down to subsequent generations?

There is absolutely no health value to white flour or white sugar. They are *substances* that are so far removed from their natural state, our bodies don't even recognize them as foods. For this reason, they are not a part of Plan-D.

HEALTHFUL WHOLE GRAINS

Refined grains are not part of Plan-D, but healthful whole grains are! In fact, you are encouraged to expand your horizons when it comes to grains, to minimize the amount of wheat you eat, and instead indulge in a variety of other whole grains. It is better to eat the whole grain, rather than flours that have been ground from the whole grains, although this does not mean that you cannot enjoy foods made from whole grain flours. It just means that you should eat more of the whole grains and less of the whole grain flours.

Whole grains are high life force energy plant foods that provide the body with energy, nutrients, and fiber for their own absorption. They contain an abundance of vitamins and minerals that are vital to health; they are also very high in fiber. Fiber is important because it helps the body to process waste efficiently and helps us to feel fuller for longer.

As you transition to eating more whole grains, there are some things you need to beware of. Many whole wheat breads and whole-wheat tortillas contain sugar or high fructose corn syrup and trans fats, in addition to a load of other additives or preservatives, so you need to read every ingredient list if you are purchasing breads. In order to avoid that problem, I recommend sprouted grain breads. A detailed description of these breads appears in chapter 11.

There are many types of whole grains: brown rice, barley, popcorn, oats, wild rice, corn, amaranth, buckwheat, bulgur, kamut, millet, quinoa, spelt, cornmeal, and whole rye.

When reading ingredient lists, look for the words "100 % whole grain" on the package. Sometimes you will see "whole wheat" or "whole of the wheat." These also mean the product is completely whole grain.

BEWARE PHRASES THAT DO NOT MEAN WHOLE GRAIN

You must also be mindful of certain phrases that do not mean whole grain. Such phrases are:

Wheat Flour – This is just refined white flour. Remember most flour originates from a wheat kernel. The product is not whole grain unless you see the word "whole."

Enriched Wheat Flour, or Unbleached Enriched Wheat Flour – Both of these are just refined white flour. Any flour that has been enriched means that it has been refined.

100% Wheat – This phrase means that the only grain in the product is wheat. It does not necessarily mean whole wheat. You must see the word "whole" if the product is actually whole grain.

Multi-Grain – This only means that the product contains more than one type of grain. All of the grains could actually be refined grains. This is usually the case. It has been my experience that most multi-grain breads are not whole grain, and most of them also contain some form of sugar.

Stoneground – This term refers to grains that are coarsely ground but may contain the germ but not the bran. Often refined flour is the first ingredient, not whole grain flour.

Pumpernickel – This is a coarse dark bread made from dark rye flour and refined white flour.[19]

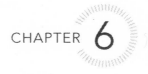

The Big "Fat" Lie

The topic of fats and oils is the topic that spins the heads of many of my nutrition students, who for the most part have all bought in to the misinformation campaign designed to boost the sales of fat-free and low-cholesterol foods. If you have never heard the provocative information you are about to read in this chapter, be warned. I'm about to break the traditional myths about fat, because you are going to find that Plan-D incorporates many healthful oils and fats as part of the daily plan. Inclusion of these fats in Plan-D has been confirmed by solid scientific studies, the testimonies and medical records of Plan-D followers, and thousands of years of history.

There is a popular trend in our culture today concerning dietary fats—reduce and eliminate as much as possible. Dieters, body builders, and concerned mothers alike confidently reach for groceries touting "low-fat" or "fat-free," in the quest for slimmer and healthier physiques. The underlying presumption is that any fat in the diet, be it olive oil or butter, will most certainly end up on our bellies, hips, and thighs.

Like almost everything in nutritional biochemistry, the story is just not that simple. The role of dietary fats in the body is complex and extensive. While some types of fat can pose serious health problems, others are absolutely vital to our survival. Most of us know this to some extent, but the problem is that nearly everything we know and believe about fat is the direct opposite of what is scientifically and historically true, despite what the U.S. government and our good friend the Food Guide Pyramid tell us.

Here are some of the big "fat" lies we've come to believe:

- Eating fat makes you fat; therefore a low-fat diet is healthy
- Canola oil is one of the healthiest oils for cooking

- Coconut oil is a dangerous saturated fat that should be avoided like the plague
- Saturated fat and dietary cholesterol are the main cause of coronary heart disease
- Real butter clogs arteries, so newfangled "healthy" margarines should be eaten in its place
- The cholesterol in egg yolks causes high cholesterol, so we should only eat egg whites or Egg Beaters

None of these widely accepted "truths" is true, and if you've been making your food choices based on these falsehoods you may be setting yourself up for some serious health problems. These fat myths have been perpetuated over the last few decades by the medical profession, nutritionists, and other health professionals, who themselves don't always have the most accurate information.

POLITICALLY CORRECT NUTRITION LEADS TO POOR HEALTH

Medical misinformation dies hard, but it is time to put an end to these false "gospel" truths. It took me years to find and decipher the *real truths* about fat by becoming an astute student of cutting edge science on the subject.

Some of that cutting edge science was published in the cover story of the July 7, 2002 issue of *New York Times Magazine*. In his article titled "What If It's All Been a Big Fat Lie?" author Gary Taubes questioned the conventional wisdom handed down by the American medical establishment that obesity and heart disease are caused by the excessive consumption of fat. He boldly asserted that what most of us have believed to be true about fats and health is actually the result of an entangled web of food industry lobbying, self-promoting medical celebrities, government intervention based on no sound science, advertising, media, and our own guilt-induced desire to redeem our health by giving up "evil" fats. The proliferation of untrue fat myths have now become so deeply entrenched in our culture that we find it difficult to believe anything else. However, when you delve into human history and the real science of it, you cannot dispute the real truth about fat.

For example, three decades of eating reduced-fat dairy products, margarines, Egg Beaters, skinless (and flavorless) chicken breasts, and about fifteen thousand low-fat and fat-free products should have rendered a healthier and slimmer nation. In 1984 the president of the American Heart Association predicted that if everyone ate low-fat, heart attacks and strokes would be rare if not eradicated by the year 2000. Because many of us jumped on the low-fat bandwagon, Americans did reduce their fat consumption from more than 40 percent of the total diet down to 34 percent by the beginning of the new millennium. However, even by 2009, the incidence of heart disease *has not declined*, and as I have already discussed, obesity is skyrocketing at alarming rates.

Why haven't we managed to achieve the optimal state of health we were promised in exchange for giving up whole milk and real cream, eggs, real butter, tropical oils, cheese, and red meat? In his widely ignored first article on the subject, "The Soft Science of Dietary Fat," published in the prestigious journal *Science* (March 30,

2001), Gary Taubes explains that the science proving a connection between dietary fat and heart disease simply was never there in the first place. Hundreds of millions of dollars of research later, *there's no proof whatsoever that eating low-fat will improve your health in any way at all.*[1] In fact, the research more accurately proves that eating a low-fat diet can be detrimental to your health.

NO SOUND SCIENCE

The fat misinformation campaign is aimed at two dietary "demons"—saturated fat and cholesterol. The lies started flying in the 1950's with a faulty hypothesis proposed by a researcher named Ancel Keys. His theory suggested that there is a direct relationship between the amount of saturated fat and cholesterol in the diet and the incidence of coronary heart disease. Despite numerous subsequent studies that put his data and conclusions into question, Keys' research became the "word" and received far more media attention than any of the opposing views.

Before 1920 heart disease in America was extremely rare. So rare that when a young internist named Paul Dudley White presented a new invention to his colleagues at Harvard University, they thought him foolish to try and market it and advised him to concentrate on a more profitable branch of medicine. The invention was the German electrocardiograph, a new machine that could detect blockages in the arteries, thus leading to early diagnosis and treatment of coronary heart disease. In the 1920's clogged arteries were such a medical rarity White had to scour the country looking for patients to try out his new machine. However, during the next 40 years White became a wealthy man as the incidence of coronary heart disease rose dramatically. By the mid 1950's when Ancel Keys was conducting his research, it was the leading cause of death among Americans.

I must admit that when it comes to heart disease, the medical establishment has made great advancements in early detection and reducing the mortality rates of people who have suffered heart attacks. In fact, my own father is still alive today because of these technological breakthroughs. But while science and technology can clear arteries once they've been severely clogged and can keep people alive once they've already suffered a heart attack—the risk and rate of our nation's leading killer continues to sharply rise. Despite the pushing of low-fat and low cholesterol diets, blood thinning drugs, polyunsaturated oils, and calorie counting, the 20th century has not made a dent in the rates of heart disease.[2] Today it is responsible for at least 40 percent of all U.S. deaths.

If, as we have been told, saturated fat and cholesterol are the leading culprits in the development of heart disease, obesity, and cancer, you would expect that during the period when the incidence of these diseases was on the rise, there would have been a correlating increase in the consumption of these dietary demons. But the exact opposite is true. From 1910 to 1970, the amount of saturated animal fat in the American diet dropped from 83 percent to 62 percent, and the consumption of butter in America decreased from eighteen pounds per person per year to four.

You may be surprised to also discover that over the past eighty to ninety years, cholesterol intake has only increased by 1 percent. What did increase sharply, by about 400 percent, was the consumption of so called "healthy" polyunsaturated vegetable oils in the form of margarine, shortening, and refined cooking oils. Also during this time, we started scarfing down more sugar and processed foods, whose consumption has increased by about 60 percent.[3]

One of the most famous research studies conducted on heart disease in America is the Framingham Heart Study. This study is often cited as "proof" of the correlation between the amount of saturated fat and cholesterol in the diet and the incidence of coronary heart disease. Begun in 1948 in Framingham, Massachusetts, researchers studied and evaluated different groups of 6,000 participants who consumed either high levels of saturated fat or low levels of saturated fat. For 40 years, participants were tested and evaluated at five-year intervals. Although the study did show that those who weighed more and had abnormally high blood cholesterol levels were slightly more at risk for future heart disease, it was not due to their fat and cholesterol intake. At the end of the 40 years, the director of the study had to readily admit:

"In Framingham, Massachusetts we found that the more saturated fat one ate, the more cholesterol one ate, the more calories one ate, the lower the person's serum cholesterol." The study also showed that the people who ate the most cholesterol and saturated fat also weighed the least and were the most physically active.[4]

Another study performed in Britain involving several thousand men asked half of them to reduce their saturated fat intake, stop smoking, and increase the amount of "good" fats such as margarine and polyunsaturated cooking oils. The other half did not make any changes to their diets but were also asked to stop smoking. After just one year, those on the "good fat" diet had 100 percent more deaths than those eating saturated fats, even though some of the men eating saturated fat continued to smoke! However, when the results were presented to the public, the study's author ignored these results in favor of the politically correct conclusion: "The implication for public health policy in the U.K. is that a preventive program such as we evaluated in this trial is probably effective. . ."[5]

DISPROVING THE LINK

Many other studies have shown similar biased and falsely presented data. And although it has been proven in laboratories that heart disease can be induced in animals if they are given massive amounts of oxidized and rancid cholesterol (about 10 times the amount in any normal human diet), there are many more compelling human studies *disproving the link* between saturated fat, cholesterol and heart disease. Consider the following:

When Dr. Weston Price documented the diets of primitive peoples all over the globe, he found all of their diets to be rich in *animal foods* containing *saturated fat* and *cholesterol* such as butter, eggs, fatty fish, wild game, and organ meats. The fats in these foods are rich in the fat-soluble vitamins A, D, E and K, which have been shown to prevent heart disease when consumed in whole foods. In fact, Dr. Price found that the primitive diets contained at least *ten times more* of the fat-soluble vitamins found in modern diets. Of the people he studied who were eating these foods on a daily basis, none of them were overweight or had any incidence of heart disease or cancer. His observations parallel the results of the Framingham Heart Study—the more saturated fat and cholesterol a person eats, the lower their weight and blood cholesterol levels. The people Dr. Price studied were indeed the healthiest people in the world, despite their high consumption of saturated fat.

Contemporary controlled studies and surveys of traditional populations echo this truth. Michael DeBakey, the famous heart surgeon, conducted a study of 1,700 patients with hardening of the arteries and found *no relationship between the level of cholesterol in the blood and the incidence of atherosclerosis.* The Medical Research Council found that men eating butter (a traditional whole food) ran half the risk of developing heart disease as those eating margarine (a laboratory-created fake fat previously thought to be healthy but now linked to diabetes, heart disease and cancer).[6]

Studies of people in northern and southern India, the Eskimos in Alaska, Mediterranean societies, and Soviet Georgia all reveal a similar pattern: the lowest rates of heart disease are found among those eating the highest amounts of animal fats.

Modern Japanese, Swiss, and French populations also eat diets high in saturated fat and have lower rates of coronary heart disease than many other western countries. Unfortunately these societies suffer from other degenerative diseases owing to their ever-increasing consumption of refined sugar, flour and processed foods.

SATURATED FATS CRUCIAL FOR HEALTH

The reason for the correlation between high saturated fat intake and healthy people is that saturated fats play a crucial role in body chemistry. You may be surprised to learn just how important they are. In their best-selling book *Nourishing Traditions*, Dr. Mary Enig, a nutritionist and biochemist of international renown for her research on the nutritional aspects of fats and oils, and Sally Fallon, a journalist and nutrition researcher, listed some key roles of saturated fats:

- Saturated fatty acids constitute at least 50 percent of all cell membranes. They are what sustain the integrity of the entire cell, providing necessary stiffness and stability.
- At least *50 percent of the dietary fat we eat should be saturated*, otherwise calcium cannot be effectively incorporated into the skeletal structure. In other words, a lack of an adequate amount of saturated fat in the diet can lead to bone density problems such as osteoporosis.
- Contrary to the fat myths, saturated fats actually *lower lipoprotein (a)*, a key substance in the blood that indicates proneness to heart disease.
- Saturated fats protect the liver from alcohol and other common toxins, such as those contained in nonsteroidal anti-inflammatory drugs (NSAIDs) like Tylenol.
- Saturated fats, especially the type found in coconut oil, enhance the immune system.
- Our bodies need saturated fats *in order to properly utilize the other fats in our diet*, especially the all-important omega-3 fats from fish oil and flax oil. Omega-3 fats are better retained in the tissues when the diet is rich in saturated fats. This means that your omega-3 supplement may not be providing its full health benefit if you are restricting your saturated fat intake too severely.

- Saturated 18-carbon stearic acid and 16-carbon palmitic acid are the *preferred fuel for the heart*, which is why the fat around the heart muscle is highly saturated. During times of stress, the heart draws on this reserve of saturated fat. If there isn't enough, the heart cannot function properly.
- Short- and medium-chain saturated fatty acids found in coconut oil, palm oil, and butter have important antimicrobial properties. They protect us against harmful microorganisms in the digestive tract.

Enig and Fallon sum up their study of saturated fats with this profound statement: "The scientific evidence, honestly evaluated, does not support the assertion that "artery-clogging" saturated fats cause heart disease. Actually, evaluation of the fat found in clogged arteries reveals that only about 26 percent is saturated. The rest is unsaturated, of which more than half is polyunsaturated." [7]

THE BIG FAT CANOLA LIE

If you are like most Americans, you believe canola oil is the best oil to use for cooking. Restaurants proudly tout they only use "healthy" canola oil. Nearly every cookbook on the market includes canola oil in its recipes. Check the ingredients of nearly every packaged food, and you will find canola oil ranking high on the list. The marketers of canola oil have claimed that it is the perfect oil, owing to its low saturated fat content, high monounsaturated fat content, and a bonus omega-3 content, making it particularly beneficial for the prevention of heart disease. Sadly, once again, we have been subjected to a twisted truth.

Canola oil has a hidden history. As mentioned earlier, the incidence of heart disease rose sharply from the 1930's on. By the mid 1980's, the high mortality rates from heart attacks had the medical community in a tizzy, and the media was having a field day. The food industry had a major problem. In collusion with the American Heart Association, numerous government agencies and departments of nutrition at major universities, the food industry had been promoting polyunsaturated oils as a heart-healthy alternative to "artery-clogging" saturated fats since the 1930's. Unfortunately, it had become increasingly clear that polyunsaturated oils, particularly corn oil and soybean oil, cause numerous health problems, including and especially cancer.[8]

The food industry was in a quandary. In the face of mounting evidence of their dangers, it was becoming hard to convince the public that polyunsaturated oils were safe to eat. The industry couldn't go back to using traditional fats like butter and tropical oils without also causing a public scare. Besides, traditional fats are way too expensive to allow for the huge profit margins the industry had been enjoying thus far. They were losing lots of money and needed to come up with a new plan.

Their plan was to convince the public to use a "new" monounsaturated oil. Studies had shown that olive oil, a monounsaturated oil, has a "better" effect than polyunsaturated oils on cholesterol levels and other blood parameters. Besides, Ancel Keys and others had popularized the notion that the Mediterranean diet—rich in olive oil—protected against heart disease and ensured a long and healthy life.[9]

Promotion of olive oil, with its long history of food use, seemed more scientifically sound to health-conscious consumers than the promotion of corn and soy oil, which had never been used in the history of humanity and could only be extracted with modern stainless steel presses and chemical processing. The problem for the industry was that there was not enough olive oil in the world to meet its needs. And, like butter and other traditional fats, olive oil was too expensive to use in most processed foods. The industry needed a less expensive monounsaturated oil. That's when the new wonder oil—canola oil—stepped on to the scene.[10]

THERE'S NO SUCH THING AS A CANOLA

The real name of canola oil is rapeseed oil (there is no such thing as a canola). The natural, untainted rape seed is high in heart healthy monounsaturated fats and also contains omega-3 fats. The problem is that about two-thirds of the monounsaturated fat in natural untainted rape seed is a type called erucic acid, that had been associated with heart lesions and other ailments. In order to remove the erucic acid, Canadian plant breeders had to genetically modify the rapeseed using a seed splitting technique to create a mutation, called LEAR, or Low Erucic Acid Rapeseed.

The new oil, called LEAR oil, was slow to catch on in the United States. In order to make it marketable, it had to be renamed. Neither "LEAR" oil or "Rape" oil were very enticing names, so the industry settled on "canola," for "Canadian oil," since most of the modified rapeseed at that time was grown in Canada.

TWISTED SCIENCE

The industry had managed to manipulate the science (genetic engineering of the rape seed) to make a perfect oil—very low in saturated fat and rich in monounsaturated fat. As a bonus, canola oil contains about 10 percent omega-3 fatty acids, which had been shown to be beneficial for the heart and immune system. Since most Americans are deficient in omega-3 fats, the oil was a dream-come-true for health-conscious consumers. But how healthy is it really?

While rapeseed has been used as a source of oil since ancient times in China and India, the way it was historically pressed from the seed (small stone presses that press out the oil at low temperatures) rendered a fresh healthy oil that was consumed immediately. It has even been proven by recent studies that the erucic acid in rapeseed oil does not create heart lesions, as long as a significant amount of saturated fat is also part of the diet. In fact, erucic acid is helpful in the treatment of the wasting disease adrenoleukodystrophy and was the magic ingredient in Lorenzo's oil.[11]

However, the way we now process canola oil, and most other oils for that matter, is a different thing entirely, rendering them *very unhealthy*. Because canola oil, and all modern vegetable and seed oils, are so unstable, it is nearly impossible to keep them from turning rancid. So they have to be highly processed and refined at high heat (400 to 500 degrees) and treated with chemical solvents like hexane, a fluid also used in dry cleaning. Traces of hexane remain in the oil, even after considerable refining. The refinement process involves bleaching and degumming, which require the use of additional chemicals of questionable safety.

Canola oil contains a good amount of omega-3 fats, which easily become rancid and foul smelling when subjected to oxygen and high heat, so the oil has to be deodorized. The deodorization process removes a large portion of the omega-3 fats by turning them into *trans-fats*. Trans-fats are formed at 320 degrees, so imagine how much damage is done at 400 to 500 degrees. Although the Canadian government lists the *trans-fat* content of canola oil at a minimal 0.2 percent, research at the University of Florida at Gainesville, found trans-fat levels as high as 4.6 percent in commercial liquid canola oil. The consumer has no clue about the presence of *trans-*fats in canola oil because they are not listed on the label.[12]

OIL REFINEMENT DESTROYS ANY ORIGINAL HEALTH BENEFITS

Similar to the refinement of sugar and flour, anything good that was in the original oil, such as vitamins, antioxidants and other nutrients are all destroyed in the oil refinement process. The remaining "pure" oil is tasteless, and by the time that bottle of oil ends up on your supermarket shelf, it's full of trans-fats and free radicals (the dangers of trans-fat and free radicals are discussed later in this chapter). The kicker is that once you buy this oil and take it home, you also *heat it very high* when you cook or bake, destroying it even further!

Liquid canola oil is easily changed by a chemical reaction into *partially hydrogenated canola oil* (a dangerous trans-fat), which is the type of canola oil used in processed foods. This canola oil contains up to 40 percent trans-fats. Almost all restaurants use the partially hydrogenated form of canola oil; so don't be fooled by those "we only use canola oil" claims. These high levels of trans-fats allow for a longer shelf life for processed foods, a crispier texture in cookies and crackers—and more dangers of chronic disease for anyone who eats those foods.[13]

The widespread acceptance of canola oil and its "heart healthy" claims come at a high price. Even those new fangled improved "margarines" made with canola oil and soybean oil are a lie. They're highly processed fake foods that have lost whatever claim they originally had to any health properties. Do yourself a favor, and avoid canola oil at all costs. Eat real butter, cook with extra-virgin coconut oil, and use extra-virgin olive oil for salad dressings.

YOU MUST EAT FAT TO LOSE FAT

Even when you are a chemist as I am, the world of fats can be confusing. However, I am going to do my best to explain it, because it is important for you to understand the essential role fats play in achieving and maintaining a healthy, slim body.

Before I delve into the chemistry, first let me say that *you must eat fat to lose fat*. And you must eat more of it than you probably realize, with one caveat—it must be the right type of fat. If you have been a low-fat dieter, you've been depriving yourself of the delicious and satisfying tastes of the good fats our ancestors ate, like avocados, olives, butter, coconuts, meats, fish, nuts, and seeds. These fats are startlingly health-protective and provide many other benefits for a beautiful well-functioning body, such as glowing skin, shiny supple hair, a good sex life, fertility, a strong vital immune system, enough vitamin E for your heart, balanced hormones, and anti-aging properties.

Vitamins A, D, E, and K (contained in many foods) are called "fat-soluble" vitamins, because they can only be absorbed into the body through fat. Fat also aids in the absorption of beta-carotene, lycopene and many other micronutrients. This is one reason why low-fat diets are dangerous. Without adequate amounts of dietary fat, you can become deficient in these important nutrients, which can then have a cascading effect. For instance, without absorption of enough vitamin D, calcium cannot be absorbed, which could then lead to poor bone health. Aside from absorbing the fat-soluble vitamins, we need fat to properly assimilate protein and minerals. Many people do not realize that proteins and fats are packaged together in nature for a reason—because we need the fat in order to utilize the protein!

Your hormones, which control every cell in your body, don't work properly without adequate fat, and neither does your immune system. Every one of the 60 trillion cells in your body relies on fat—to keep its membranes flexible so that nutrients can enter and toxins can exit, and so it can communicate with the other cells in the body.[14]

Fat is important for proper growth and development and provides insulation for our internal organs and nerves. Fat provides taste, consistency, and stability in our foods. Because of its high energy content, fat quickly satisfies hunger, so you will tend to eat less when you have enough fat in your diet.

According to Dr. Ron Rosedale of the Colorado Center for Metabolic Medicine, fat is the body's preferred fuel, not sugar (the metabolic breakdown product of carbohydrates). He points out that when the body stores excess sugar, it's stored as fat, in a good usable form. Fats not only don't make you fat (unless you eat them to huge excess—and even then, only if you also ingest enough sugars and starches to stimulate your fat-storage system), they're good weapons against obesity.[15]

THE WORLD OF FATS "DEE-MYSTIFIED"

I put together this section for my followers who want to know the science behind healthy and unhealthy fats. You don't absolutely have to know all of this information in order to lose weight and be healthy, but if you're interested in how it all works, I think it will help clear up some of the "mystery" shrouding the world of fats. If it's too technical for you, you can skip it, but make sure you read the next chapter on trans-fats, because you do need to know about those to save yourself from serious health problems.

Chemists have a whole language of their own to describe molecules and their structures. This language is called "nomenclature." In recent years, some of this nomenclature has trickled out to the public by way of food descriptions, particularly fats. The terms "saturated," "trans-fat," "omega-3," "fatty acid," "free radical," "monounsaturated" and "polyunsaturated" are all chemical terms that describe how the carbon atoms and hydrogen atoms within the fat molecules are attached to each other and how they react with other substances.

In general, all fats are substances that are not soluble in water (meaning they don't dissolve in water). This is why your oil and vinegar salad dressing separates. In chemistry, fats are classified according to their molecular structures and physical properties. So, in order to understand what constitutes a good fat or a bad fat, you have to know a little something about the chemistry of fats.

In simple terms, fat molecules look like chains with two little balls attached to one end. The "chains" are made up of strings of carbon (C) atoms bonded, or linked, together. Each carbon atom has four bonding sites. Two of the bonding sites are linked to another carbon atom, and the other two bonding sites are linked to hydrogen (H) atoms, with the exception of the carbon atom at the very beginning of the chain, which is bonded to three hydrogen atoms (see figure 6.1). This is often referred to as a "hydrocarbon" chain.

The "balls" at the end of the chain is actually a group of atoms called a "carboxyl group". It consists of one carbon atom, two oxygen atoms, and one hydrogen atom (COOH). In chemistry, the carboxyl group functions as an acid, therefore fats are interchangeably called "fatty acids." Figure 6.1 is a simple depiction of a fatty acid:

Figure 6.1 A simple chemical structure of a fatty acid chain

Carbon atoms are linked together with hydrogen atoms filling in the bonding sites.

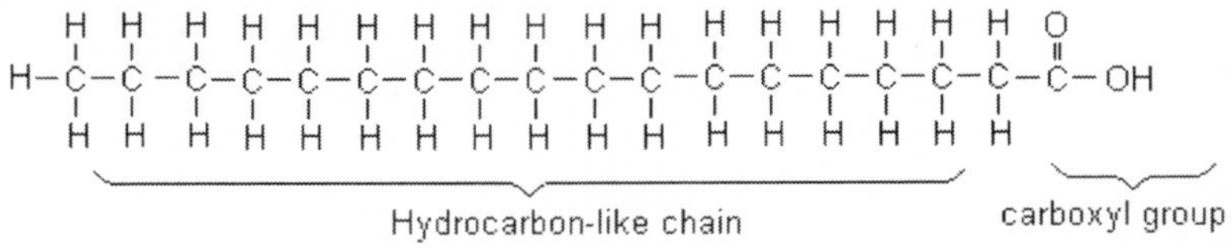

Hydrocarbon-like chain   carboxyl group

Image Source: http://www.chem.csustan.edu/chem1102/stearic.html

Most fats are very long chains (containing anywhere from 14 to 24 carbon atoms linked together), some are medium length chains (8 to 12 carbon atoms), and some are short chains (4 to 6 carbon atoms). Some fat chains are straight, while others are bent. Their length and their shape determine their physical and chemical properties.

As mentioned before, each carbon atom in the chain has "bonding" sites where hydrogen atoms are attached. The bonding sites can either be all filled with hydrogen atoms or only some of the sites are filled. When all the bonding sites are filled with hydrogen atoms, the fat is called "saturated." If some of the bonding sites are empty, or missing hydrogen atoms, the fat is called "unsaturated." The fat in figure 6.1 is an example of a saturated fat because all the bonding sites are filled.

SATURATED FATS

The Webster's dictionary definition of the word "saturated" means *to treat, furnish, or charge with something to the point where no more can be absorbed, dissolved, or retained.* Think of a towel that has soaked up all the water it can, to the point where it is sopping wet and cannot absorb any more water. Sometimes people will say that their brains are "saturated" when they feel they can't retain any more information in a given amount of time.

In the chemistry of fats, a "saturated" fat has all of its bonding sites filled with hydrogen atoms and nothing else can attach to it. Because of this saturation, the fat molecule is highly stable. This means that saturated fats do not normally go rancid, even when heated for cooking purposes. All of the carbon bonds within the fat chain are single bonds, giving the molecule a straight shape; therefore they pack together easily, so that they form a solid or semisolid fat at room temperature.

The most common saturated fats are found in butter, mother's milk, coconut oil, palm oil, cocoa butter, goat's milk, cow's milk and its dairy products, and meat. Typically the saturated fats in animals are made up of long chain saturated fats, whereas the saturated fats in plants like coconuts and palm fruit are made up of medium chain or short chain saturated fats. An exception to this is one of the fats in butter, which is a short chain saturated fat called butyric acid responsible for its yummy butter flavor. Our bodies can also make saturated fats from carbohydrates, which is why you store lots of fat if you eat too many carbohydrates. Figure 6.2 is a molecular structure of a long-chain saturated fat, called stearic acid.

Figure 6.2 Saturated Fat Molecular Structure

3-Dimensional molecular structure of stearic acid, an 18-carbon saturated fat found in animal fats.

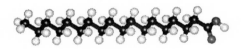

The dark balls represent carbon atoms and the light balls represent hydrogen atoms. All bonding sites (carbon atoms) are filled with hydrogen atoms and the molecule has a straight shape.

Image Source: http://www.chem.csustan.edu/chem1102/stearic.html

UNSATURATED FATS

The other types of fats are called "unsaturated," meaning that there are bonding sites on two adjacent carbon atoms that are not filled. Each adjacent carbon atom is missing one hydrogen atom, which causes them to form a "double bond" to each other, but this double bond is not as stable as the single bonds in saturated fats. Therefore, unsaturated fats are more reactive and susceptible to being changed by heat, oxygen, and light—meaning they go rancid more easily. There are two types of unsaturated fats: "monounsaturated" and "polyunsaturated."

Monounsaturated: The prefix "mono" means one, hence monounsaturated fats have one empty bonding site (one double bond). Monounsaturated fats have a kink or bend at the place in the molecule where the double bond occurs, making them "V-shaped" (see figure 6.3). This V-shape prevents them from packing together easily like the saturated fats do, so monounsaturated fats tend to be liquid at room temperature, but can turn solid, like butter, if refrigerated (this is why your olive oil salad dressing solidifies when you put it in the refrigerator.)

Like saturated fats, the monounsaturated fats are relatively stable. They do not go rancid easily and therefore they can be used in low heat cooking. The most common monounsaturated fat found in our food is called "oleic acid." It is the main component of olive oil and the fat found in avocados, almonds, pecans, cashews, and peanuts. Our bodies can make monounsaturated fats from saturated fats and use them in a number of ways. Monounsaturated fat, if it has not been heated too hot, is known to protect against heart disease.

Figure 6.3 Monounsaturated Fat Molecular Structure

3-Dimensional molecular structure of oleic acid, an 18-carbon monounsaturated fat with one double bond commonly found in olive oil

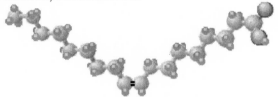

The big balls represent carbon atoms and the small balls represent hydrogen atoms. Two adjacent carbon atoms are each missing one hydrogen atom, so they have formed a double bond (=) with each other and the molecule has a "V-shape."

Image Source: http://scientificpsychic.com/fitness/fattyacids.html

Polyunsaturated: The prefix "poly" means many, or more than one, hence polyunsaturated fats have more than one empty bonding site (two or more double bonds). They have kinks or turns at the positions of each double bond, making them "V-shaped" or "U-shaped," therefore they do not pack together easily. They are liquid, even when refrigerated.

Our bodies cannot make polyunsaturated fats; hence they are called **"essential fats"**, or "essential fatty acids" (EFAs). We must obtain these essential fats from the foods we eat. The two polyunsaturated fats found in many of our foods are linoleic acid, with two double bonds—also called omega-6; and linolenic acid, with three double bonds—also called omega-3. (If you count the carbon atoms in the chain from left to right, the omega number refers to the position on the carbon chain where the first double bond occurs.)

Polyunsaturated fats (both omega-3 and omega-6) are found in such foods as fish, whole grains, nuts, seeds, eggs, and vegetables.

The double bonds in these fat molecules make them extremely fragile and susceptible to becoming rancid, especially the omega-3s. They must be treated with great care so as not to expose them to oxygen, heat, and light for too long. Because of this, polyunsaturated fats *should never be heated or used in cooking.*

This may confuse you because the supermarket shelves are full of polyunsaturated cooking oils. They are derived mostly from soy, as well as from corn, safflower and canola (rapeseed). They are also widely used in restaurants and food production (either soybean oil or canola oil appear on the ingredient list of nearly every packaged food). While polyunsaturated oils contain essential omega-6 and omega-3 fats that are crucial to our health, these fats are only healthy for us when we eat them in their natural state, not as oils that have been extracted from the foods and then highly processed. In other words, we need to obtain these oils from eating raw nuts and seeds, whole grains, and fish, not from processed oils. An exception to that is the omega-3 oils that are cold pressed from flax seeds, hemp seeds and fish. Flaxseed oil and fish oil are pressed from the foods and stored in such a way as to not destroy their fragile omega-3 fat.

Figure 6.4 Polyunsaturated Fat Molecular Structure

3-Dimensional molecular structure of linoleic acid, an 18-carbon polyunsaturated fat with two double bonds commonly found in vegetable oils, whole grains, nuts and seeds.

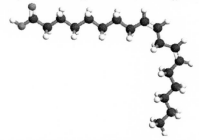

The big black balls represent carbon atoms and the small white balls represent hydrogen atoms. Two double bonds (=) in the molecule give it a bent "U-shape."

Image Source: http://www.raw-milk-facts.cim/CLA_T3.html

DANGERS ASSOCIATED WITH POLYUNSATURATED OILS

Polyunsaturated vegetable oils were never part of the human diet prior to the 1930's. Today the Western diet can contain up to 30 percent of calories from these oils, derived mainly from soy, corn, safflower, and rapeseed (canola oil). But scientific research indicates that this amount is way too high.

In native populations, intake of polyunsaturated oils comes from the small amounts found in legumes, grains, nuts, green vegetables, fish, olive oil and animal fats, but not from commercial vegetable oils. As I described earlier, the processing of these oils is extremely damaging to the healthful qualities found in the natural plants. For instance, if you eat raw sunflower seeds, you get healthy, unadulterated polyunsaturated oil. But if you eat a tortilla chip that has been deep-fried in processed sunflower oil, you get nothing but poor health.

Overconsumption of polyunsaturated oils has been shown to contribute to a large number of diseases including cancer and heart disease; compromised immune system; liver damage; digestive disorders; diseases of the reproductive organs and lungs; and weight gain.[16]

A FREE RADICAL IS NOT A HIPPIE DUDE FROM THE 60'S

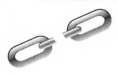 There is a reason why polyunsaturated oils cause so many health problems. The double bonds in unsaturated fats are sites on the fat molecules where a pair of electrons is being shared between two adjacent carbon atoms. When subjected to heat, oxygen and moisture as in cooking and processing, the bond becomes unstable and loses one of its electrons, leaving a carbon atom with an unpaired electron. In simple terms, one of the chain links has been broken open, leaving a gap, or loose link. In chemical terms, this is called a "**free radical**." Free radicals are basically rancid, or oxidized molecules, also known as "oxidants."

A free radical is an unstable molecule with an unpaired electron that is highly reactive. It wants to become stable again, and so it will try to steal an electron from another molecule so that it can close up the chain. The problem is that when we ingest a free radical, it acts like a little terrorist Pac Man racing through our body looking to replace its missing electron by gobbling up an electron from a healthy cell, which then in turn becomes a free radical itself. This cascading domino effect can do a huge amount of damage.

Because we typically don't ingest just one free radical—we ingest an army of them—the result is an exponential amount of altered cells. And remember, polyunsaturated fat molecules have two or more double bonds, so it is possible there are two or more free radical sites acting from just one fat molecule. Free radicals not only attack cell membranes, they can also damage the cell's DNA—the basic building block of cells—thus triggering mutations in tissue, blood vessels, and skin. Free radical damage to the skin causes wrinkles and premature aging; free radical damage to the tissues and internal organs is the precursor for tumors; free radical damage in the blood vessels initiates the buildup of plaque.

It should not be any surprise that numerous studies have repeatedly shown a high correlation between cancer and heart disease with the consumption of polyunsaturated oils. Evidence now links free radical damage with premature aging, autoimmune diseases such as arthritis, Parkinson's disease, Lou Gehrig's disease, Alzheimer's and cataracts.[17]

ANTIOXIDANTS ARE THE ONLY DEFENSE

Food is not our only exposure to free radicals, but it is certainly one of the most prevalent in modern times. Free radicals also come from pollution and other sources. Throughout human history, we have always been exposed to free radicals. However, that exposure was quite low because we did not eat processed oils and environmental pollution was minimal. Our bodies were able to deal with free radicals easily because our traditional diets contained significant amounts of *antioxidants*. Today, we are exposed to millions of free radicals without also supplying our bodies with sufficient amounts of antioxidants. As a result, free radicals multiply to a point called oxidative stress, a point beyond the body's ability to neutralize them. When this occurs, premature aging and disease takes over.

Antioxidants are the body's only defense against free radicals. Antioxidants are special types of phytochemicals found in plant nutrients—yes, that's right, from fruits, vegetables, legumes, and whole grains. And much to your surprise, another very potent antioxidant is cholesterol, the very element we've been told to banish from our lives to preserve our health.

Antioxidants stop free radicals (oxidants) in their tracks, before they can do serious damage. They are like the ghosts in the Pac Man game, swallowing up and stopping the hungry Pac Man from stealing any electrons from healthy cells. They do this in a philanthropic way: by simply donating one of their own electrons. In fact, this is an antioxidant's sole purpose; they don't need their extra electron and so they don't even miss it. Another way of looking at it is to think of a philanthropist who has an abundance of money donating just one dollar to someone who has no money and who would otherwise have to steal that dollar from someone else in order to survive. The philanthropist donating the dollar never misses it, and the donation stops the recipient from stealing.

The Bono's and Bill Gates' of the antioxidant world are vitamins A (as beta-carotene and other carotenoids), C and E, the minerals selenium and zinc, phytonutrients lycopene and squalene found in olive oil, and alpha-lipoic acid. With the exception of alpha-lipoic acid (an important compound found in every cell of the body that helps turn glucose into energy), our bodies cannot make these antioxidants; they all need to come from foods. This is why it is so important to eat plenty of vegetables, fruits, and other foods that contain these antioxidants (see the side box for a list of antioxidant-rich food sources).

THE ESSENTIAL FATS

In my initial stages of weight loss in the early 1990's, I bought in to the "fat" lies. I reduced my fat intake to 10% of my calories using all the wrong fats. Like most Americans, I ate salad dressings made from soybean and canola oils and used margarine instead of butter. And while I did lose weight (mainly from a reduction of overall calories and the elimination of sugar and flour), a few years after my weight loss, my joints were stiff and I was very cold all the time. I hadn't yet learned about the essential fats, which keep our joints lubricated and regulates our body temperature. Essential fats are now recognized as crucial to our good health, but we also have to be aware of the important delicate balance of these fats in our foods and in our diets.

As mentioned before, polyunsaturated fats are called "essential" because our bodies cannot make them, but we must have them, therefore we have to get them from our food. And while we must avoid processed polyunsaturated vegetable oils at all costs, we absolutely must eat real whole foods that contain these polyunsaturated essential fats. Without essential fats, we literally begin to die; virtually every cell function in the body shuts down and degenerative disease takes over.

FOOD SOURCES OF ANTIOXIDANTS

Vitamin A as Beta-carotene and other carotenoids	Apricots, asparagus, beets, broccoli, cantaloupe, carrots, corn, green peppers, kale, mangoes, turnip and collard greens, nectarines, peaches, pink grapefruit, pumpkin, squash, spinach, sweet potato, tangerines, tomatoes, and watermelon.
Vitamin C	Berries, broccoli, Brussels sprouts, cantaloupe, cauliflower, grapefruit, honeydew, kale, kiwi, mangoes, nectarines, orange, papaya, red, green or yellow peppers, snow peas, sweet potato, strawberries, and tomatoes.
Vitamin E	Broccoli, carrots, chard, mustard and turnip greens, mangoes, nuts, papaya, pumpkin, red peppers, spinach, and sunflower seeds.
Selenium	Brazil nuts, tuna, beef, poultry and whole grains.
Lycopene	Tomatoes, red bell peppers, grapefruit, and watermelon. Lycopene in tomatoes is better absorbed into the body when it has been heated, as in cooked tomato products like stewed tomatoes, tomato sauce and tomato paste, which can be used to make sauces, soups, and chili.
Squalene	Olive oil, rice bran, wheat germ, and amaranth seeds.
Alpha Lipoic Acid	A healthy body makes enough alpha-lipoic acid, however it is also found in red meat, organ meats (such as liver), and yeast (particularly Brewer's yeast), as well as dietary supplements.
Other super foods that are rich in antioxidants include:	Apples, all berries, alfalfa sprouts, beans, eggplant, onions, plums, prunes, raisins and red grapes.

There are two essential fat groups, **omega-3** and **omega-6**. Both are in the polyunsaturated family. It is the omega-3s that are truly the miracle workers in the family of fats, and they are found in cold-water fish like salmon, tuna, mackerel, and sardines, walnuts, meat, and leafy green vegetables (once again those leafy greens are loaded with nutrients). Of the meats, lamb has the most omega-3s (perhaps this is why Edgar Cayce often recommended including lamb in the diet.) Flaxseeds, hempseeds, and chia seeds also contain a high amount of omega-3s. Likewise flaxseed oil and hempseed oil are also excellent sources of omega-3s.

THE AMAZING HEALTH BENEFITS OF OMEGA-3s

Omega-3's provide us with some amazing health benefits. They reduce plaque build-up in the arteries, increase levels of HDL (the good cholesterol), and drastically reduce triglycerides. According to a study published in the medical journal *The Lancet*, researchers at Southampton University found that omega-3 fat stops the build up of fatty deposits in the arteries.[18] It has been said that omega-3 acts like a Teflon coating in the arteries, preventing other fats from sticking. Omega-3s also keep our cell membranes fluid for optimum functioning, protect against stroke by preventing platelets from sticking together to form blood clots, lower blood pressure, inhibit erratic heartbeat (a primary factor in fatal heart attacks), improves Attention Deficit Disorder (ADD) symptoms, eliminates osteoporosis, keeps joints lubricated, discourage gout and arthritis, facilitate weight loss, and protect memory and brain function. A daily dose of omega-3 fats have also been shown to correct mood disorders such as depression and bipolar disease better than any known medication. Omega-3s have anti-inflammatory properties; in fact all of my arthritic clients experience a relief in symptoms after adding the right amount of omega-3 fat to their overall healthy diets.

At this point the classification of omega-3s gets a little confusing. Some omega-3s are short chain fats and some are long-chain fats. The short chain omega-3s are found in plant foods such as flax seeds, hemp seeds, and some green leafy vegetables. The long chain omega-3s are found in marine algae and in fish, who eat the algae. When we eat the short chain omega-3s, they have to be converted in our bodies to the long chain omega-3s in order for us to experience their amazing health benefits.

The long-chain omega-3s come in two forms: EPA (eicosapentaenoic acid) and DHA (docosahexaenoic acid). EPA is more involved in the functioning of the heart, while DHA is associated with brain function, but obviously we need both. Fatty fish contain both EPA and DHA (though only about 20 percent of the fish's fat contains these two oils; the rest is saturated fat—another example of the perfection of whole foods. Remember our bodies need saturated fats in order to properly utilize the other fats in our diets, especially the all-important omega-3s. Omega-3 fats are better retained in the tissues when the diet is rich in saturated fats.)

The neurological significance of omega-3s can hardly be overestimated. Omega-3s are one of the few substances that can cross the blood-brain barrier. The brain is close to 70 percent fat, so we're literally fatheads, and although it's in every cell in the body, most of the omega-3 is concentrated in the brain and the retina. To promote optimal brain function and visual acuity, you need a steady supply of omega-3s, which also increase blood flow (the brain gets 25 percent of the body's blood). Omega-3s have a profound role to play in Alzheimer's, dementia, memory loss, mood disorders, and a healthy nervous system.[20]

WOEFULLY DEFICIENT IN OMEGA-3s, GROSSLY ABUNDANT IN OMEGA-6s

Most Americans are deficient in omega-3 fat, mainly because fish and leafy greens are no longer the staple foods they once were. Historically, humans obtained adequate amounts of omega-3 fats from eating cold-water fish and dark green leafy vegetables on a regular basis. Today we get only about 125 milligrams of omega-3 fat per day, whereas our grandparents got 2,500 milligrams by taking a daily spoonful of cod liver oil (sometimes your grandmother made you take it too!) A traditional practice that is nearly extinct in our modern times, a spoonful of cod liver oil was taken just because, for some reason everyone knew it was good for us. The Japanese, who eat lots of fish and seaweed, have omega-3 levels about ten times higher than Americans.

Most Americans get plenty of omega-6 fats; in fact we get too many of them (mainly from those nasty processed vegetable oils found in most of our processed foods, fast foods, and restaurant foods). Omega-6 fats are also found in smaller amounts in whole foods like eggs, whole grains, sunflower seeds, pumpkin seeds, sesame seeds, corn, soybeans, and other plant sources. Eating these foods in their natural form ensures that the oils contained within them are not oxidized.

Other not so well known sources of omega-6 fats are evening primrose oil, black currant seed oil, and borage seed oil—usually only available in supplement form. These oils provide a good source of a type of omega-6 fat called gamma-linolenic acid (GLA), which has been used to help heal arthritis, allergies, multiple sclerosis, cancer, and PMS.

When we have too many omega-6s in our bodies, they have the opposite effect as the omega-3s. Research shows that an excess of omega-6 in the diet creates a disruption in the body that results in an increased tendency to form blood clots, inflammation, high blood pressure, irritation of the digestive tract, depressed immune function, sterility, cancer and weight gain.[19] Yet, omega-6s are still essential, without them we die. Like the helpful qualities of GLA, omega-6s have some important functions in the body (such as blood clotting for wounds), but we have to make sure that we keep them in an ideal ratio with omega-3s.

THE IDEAL RATIO OF OMEGA-3 FATS TO OMEGA-6 FATS

Good health requires the right ratio of omega-3 fats to omega-6 fats in the overall diet. The ideal ratio is about **1:1** (1 omega-3 to 1 omega-6), or the Japanese ratio of **2:1** (2 omega-3s to 1 omega 6). However the modern American eats a ratio of about 1:20 or 1:50, with way too much omega-6 and not enough omega-3.

Recent statistics indicate that nearly 99 percent of people in the United States do not eat enough omega-3 fat. However, the symptoms of omega-3 deficiency are very vague, and can often be attributed to some other health conditions or nutrient deficiencies. The symptoms of omega-3 deficiency include fatigue, dry and/or itchy skin, brittle hair and nails, constipation, frequent colds, depression, poor concentration, lack of physical endurance, and/or joint pain. Chronic deficiency leads more serious symptoms such as cancer, arthritis, heart disease, artherosclerosis, and type 2 diabetes. Studies have shown that consuming enough omega-3s and reducing consumption of omega-6s could prevent, treat, or reverse all of these health conditions.

The average American intake of omega-3 fats is a shockingly low 125 milligrams per day. But even if a person is taking in omega-3s, sugar consumption, trans-fats, and alcohol can interfere with the enzymes that convert the short chain omega-3s into the useable long-chain omega-3s, creating an even greater deficiency. **The recommended intake of omega-3s is 3,000 milligrams per day.** You can increase your intake of omega-3s by eating some of the recipes in this book, by eating cold-water fish several times each week, and through supplementation.

I recommend taking a high quality supplement in addition to dietary sources of omega-3 to make sure you are getting enough. The absolute best source of omega-3 fat is fish or a pharmaceutical grade fish oil or cod liver oil (it will say pharmaceutical grade on the label). Pharmaceutical grade means that all toxins, such as heavy metals, have been safely removed from the oil without destroying the oils healthful qualities. The second best source is organic flaxseed oil with lignans (phytochemical compounds found in the fiber of flaxseeds that are effective in fighting breast cancer), about 1 tablespoon for every 100 pounds of body weight. Flax seeds are also a good source, but it takes about ¼ cup of ground seeds to get the equivalent amount of omega-3 fat in 1 tablespoon of flax oil or a piece of fish. I recommend a combination of oil and ground seeds.

THE ROLE OF OMEGA-3s IN WEIGHT LOSS

Omega-3 fats play an integral role in weight loss. At the very least, eating foods that contain omega-3 fat creates a feeling of satiety, meaning you feel full and satisfied for a longer period of time. A tablespoon of flaxseed oil or a capsule of fish oil will keep you feeling satiated for 3 to 4 hours. When you feel full, you don't snack between meals. However, more importantly, omega-3 works in a very unique way in regards to its affect on weight loss. Studies have shown that omega-3 burns fat even without a reduction in caloric intake. Omega-3 promotes circulation, so your fat-burning ability is enhanced because of increased blood flow to the muscles. Omega-3 also assists fat-transporting enzymes, enabling fat to be better used for energy. This is especially beneficial for liquefying and eliminating the stored hard fats often found in overweight people.

FINAL NOTES ON FAT

A common misconception that many people have is that all substances that contain fat such as avocados, butter, cream, or coconuts, are only made up of one type of fat. Actually, all fat substances contain mixtures of the different types of fats—so there's no such thing as a completely saturated or completely unsaturated fat. It depends on the ratio of saturated to unsaturated that determines its classification. Coconut oil, for example, is 92 percent saturated, whereas butter is about 40-60 percent saturated. Olive oil is about 85 percent monounsaturated. Bacon, the seemingly quintessential saturated fat, actually contains a good percentage of the same monounsaturated fat that olive oil contains. In a one ounce serving of bacon, 42 percent is monounsaturated, while 32 percent is saturated. Perhaps this is why Edgar Cayce recommended occasional crisp bacon in the diet. This makes sense, because the combination of monounsaturated and saturated fats makes it 75 percent heart healthy types of fat. However, I want to repeat the word *occasional*, because Cayce's recommendation is quite an anomaly. Just as Edgar Cayce also advised, with the exception of occasional crisp bacon, pork and pork products are not recommended in Plan-D.

I hope that this chapter has given you a true understanding of the important role fats play in keeping our bodies healthy. Following Plan-D will ensure that you are eating the right types of fat in the proper amounts. In addition to enjoying the wonderful flavor and satiety that fats provide, you will also experience glowing skin, pain-free joints, and loads of energy.

There is one type of fat that I didn't mention in this chapter because I felt it required separate mention. In the next chapter you will learn why trans fats are the *real* dietary demons and should never have been approved for human consumption.

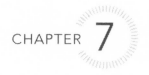

Trans Fats:
THE WORST NUTRITIONAL DISASTER IN HISTORY

In the last chapter I discussed how the public scare over the use of polyunsaturated corn and soy oils forced the food industry to come up with a new cooking oil. Through genetic engineering and chemical processing, canola oil became America's new wonder oil. The same type of twisted science allowed them to come up with a new solid oil to use in processed foods—the trans fat. Canola oil is not the wonder oil it has been touted to be, and we now know that trans fats are extremely detrimental to our health.

Up until the mid-1980s, most of our commercial food supply contained ample amounts of real butter and the tropical fats, namely coconut oil and palm oil. As discussed in the previous chapter, these types of saturated fats are extremely stable, in addition to being very tasty, so they were extensively used to make cookies, breads, crackers, pastries, other baked goods, fried foods, and many other packaged and prepared foods. As saturated fats were becoming unpopular due to the "fat lies" surrounding saturated fat, in 1986 the soy industry saw a chance to claim this strong market for itself. Since soybean oil was cheap and plentiful, food chemists tinkered with a way to turn the liquid oil into a stable solid fat. Thus was born the trans fat—a cheap and stable chemically altered oil that provides yummy flavor and long shelf life to food products. The problem is, like with high fructose corn syrup and artificial sweeteners (and most everything else that food scientists come up with), it's an artificial oil that our body doesn't recognize as food.

QUINTESSENTIAL TWISTED SCIENCE

Trans fats are made through a process called "hydrogenation." The process of hydrogenation turns a polyunsaturated natural oil, which is normally liquid and fragile at room temperature, into a fat that is more solid and stable at room temperature. The result is an unnatural fat that looks, tastes and behaves like the saturated fats—butter and tropical oils—it was designed to replace. The margarines and vegetable shortenings (Crisco, for example) we've all been eating for the last 30 years contain trans fats. Like saturated fats, trans fats will keep for a very long time, which is why cookies and baked goods like Twinkies have such a long shelf life!

To produce trans fats, manufacturers begin with the cheapest oils—soy, corn, cottonseed or canola, already rancid from the extraction process—and mix them with a metal catalyst, usually tiny metal particles of nickel oxide. This oil-nickel mixture is then subjected to hydrogen gas in a high-pressure, high-temperature reactor. Next, soap-like substances, called emulsifiers, and starch are squeezed into the mixture to give it a better consistency; the oil is yet again subjected to high temperatures when it is steam-cleaned. This removes its unpleasant odor. At this point the color of the oil is an unappetizing gray (unbecoming of anything we'd want to spread on our toast), so the gray color is removed by bleach. Dyes and strong artificial flavors must then be added to the oil to make it look and taste like butter (they do such a good job of it that manufacturers were able to come up with gimmicky names like "I Can't Believe It's Not Butter"). Finally, the mixture is compressed and packaged in blocks or tubs and for many years was sold as a healthy alternative to real butter![1]

CHOOSY MOTHERS SHOULD NOT CHOOSE TRANS FATS

If you read the ingredient list of any packaged food, you won't see the term "trans fat." Because the process of creating trans fats is called "hydrogenation," the fats themselves are called "hydrogenated oils", or "partially hydrogenated oils." The most common ones you'll see in ingredient lists are "partially hydrogenated soybean oil" and "partially hydrogenated cottonseed oil or safflower oil." Vegetable shortenings and margarines are hydrogenated, so virtually all commercial baked goods like cookies, crackers, breads, pastries, cake mixes, pancake mixes, dough mixes like pizza dough and pie crusts, biscuits and rolls, and tortillas (even the whole wheat versions) contain trans fats. According to Dr. Mary Enig, a leading American lipid researcher, extensive studies of the food supply have found that the most trans fats turn up in sandwich cookies, vanilla wafers, animal crackers, and honey graham crackers—favorite treats for kids. Almost all frozen food includes partially hydrogenated oils, and microwave popcorn and movie popcorn are popped in trans fats. Even peanut butter, unless it is completely natural, contains trans fats (especially the one that choosy mothers choose).[2]

In her book, *The Good Fat Cookbook*, an extensive expose on the good and bad fats, Fran McCullough details the extent and pervasiveness of trans fats:

> Virtually all fake fat, from margarine and Olestra, to imitation cheese (processed cheese) to anything labeled "lite" or "fat-free," is loaded with trans fats. Powdered fats, such as the powdered milk that gets added back into skim and low-fat milk (to give it better color and flavor), or the powdered eggs that go into baked goods, belong in this category too. Another great source of trans fats are the artificial creamers that everyone adds to their coffee, the powdered ones and the liquid ones. The great

irony, of course, is that we choose these products to protect our health, while the very act of consuming them jeopardizes it more than any other food we could eat, including pure sugar and pure natural fat. Dr. Mary Enig reports a claim that birds will not eat margarine; they're apparently much better at spotting potential toxins than we are, good canaries in the coal mine. Or possibly margarine just doesn't please the avian palate, as it shouldn't please ours.[3]

Prior to the recent 2006 FDA ruling that trans fat counts be listed on nutrition fact panels, Americans were consuming 2,500 percent more of them than we did seventy-five years ago—a whopping statistic that applies to no other food, even sugar. Some researchers believe this fact alone accounts for the skyrocketing rates of heart disease and cancer.[4]

IT'S NOT NICE TO FOOL MOTHER NATURE

Trans fats are even worse for you than the highly refined polyunsaturated vegetable oils from which they are made. The reason for this has to do with the chemical changes that occur during the hydrogenation process. Referring back to my discussion in the previous chapter, unsaturated fats have one or more double bonds. Before hydrogenation, at the site of the double bond, a pair of hydrogen atoms occur together on same side of the double bond, causing the molecule to bend slightly. This is called the **cis** configuration.

The Latin prefixes Cis and Trans describe the orientation of the hydrogen atoms with respect to the double bond. Cis means "on the same side" and Trans means "across" or "on the other side." The Cis configuration is the one that generally occurs in nature and makes oils liquid at room temperature. The Cis configuration can only be changed through a forced chemical reaction that breaks the double bond and rearranges the hydrogen atoms.

This forced chemical reaction is called *hydrogenation*. Under high temperatures, the nickel catalyst causes the hydrogen atoms to change position at the double bond. One hydrogen atom of the pair is moved to the other side of the double bond so that the molecule straightens. This is called the **trans** configuration, a molecular structure rarely found in nature. Because of this change in configuration, the chemical properties of the trans fat are quite different from the chemical properties of the naturally occurring cis fat.

Trans fats resemble saturated fats because of their straight molecular shape and because they are solid at room temperature. But that's about all that's similar about these two fats. First of all, a trans fat is *not* a saturated fat. Remember, saturated fats do not contain double bonds, while trans fats do. Secondly, saturated fats, while solid at room temperature, get broken down easily by body heat and do not stay hard at body temperature. They do not oxidize in the body and are not easily susceptible to becoming free radicals.

Trans fats on the other hand, are so solid they can't be broken down by body heat, thus they stay very solid and hard once they get into our bodies. The body doesn't quite know what to do with trans fats, because it doesn't recognize their altered structure. They become toxins to the body, but unfortunately our digestive system invites them in as if they were real fats. Instead of being rejected as toxins, trans fats are incorporated into our cell membranes as if they were natural cis fats. Because of their solid nature, trans fats make our cell membranes stiff and hard, while cis fats allow our cell membranes to be supple and pliable.

Figure 7.1

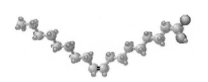 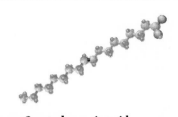

Cis-9-octadecenoic acid
(natural olive oil)
The two hydrogen atoms occur on the same side of the double bond in the **cis** formation, causing the molecule to bend and form a V-shape. The **cis** formation is the one that occurs the most in nature, giving oils a liquid texture.

Trans-9-octadecenoic acid
(hydrogenated olive oil)
The two hydrogen atoms occur on opposite sides (across from each other) of the double bond in the **trans** formation, causing the molecule to straighten and the oil to become solid. The trans formation rarely occurs in nature.

Through the process of hydrogenation, the V-shape of the naturally occurring cis fat is converted to a straight shaped trans fat. This changes the oil from a liquid to a solid, and changes how it behaves in the body.

Image Source: http://scientificpsychic.com/fitness/fattyacids.html

WOLVES IN SHEEP'S CLOTHING

Trans fats are like wolves in sheep's clothing for this reason: our cell membranes have V-shaped receptor sites in them that are specifically designed to accept the bent V-shape of natural cis fats. When we eat natural cis fats, they fit nicely into the perfectly designed receptor sites in our cell membranes. Once there, the cis fats act as conduits for nutrients and other substances to move into the cell for important biochemical reactions to occur. For example, glucose (blood sugar) is converted to energy on the inside of our cells. But the sugar has to be transported into the cell by way of the conduit—the cis fat. This occurs easily when natural cis fats occupy the receptor sites. When sugar is converted to energy inside the cell, it does not build up outside of the cell in the bloodstream, thus preventing high blood sugar that leads to diabetes.

Another reaction that occurs on the inside of cells is the conversion of bad cholesterol to good cholesterol. Once again, if the bad cholesterol can get inside the cell by way of the cis fat conduit, it can be converted easily, and bad cholesterol does not build up in the bloodstream.

However, since the body thinks the trans fats are real fats, the straight trans fats can actually force their way into the bent V-shaped receptor sites. But trans fats do not act like conduits, and once they are incorporated into the cell membrane, they get stuck there because they don't fit properly. Unlike natural cis-fats that allow nutrients to freely flow in and out of the cell, trans fats just block the receptor sites and nothing can get in, not even the good fats.

It's kind of like when you have a key that looks like it's the right key for your keyhole. You can actually fit the key into your keyhole, but once you turn the key, it breaks off in the lock. Now you can't even get the right key into the keyhole because it is completely jammed up. That's what trans fats do to our cell membranes. They jam up the receptor sites and important body chemistry is completely disrupted. Sugar cannot be converted to energy, so it builds up in the blood stream and eventually becomes diabetes. Bad cholesterol builds up in the blood stream and leads to high cholesterol levels and heart attacks. What's worse is that even when we are eating the good essential fats, they don't get utilized properly because the trans fats block them from being incorporated into the cells.

The blockage of cell receptor sites leads to many problems. Trans fats have now been implicated in cancer, heart disease, multiple sclerosis, diverticulitis, and diabetes, among other diseases. Trans fats also interfere with the reproductive system, producing abnormal sperm and decreasing the amount of cream in human milk. They weaken the immune system and inhibit enzymes that metabolize toxic chemicals, carcinogens, and medications. They decrease the response of cells to insulin, setting the stage for insulin resistance and all the terrible things it brings in its wake, from obesity and diabetes (which are now epidemic in our country) to heart disease.[5]

There are a host of other problems with trans fats. When our body tries to metabolize trans fats, normal biochemistry is blocked and enzymes are inhibited from the natural production of the body's own fatty acids (remember, our bodies can produce their own saturated and monounsaturated fats).

Trans fats also affect our body's electrical circuitry. The good fats (cis fats) are necessary for electrical and energy exchanges that involve proteins, oxygen, and light. These electrical currents are responsible for all body functions, from the way our minds work, to our heartbeat, cell division, muscle coordination, and energy levels. Tran's fats are not suitable in these processes and jam the "plug" for the cis fats.

Trans fats are stickier than cis fats, increasing the likelihood of a clot in a small blood vessel causing strokes, heart attacks, or circulatory occlusions in other organs, such as lungs, extremities, and sense organs. Our hearts use fatty acids as their main fuel source. Trans fats are less easily broken down by enzymes and have slower use as an energy source, which could have serious consequences in a high-stress situation. Trans fats also interfere with our liver's detoxification pathways. They're just bad news all around!

ZERO GRAMS TRANS FAT NOT NECESSARILY TRUE

To escape the havoc trans fats play in our bodies, our best defense is to avoid them like the plague. We need to eliminate them as much as possible from our diets by avoiding margarines, vegetable shortening, fried foods (especially French fries), and other obvious sources like popcorn and foods cooked in oil. **You must read every ingredient label**, looking for the words "hydrogenated oil" "partially hydrogenated oil," "soybean oil," and "canola oil" (remember that even liquid canola oil contains trans fats). Never buy anything labeled "lite," "low calorie," or "fat-free."

In 2006 the U.S. Food and Drug Administration (FDA) tried to help us out by making it mandatory for food manufacturers to list on their nutrition fact panel the amount of trans fat in their products. As usual the FDA didn't go far enough. A manufacturer is only required to list trans fats if the food contains 0.5 gram (one half gram) or more per serving. Therefore, if a serving contains 0.4 grams, it does not have to be listed on the nutrition fact panel. This misleads the unsuspecting consumer into thinking that the product does not contain trans fats. The tricky food industry even boasts claims on the front of the packaging "0 grams trans fat," but if you read the ingredients and still see "hydrogenated oil" listed, it is not trans fat free.

You may also be interested to know that 1 tablespoon of stick margarine contains 3 grams of trans fats, and that a medium order of fast-food French fries contains 8 grams of trans fats (when cooked in partially hydrogenated oil).

Before the FDA approved the requirement of listing trans fats on nutrition fact panels, they asked the Institute of Medicine (a branch of the National Academy of Sciences) to prepare a report. Three years later, in July 2002, the institute declared that *there is no safe level of trans fats in the diet*. You have to realize that trans fats are harmful even in tiny amounts, like less than 0.5 gram per serving (most people eat more than one serving of processed foods anyway, so those partial grams of trans fats can add up to anywhere from 1 to 5 grams). Even in tiny amounts, they jam up the receptor sites in our cell membranes, making cells hard and stiff. Our friend Dr. Walter Willet, professor of epidemiology at Harvard School of Public Health, has called the introduction of trans fats into the food supply "the worst food-processing disaster in human history."

The good news is that by following Plan-D, you can completely eliminate trans fats from your life. No recipes or food products recommended in this book contain trans fats!

CHAPTER 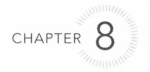 8

Living Processed-Free in a Processed Food World

In the incredible pace of our lives and with the availability of every prepackaged food imaginable, we have lost the connection between what we eat, why we feed ourselves, and how we feel.
    —Halé Sofia Schatz, If the Buddha Came to Dinner

According to recent statistics, about 90 percent of the money Americans spend on food goes toward purchasing processed food. Ninety percent! We now know that most of the food available to us has been processed in some way, mainly sugars, flours and oils. So how are we supposed to live processed-free in world that hardly supports us in doing so?

We have to become conscious and aware shoppers and diners, and take responsibility for everything we put into our bodies. Until the food industry catches up to our high level of awareness, we have to be our own advocates.

The first step in making sure we are getting the best food available is to learn how to shop. Even if you don't have access to a natural food market, you can still buy healthy foods in a mainstream grocery store. Besides, natural food stores also contain many items that are not necessarily healthy. This chapter will help you live processed free in a processed food world.

MAKING OVER YOUR SHOPPING CART
Shop the Perimeter
The most common mistake people make when trying to shop healthily at the grocery store is that they scour the packaged food aisles looking for supposedly healthy options. Usually they wind up with way too much junk in their carts. You will do far better avoiding the store's central aisles altogether. That's where all the processed-food temptations hang out.

Shopping the perimeter of the grocery store is a much better strategy. The perimeter is where all the perishable food is – things like fruits and vegetables, fish and chicken, and dairy. Basically, the vast majority of whole foods are located at the perimeter, so do what you can to stay out of the center aisles.

Avoid Low-Fat, Fat-Free, Sugar-Free, and Low-Carb Items

Butter is better for you than margarine. Real eggs are better for you than Eggbeaters. Whole grains are better for you than low-carb items with added artificial sweeteners. For the most part, products claiming to be fat-free or sugar-free are designed to mislead people and give them a false sense of security. They're attention-getting, but they rarely tell the whole story.

For example, a fat-free item may not have any fat in it, but it will probably have more sugar in it than the regular version of that item. This is particularly true of salad dressings. Sugar is converted into fat in your body, so the claim of fat free is very misleading.

A soda might have "no fat" on it, but that doesn't make it good. You can take a food that says "low carb," but it could be full of trans fats and other processed chemicals that work against you. Most foods that have marketing claims on them are loaded with chemical ingredients.

Read Ingredient Lists

The single most important tool you have for going processed-free is the ability to read and decipher ingredient lists. It's important to read the ingredient list carefully. This may take you longer the first few times you go shopping, but once you know what you're looking for, you'll be zipping through the store with your newfound ingredient reading ability.

The basic rule of thumb is this: If you have to buy something with a label, make sure you know what all the ingredients are and that you're comfortable putting them in your body. If there are chemical names on the ingredient list that you can't pronounce, it's a pretty sure bet that it isn't real or healthy. For the most part, unless you know what it is, you should avoid foods with more than five or six ingredients.

Finding the ingredient list on a food package and also being able to read it can sometimes be a challenge. Ingredient lists are often in very small print or under the flap of the packaging material. If you need glasses to read, you should always bring them with you to the grocery store.

Packages may have statements like "Natural Fruit Flavors, "Made with Real Fruit Juice", "All Natural Ingredients" and "No Preservatives Added." These statements do not mean that there are no harmful chemicals in the product. Manufacturers bank on the hope that you'll think these are healthy natural products. One thing you need to know is that there is no regulation on the word "Natural." Manufacturers are really stretching it these days by trying to convince the public that their product is natural just because it was derived from a real food. For instance, the Splenda company claims that their product is more natural than other artificial sweeteners, just because they use sucrose as the starting ingredient.

Ingredients are listed in order of the weight of the ingredient in the recipe. Therefore, the ingredient that weighs the most is listed first; the ingredient that weighs the least is listed last. Take note: you will often see the statement "Contains less than 2% of the following ingredients:" Do not be fooled by this. If a food contains less than 2% of arsenic or other poisonous substance, you will still be poisoned.

As a general rule, if the ingredient list is long and contains names of chemicals that you cannot pronounce, you are probably risking your health by eating it. If the ingredient list is short, it may or may not have harmful additives in it, so read ingredients carefully before you decide to purchase the product.

The top ingredients to avoid are:

- Sugar
- Enriched wheat flour
- Unbleached enriched wheat flour
- Wheat Flour
- High Fructose Corn Syrup
- Partially Hydrogenated Oil (usually soybean oil) –also known as trans-fats
- Hydrogenated Oil – also known as trans-fats
- Canola Oil and Safflower Oil – contains trans fats
- Mono and Diglycerides – these are similar to trans-fats and have many harmful effects
- Monosodium Glutamate (MSG)
- Sucralose (Splenda)
- Aspartame (Equal)
- Saccharine
- Acesulfame K
- Maltodextrin
- Anything with a number after it (i.e. red dye #40, polysorbate 80, etc.)
- Artificial colors
- Artificial flavors – these may contain up to 30 different chemical ingredients

Choose local, fresh and as close to natural as possible

Local foods, meaning foods that are grown in the proximity to where you live, will have the highest life force energy and the highest level of nutrients. Shop farmer's markets or grocery stores that carry locally grown produce.

Eat loads of fresh fruits and vegetables, whole grains and high quality fresh meats and poultry. Following Plan-D helps you do this. But does this mean that there aren't *any* good foods in the canned, boxed, bagged or frozen-food aisle? No, it just means they're few and far between. Things like frozen fruits and canned beans can still be good for you, as long as they don't contain a bunch of unhealthy and unnecessary ingredients. There are now many healthy organic and frozen food items available in natural food markets, but try to eat more of your foods fresh.

I realize that's not always realistic to eat everything fresh all of the time. We need to have convenience foods and we need to eat out to help us deal with time crunches. I do it all the time, but I read every label and am very picky about what and where I eat. Choose packaged foods that are made with real-food ingredients over those with factory-created components. Be a smart consumer and look for things that are going to help your body thrive. When you pick something up, ask yourself the question: "Is this something my great grandmother would have eaten?" If the answer is "no," you should probably put it back.

STOCKING A HEALTHY PANTRY

Now that you know what to avoid, go to your cabinets, refrigerator, and freezer and toss out or phase out any foods that contain the ingredients on the avoid list.

The following is a table of foods that you can replace in your pantry with healthier foods.

UNHEALTHY PROCESSED ITEM	REPLACE WITH HEALTHY ITEM
Refined White Sugar	Stevia, agave nectar, honey, brown rice syrup, or Rapadura Whole Cane Organic Unrefined Sugar
Margarine and Shortening	Organic real butter or extra virgin coconut oil
Commercial Peanut Butter containing sugar or trans fats	Natural peanut butter, or other nut butters such as almond butter or cashew butter, with only one or two ingredients: nuts and salt
Table salt (iodized salt)	Natural Celtic Sea Salt
Canned vegetables/fruit	Fresh or frozen fruits and vegetables
Soft drinks	Good clean water, herbal teas
Pasta made from white flour	Pasta made from whole grains such as brown rice, quinoa, spelt, corn, and whole wheat
White Flour	Whole grains like brown rice, oats, quinoa, and spelt, wild rice, buckwheat, barley, rye, millet, kamut, amaranth, and whole wheat
White Bread	Flourless sprouted bread or a good 100% whole grain bread. The ingredient list should be short with only a few ingredients such as whole grain flour, yeast, honey, and sea salt.
Crackers	Whole grain crackers –Ak-Mak, Mary's Gone Crackers, or Flax Seed Crackers
Breakfast Cereals	Whole grain cereals such as Ezekiel, Nutty Brown Rice, Uncle Sam Cereal and others. Look for short ingredient lists.

EATING ORGANIC ON A BUDGET

I didn't start out my weight loss journey eating organic, but I have since converted as much as I can to making sure the food I eat is clean and free of chemicals. You will do well to start eating more organic food as you adopt a processed-free lifestyle.

Even small doses of pesticides and other chemicals can cause lasting damage to human health. Pesticides have been linked to various disorders and diseases, including cancers of the reproductive, endocrine and immune systems. Pregnant women and children are especially vulnerable, as pesticides have also been linked to developmental and behavioral disabilities and impairment.

The specific effects of many pesticides are unknown. Pesticide manufacturers claim their products are safe, but the studies on these products are usually done with high doses, rather than testing the chronic low doses that people typically experience. Companies used to claim that DDT (a classic example of an endocrine-disrupting pesticide) was safe, right up to the day it was banned.

This reason alone should convince you to eat organic food, however, most of us have budgets that dictate our food choices. But eating organic is doable, even on a modest budget. A common perception is that organic food is so expensive that it is out of the budget for the average family or even for the average single consumer. It is also commonly perceived that the average grocery purchase of processed foods at a neighborhood supermarket, using the store discounts, makes the processed food diet within the budget of most families. If you go along with those who accept that hypothesis, you may be surprised to learn how you can eat a mainly organic diet for about the same amount of money as a typical processed food diet. The key is to learn how to shop and what to choose in order to stay within your food budget.

The benefits of eating organic foods are many. They have been proven to contain a higher percentage of nutrients, have no pesticide residue, generally taste better and have positive benefits on the environment and the people who farm them. When you eat organically, you can rest assured that what you are eating has not been processed.

In order to keep food costs within your budget, you can buy more organic foods by employing smart shopping tactics. Here are a some tips and resources I have found to help make eating organic a healthy and affordable choice:

Decide which foods you consume the most, then prioritize. Whether it's produce, milk, cereal or bread, decide which products makeup the core of your diet. For instance, if you drink milk, eat yogurt, or breads on a daily or regular basis, you should buy those organic. If you only eat radishes every once in a while, then you don't have to worry so much about buying those organically grown.

Once you've decided on your core items, try these ideas:

- Buy in season and be flexible. Purchase what is in season and you can save big on your produce purchases. Find out if your city has a local farmer's market. This is a great source for in-season, fresh produce that if not certified organic, may still be pesticide-free since it does not travel far. Many cities have farmers' markets year-round, rain or shine.
- Check for local food-coops. You can become a member for very little money and you then have access to all types of organic foods at great prices. Many times, if you can find about eight hours a month to donate at the co-op you can save an additional 10-12% off your purchases. To find a local co-op or learn how to organize one, contact the coop directory service at www.

thegang@coopdirectory.org.
- Be on the lookout for coupons. Many natural products have coupons right on the package to be redeemed at checkout. Many magazines also have coupons for healthy products, or visit company websites. Many offer coupons and or incentives to try their products.

Keep an eye out for sales. Yep, organic products go on sale the same as anything else. This is where you can scoop up some great deals. Many local natural foods markets have sales on organic produce and products. The general idea here is to be flexible and stock up when something you like goes on sale.

Buy Bulk. This is one area that many people ignore and can save you quite a bit of money. You can purchase nearly all of your grains, pastas, dried fruits and nuts from the bulk bins. You can purchase ¼ lb or 5 lbs - the difference is that you are not paying for packaging. Your local grocery store and natural foods stores have bulk aisles where you simply fill a bag, write the price on the twist tie and they'll weigh it at the register. You can buy organic brown rice for $.99 a pound or fresh, shelled almonds for $4.99 a pound. Re-use your plastic bag and you'll help preserve the environment and natural resources too.

Give up your dependence on conventional supermarkets. Limiting yourself to the organic section or natural foods section of your local grocer is a great way to pay too much for organic products. These days there are tons of places to buy organic foods. Besides the supermarkets, you can find them in health food stores, specialty stores, co-ops, gourmet delis, farmers' markets, community-supported agriculture programs, convenience stores and even vending machines.

Shop Online. If you can't find a local source for the organic food you want, don't give up. Hop online. You may be able to order the organic foods that you want online.

Rearrange your food budget. Free up more dollars for organic food by trimming the fat from your conventional food budget. Add up all the dollars you spend every month on food, including fast food meals, morning cups of coffee, bagels and even trips to vending machines. A small change in your eating habits could free up the money you need to buy the organic foods that you really want.

Ease into organic. Begin the transition to eating organic with some of your favorite foods. Pick a product or two that you decide you really notice a difference in taste and that really excites you. If you have young children you may want to start by buying organic baby food and dairy products. Whatever your kids eat the most of is where you start.

THE CASE FOR ORGANIC POPCORN

Popcorn is a food that most people consider to be relatively harmless and safe during dieting. Its high fiber and low calorie content are espoused on websites and diet books galore. But dieters take note: popcorn has a darker side.

If you eat popcorn that is not organically grown, you could be eating yourself sick. According to studies conducted by the US Food and Drug Administration (FDA), non-organic popcorn is among one of our nation's most heavily contaminated food crops. The pesticides, herbicides, and other chemicals that are sprayed on the crops remain on the food in small or large quantities even after being packaged and shipped to your local market.

The 2008 Agri-Chemical Handbook of the Popcorn Board (yes, there is such a thing) lists 28 insecticides (including malathion), 44 herbicides, 5 fumigants, 15 fungicides, and 8 "miscellaneous" chemicals that are approved for use on non-organic popcorn crops.[1]

HAD I NOT BEEN A CHEMIST, I WOULD NEVER HAVE KNOWN

During my years as an environmental chemist, my primary job in the laboratory was to perform analytical testing on water, soil, air, and sometimes crop samples to determine the concentrations of residual environmental pollutants in the samples. Popcorn is among the food crops that are routinely tested for residues of persistent organic pollutants (POPs). These pollutants are approved for use by the United States Food and Drug Administration (FDA) and are commonly used in agriculture, electronics manufacturing, water treatment, exhaust from the combustion of fossil fuels, and many other industrial uses. I became intimately familiar with the names and chemical properties of many of these environmental pollutants, as I handled them in a controlled laboratory setting on a daily basis.

The samples I tested often contained high levels of volatile organic compounds (VOCs) used in electronics manufacturing such as such as toluene, benzene, xylenes, trichlorothene, and methylene chloride. I also tested for herbicides and pesticides such as endrin, dieldrin, chlordane, DDE, DDT, and toxaphene among others. All of these compounds are known carcinogens (cancer-causing agents).

Although I mainly tested water and soil samples, I specifically remember a batch of cantaloupes that were brought to the lab for testing. The results were so extraordinarily high in herbicides that I had to serially dilute the samples numerous times just to get the readings within the detectable range of the analytical instrument. The lab smelled sickeningly of cantaloupes for days, and all of the chemists in my department vowed to never eat another cantaloupe!

Unfortunately, diluting samples to obtain usable readings is not an uncommon practice in environmental testing laboratories. After such a horrifying experience with the cantaloupes, I decided to investigate what other common food crops were contaminated with high levels of POPs. To my surprise and ultimate disgust, I discovered that my all-time favorite comfort food—popcorn—was among the top ten foods most contaminated with pesticides and other toxic organic chemicals in the FDA's 2003 Total Diet Study (TDS).

A webpage updated July 2008 of the USFDA Center for Food Safety and Applied Nutrition/Office of Food Safety describes the Total Diet Study:

The Total Diet Study (TDS), sometimes called the market basket study, is an ongoing FDA program that determines levels of various contaminants and nutrients in foods. From this information, dietary intakes of those contaminants by the U.S. population can be estimated. Since its inception in 1961 as a program to monitor for radioactive contamination of foods, the TDS has grown to encompass additional contaminants, including pesticide residues, industrial chemicals, and toxic and nutrient elements. A unique aspect of the TDS is that foods are prepared as they would be consumed (table-ready) prior to analysis, so the analytical results provide the basis for realistic estimates of the dietary intake of these analytes.[2]

Very important note—*a unique aspect of the TDS is that foods are prepared as they would be consumed (table-ready, i.e. washed and prepared) prior to analysis, so the analytical results provide the basis for realistic estimates of the dietary intake of these chemicals by humans!*

Yes, that's right folks. The FDA tests foods and *knows they are contaminated* and does nothing to inform the public that these foods might better be consumed organically grown. Non-organic popcorn—one of America's most beloved snack foods—was found to contain 33 toxic organic compounds, including some that have been linked to serious health consequences. Even when exposure is extremely low, these chemicals are known to cause cancer, reproductive disorders, birth defects, lower IQ in children, and the decline of bird and aquatic species. This occurs because many of the chemicals mimic human and animal hormones and are capable of crossing the placenta during pregnancy.[3]

Perhaps you'll think twice the next time you cuddle up with a bag of popcorn at the movies. As for me, I make mine organic!

List of chemicals and their maximum concentration found in non-organic popcorn popped in oil, from the USFDA September 2003 Total Diet Study, pages 14-15:

Compound Name	Maximum Concentration in micrograms per Kilogram (μg/Kg)
1,1,1,2-tetrachloroethane	16
1,1,1-trichloroethane	27
1,2,4-trimethylbenzene	14
benzene	58
bromodichlorobenzene	5
n-butylbenzene	7
sec-butylbenzene	1
chlordane	80
cis-chlordane	2

trans-chlordane	3
chlorobenzene	2
chloroform	18
chlorpyrifos	10
p,p'-DDE	2
diazinon	10
p-dichlorobenzene	292
dieldrin	2
endosulfan sulfate	1
ethylbenzene	4
lindane	2
malathion	110
p,p'-methoxychlor	300
cis-permethrin	7
trans-permethrin	7
methyl pirmiphos	240
polychlorinated biphenyls	30
n-propylbenzene	3
styrene	11
tetrachloroethene	4
toluene	74
toxaphene	20
trichlorethene	26
m,p-xylene	33
o-xylene	7

Source: www.cfsan.fda.gov

THE MOST IMPORTANT FOODS TO BUY ORGANIC

If you are just starting out with buying organic, the foods that are the most important to consider are dairy products and produce. Meats, eggs, and poultry should also be a concern. Milk that is conventionally produced often comes from cows that are raised under disturbing farm conditions. They may graze on pastures that have been treated with pesticides, herbicides, and sewage sludge. When the cattle are not let outside, they feed on less nutritious dried grass and hay, grains that may be genetically modified, and fishmeal which may contain PCBs and mercury.

When cows ingest toxins, those toxins concentrate in their milkfat. Therefore, if you do drink conventional milk, it is best to drink fat-free milk. Fat free milk is less likely to contain toxins, such as dioxin, an industrial by-product and a known carcinogen that's ingested by cows when they eat contaminated grass. However, the double-edged sword is that fat free milk is not healthy anymore. When I was first losing my weight, I used skim milk. It had a kind of blue color to it, making it somewhat weird and unappealing to most consumers. I've since given up drinking milk, but on the few occasions when I have purchased it, I notice that the blue cast that fat free milk once had is no longer there. That's because now it's artificially colored. Low fat milks, 1% and 2%, have dried milk powder added to bulk them up. This milk powder contains rancid fats, oxidized cholesterol, and lots of nitrites. There are a few ethical dairy farms that do not do this to their milk, but they are few and far between. You're better off drinking organic milk and eating organic milk products.

Cows on conventional farms are often given antibiotics--even when they are healthy—to prevent them from getting sick. Although the milk supply is tested before it reaches consumers to make sure it does not contain antibiotics, the overuse of these medications might contribute to a rise of drug-resistant bacteria, making some diseases more difficult to treat.

In some factory farms, thousands of cows are crammed inside barns to allow easy access for milking. Their milk production can be forced beyond normal capacity through injections of a synthetic growth hormone called rbST (also called rbGH). Studies show that these cows are more susceptible to diseases because their natural life cycle is being distorted.

Conventional milk may be cheaper than organic, but the savings may be hard to justify if you're concerned about health issues. For instance, researchers are analyzing the effect rbST has on natural hormones that are transferred from the cow into the milk. One of these, called insuline-like growth factor 1 (IGF-1), may, at high levels, be associated with an increased risk of breast, colorectal, and lung cancers in people, according to studies by Brigham and Women's Hospital and other medical centers.

ORGANIC PRODUCE – BELOW GROUND VEGETABLES AND THE DIRTY DOZEN

As to what produce to eat organic or not, there's some general guidelines. If it grows below the ground, you should buy organic, because foods that grow below the ground absorb more toxins. Common foods that grow below the ground are potatoes, carrots, beets, parsnips, rutabagas, and radishes. If it has an outer protective peel or shell, it is likely less contaminated and OK to eat conventionally grown. Examples are bananas, coconuts, avocados, pineapples, and citrus (unless you are eating the peels).

There is a non-profit organization called The Environmental Working Group (EWG) (www.ewg.org) that has produce tested for residues of pesticides and herbicides. Each year they publish an extensive list of the most contaminated produce. Their studies show that we can lower our pesticide exposure by 90 percent if we avoid the *Dirty Dozen*—the 12 most contaminated conventionally grown fruits and vegetables—and substitute organic produce instead. The EWG publishes another list called *The Clean 15*, which lists the 15 least contaminated fruits and vegetables.

According to the 2009 list put out by the EWG, the 12 most contaminated produce are: peaches, apples, sweet bell peppers, celery, nectarines, strawberries, cherries, kale, lettuce, grapes (imported), carrots, and pears. *These you should definitely eat organic.* The 15 least contaminated are: onions, avocados, sweet corn, pineapples, mangoes, asparagus, sweet peas, kiwi, cabbage, eggplant, papaya, watermelon, broccoli, tomato and sweet potato. *These are OK to eat conventionally grown if you are on a budget and cannot afford to buy all organic.*

You can download a printable wallet guide of The Dirty Dozen and The Clean 15 at www.foodnews.org. Carry the list in your purse or pocket when you go shopping.

HOW TO IDENTIFY ORGANIC PRODUCE

Grocery stores are required by law to keep the organic produce separate from the conventionally grown produce, but if you're wondering how to tell if the produce you are buying is organic, look at those annoying little stickers that they put on it. The stickers are part of an international PLU (price look-up) system grocers use to make check-out and inventory control easier. If the item does not have a sticker on it, just look at the sign for a four or five digit PLU number.

If the item is conventionally grown, the number has four digits (for example, 4060 stands for broccoli). If the item is organically grown, the number has five digits starting with a 9 (so its "94060" for organic broccoli).

There's also a third PLU option. A five digit number beginning with an "8." That would indicate that the produce you are holding has been genetically modified. If you're eating non-organically grown food, you're probably eating some genetically modified food without even knowing it. Genetically modified food has been in the food supply for many years now (the rapeseeds used to make canola oil are genetically modified). Unfortunately, at this time, there is no way of knowing if the ingredients in packaged or canned foods have been genetically modified, unless they are organic. Organically grown foods are not genetically modified.

BUY GRASS-FED, HORMONE FREE MEATS,
HORMONE-FREE AND ANTIBIOTIC-FREE
POULTRY AND EGGS, AND WILD CAUGHT FISH

Our livestock and poultry are prone to contamination from pesticides, herbicides, and chemical fertilizers as well as massive amounts of antibiotics and growth hormones, making them extremely harmful for human consumption. They are also fed grains, which is not the natural diet for livestock. Cows are designed to eat grass, not grains. Grains make animals fatter (and people too), which makes the meat fattier and unhealthy for us. It is no wonder so many people are fat and sick!

Unfortunately organic meats, poultry and eggs are much more expensive than their conventionally raised counterparts. For this reason alone, it is best to consume meats occasionally rather than often, and when you do consume them, they should be in smaller quantities than what you may typically be accustomed to. Plan-D recommends 3- to 4-ounce portions of meats and poultry, quite a stark difference to the 6- to 8-ounce portions you get in restaurants.

The eggs you eat should be either organic or free range and free of hormones and antibiotics. You will notice the difference in the taste, as well as the difference in the color of the yolk. Organic eggs have a nice brightly colored yolk that is brimming with nutrients.

With the rising popularity of eating fish, grocery stores and food establishments have turned to farm raised fish to meet the demand. Farm raised fish are not fed their natural diet either. They are also fed grains, which upsets the ratio of their fat content. Research has shown that farm raised fish contain higher ratios of omega-6 fats, which creates a harmful imbalance for our bodies. Wild caught fish eat their natural diet of smaller fish and sea creatures, making them leaner with higher levels of the healthy omega-3s.

HOW TO READ USDA ORGANIC LABELS

The U.S. Department of Agriculture (USDA) approved four categories of organic labels, based on the percentage of organic content. The organic labels began to appear on store shelves on October 21, 2002:

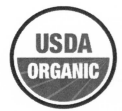 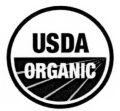

If you see either of these labels, you can be sure the product is at least 95% organic.

100 Percent Organic – Must contain 100 percent organically produced ingredients, not counting added water and salt. May carry USDA Organic Seal

Organic – At least 95% of content is organic by weight (excluding water and salt) and cannot contain added sulfites. May carry the USDA Organic Seal.

Made With Organic Ingredients - At least 70% of content is organic and the front product panel may display the phrase "Made with Organic" followed by up to three specific ingredients. Cannot contain added sulfites, with the exception of wine, which may contain a certain level of added sulfur dioxide. (May *not* display new USDA Organic seal)

Less than 70 % of content is organic and may list only those ingredients that are organic on the ingredient panel with no mention of organic on the main panel. (May *not* display new USDA Organic seal)

CHAPTER 9

Food Additives – What's Safe and What's Not

Living processed-free has become a way of life for me. Learning about what food companies add to food has astounded me. What's even more astounding is the sheer number of food additives that exist. There are more than 3,000 different chemicals that are purposefully added to our food supply. The testing for the safety of these chemicals is usually funded or performed by the company that wants to produce the chemicals or to use the chemical additives in the foods they produce. This is why the studies on chemical additives are often biased and unchallenged.

Back in 1958, Food Additive laws prohibited any additives (including pesticides) that were proven to cause cancer in humans or animals from being added to our food. However, just like with the Food Guide Pyramid, economic pressure from industries caused our friend, the Food and Drug Administration (FDA), to relax these standards and allow some cancer causing and otherwise harmful substances to be used in foods. For instance, the laws were amended in 1996 so that they no longer apply to pesticides.

GENERALLY REGARDED AS SAFE (GRAS)

The FDA has come up with a classification list of foods and food additives that it has deemed safe for human consumption. This list is called the Generally Regarded as Safe (GRAS) list. However, if an additive makes it onto this elite list, it is not a guarantee that the additive is safe. The FDA evaluates additives only based on whether or not they cause cancer and harmful reproductive effects. The FDA *does not* evaluate, and in fact ignores, other harmful reactions or outcomes from ingesting a food additive, such as migraines, weight gain, or neurological disorders. Many additives have not undergone any testing, but they are regarded as safe by the scientific community. These substances are put on the GRAS list, which contains approximately 700 items. You may be surprised to learn that coconut is on this highly exclusive list; soy is not. Some other items on this list are: guar gum, sugar, salt, and vinegar. The list is evaluated on an ongoing basis.[1]

A number additives that were once on the GRAS list have been removed *after they were found to be harmful*. Due to the fact that most additives are toxic, it is with virtual certainty that some additives that are now being commonly used in foods and are considered to be safe, will be taken off the GRAS list at some point in the future. Furthermore, additives that are individually safe may be harmful in combination with other additives. Testing for additive safety is performed for individual additives only, not for combinations of additives. It is rare that any food has only one additive in it.[2]

The effects on human health of the many different additives used in the thousands of different combinations is unknown. However, more research is showing the harmful effects of eating multiple additives in foods. Numerous studies over the past 50 years have tracked the increased consumption of additives in the western diet and the corresponding negative effect on health.

One study indicated, "The average American consumes about 5 pounds of additives per year. If you include sugar—the food-processing industry's most used additive—the number jumps to 135 pounds a year."[3]

In another report, "The Adverse Effects of Food Additives on Health", it is estimated that the amount of additives ingested annually per person is even higher with proven negative effects on physical and mental health. It is reported:

> The use of food additives has increased enormously in the last few decades. As the result, it has been estimated that today about 75 percent of the Western diet is made up of various processed foods, each person consuming an average 8-to10 pounds of food additives per year, with some possibly eating even more. The following 16 adverse effects have been attributed to the consumption of food additives: eczema, urticaria, angioedema, exfoliative dermatitis, irritable bowel syndrome, nausea, vomiting, diarrhea, rhinitis, bronchospasm, migraine, anaphylaxis, hyperactivity and other behavioral disorders. With the great increase in the use of food additives, there also has emerged considerable scientific data linking food additive intolerance with various physical and mental disorders, particularly with childhood hyperactivity.[4]

BEWARE MSG

One of the most common and harmful food additives is monosodium glutamate or MSG. MSG has been called the nicotine of food additives because, in addition to its harmful effects on the body, it is highly addictive. Comprised of sodium and glutamic acid, MSG is a flavor enhancer that triggers our taste buds and makes us eat more and eat faster. Nearly every fast food and chain restaurant uses MSG in some form, and it is added to thousands of prepared and processed foods. The foods that contain the most MSG are processed fat-free foods and sugar-free foods, mainly because when fat and sugar are absent, the food is nearly flavorless, so MSG is added to enhance their flavor.

When I was a teenager, there was a commercial on TV with a guy munching down a whole bag of Doritos Nacho Cheese Tortilla Chips, claiming that they were so good, he couldn't stop. I had the same problem when I ate Doritos, I just couldn't stop. In fact, I had the same reaction to many other processed foods, especially the sweet and salty ones. Later, after I stopped eating those types of foods, I read the ingredient labels, and sure enough, MSG was prominently listed.

Use of MSG has doubled every decade since it was first introduced to the United States in the 1940s, and in 2001, three billion pounds were manufactured. It is used in hospitals, nursing homes, school cafeterias, and everywhere else food is served. MSG is found in everything from ketchup, soups, and mashed potatoes to chips and ice cream. Most sauces, dressings, canned soups, and seasoning products like bullion and broth contain MSG or free glutamic acid, a similar product. It is the main ingredient in additives called "seasonings."[5]

MSG is a horrible thing. It works on our brains and fools our taste buds into thinking we are eating something that tastes better than it actually does. The Doritos are not really that good, but the MSG alters our perception. It stimulates the taste buds on our tongues, so our brains think the food tastes better. This allows food manufacturers to use cheaper quality ingredients yet allow the crappy food to seem to taste good.

HIDDEN MSG

The real scary thing about MSG is that it can be hidden in other food additives and won't show up on food ingredient lists. If an additive contains less than 79 percent MSG, the FDA does not require food manufacturers to list MSG as an ingredient. So, an additive could contain 78 percent MSG, and we would never know there was MSG in the food. But smart scientists and other food detectives have caught on to this, and have figured out which additives contain high percentages of MSG. The following all contain plenty of MSG:

- Hydrolyzed yeast
- Hydrolyzed protein
- Textured protein
- Sodium caseinate
- Yeast extract
- Maldtodextrin
- Textured soy protein
- Autolyzed yeast
- Natural flavorings

Other food ingredients that contain MSG but are not required to say so include stocks, broths, and seasonings. Also, any food that contains aspartame, Nutrasweet or Equal may cause the same effect as MSG because aspartame is converted to glutamic acid by the body.

MSG CAUSES HEADACHES AND OBESITY

The effects of MSG were first documented in 1968 when a Chinese doctor developed numbness, tingling and tightness in his chest after eating in certain Chinese restaurants. This is why so many Chinese and other restaurants now boast that they don't use MSG. But don't be fooled by those claims. While the restaurant may not add any MSG to their food, if they are using prepared items (as most restaurants do) like sauces, egg rolls, dressings, and broths, then their food will still contain plenty of MSG.

Another common MSG-related symptom is a headache that feels like a tight band around the head. But the most alarming effect of MSG is its link to obesity. MSG is used in laboratory studies to induce obesity in animals. Scientists observe that animals fed MSG become grotesquely obese very quickly. They do this to get the animals fat quickly in order to study pre-diabetes and obesity.[3]

MSG is an excitotoxin, meaning it affects the mechanism in the brain that controls our appetite. When we eat foods containing MSG, we eat more than we need to. If the lab rats are getting grotesquely obese, doesn't it make sense that humans are too?

SODAS KILL OUR DNA

Another nasty additive is sodium benzoate. Derived from benzoic acid, it is used as a preservative by the carbonated drinks industry to prevent mold in soft drinks. To understand the effects of sodium benzoate on human cells, Peter Piper, a professor of molecular biology and biotechnology at Sheffield University who is considered an expert in aging, conducted research to examine the effect of sodium benzoate on the mitochondria DNA in cells. After testing the effect of sodium benzoate on living yeast cells in his laboratory, Professor Piper reported,

> These chemicals have the ability to cause severe damage to DNA in the mitochondria to the point that they totally inactivate it: they knock it out altogether. The mitochondria consumes the oxygen needed to produce energy and if it is damaged—as happens in a number in diseased states—then the cell starts to malfunction very seriously. There are now a whole array of diseases that are being tied to this type of damaged DNA—Parkinson's and a host of neurodegenerative diseases, but above all the whole process of aging.[6]

NITRATES AND NITRITES

Nitrates and nitrites are used as coloring agents and preservatives, mainly in processed meats such as hot dogs, bacon, bologna, salami, and other packaged or canned meats like Spam and corned beef hash. The FDA requires pre-packaged, processed meats to contain nitrites to preserve them.

Unfortunately, nitrites have been shown to cause cancer and other health problems in laboratory animals. More recently they have been linked to lung disease. As with all additives, toxicity depends on how much of them one eats and for how long. The best way to avoid nitrites and nitrates is to stay away from pre-packaged processed meats. Look for nitrate-free and nitrite-free versions, however you are much better off not eating these types of foods.

OTHER COMMON FOOD ADDITIVES

In order to avoid some of the negative consequences of food additives, you should become familiar with the names of some of the most common food additives and their documented health effects on humans. In her booklet *Food Additives, A Shopper's Guide to What's Safe & What's Not*, author Christine Hoza Farlow lists 800 of the most common food additives with brief descriptions of their documented health effects. The following is a short list of some of the ingredients you need to look out for.

- **Acacia gum**– may cause skin rashes.
- **Acesulfame K (also called Acesulfame Potassium)**– a high potency artificial sweetener that is that is definitely NOT safe. Even compared to aspartame and saccharin (which are afflicted with their own safety problems), Acesulfame K is the worst. The additive is inadequately tested—the FDA based its approval on tests of Acesulfame K that fell short of the FDA's own standards. But even those tests indicate that the additive causes cancer in animals, which means it may increase cancer risk in humans. In 1987, the Center for Science in the Public Interest (CSPI) urged the FDA not to approve Acesulfame K, but was ignored. After the FDA gave the chemical its blessing, CSPI urged that it be banned. The FDA hasn't yet ruled on that request.
- **Aluminum**– may be associated with senility, memory problems, kidney problems, neurological problems, mouth ulcers, mineral malabsorption. Other names: Aluminum ammonium sulfate, aluminum calcium silicate, aluminum chloride, aluminum potassium sulfate, aluminum sulfate.
- **Benzoic Acid, Benzoate of Soda, Calcium Benzoate**– the benzoate can convert into benzene, a toxic and carcinogenic compound. May cause skin rashes, stomach upset, neurological disorders; has caused birth defects in animals.
- **BHA (butylated hydroxyanisole)**– can cause liver and kidney damage, behavioral problems, infertility, weakened immune system, birth defects, cancer; should be avoided by infants and young children.
- **BHT (butylated hydroxytoluene)**– same problems as BHA. Has been banned in England.
- **FD&C Red, Green, Blue, Yellow**– may contain aluminum, may be contaminated with carcinogens, causes thryoid tumors.
- **Potassium Bromate, Bromated Flour**– used to enhance enriched flours to make bread more fluffy; causes cancer in lab animals. Banned worldwide except Japan and U.S.
- **Benzaldehyde, Butyl Acetate**– may cause central nervous system depression, decreased sex drive, immune system stress.
- **Calcium Casseinate**– may contain free glutamic acid or MSG, harmful to anyone with milk allergies.
- **Calcium Disodium EDTA**– may cause skin irritation, stomach upset, liver

and kidney damage.

- **Calcium Chloride**– may cause heart problems, stomach upset. Calcium chloride tastes extremely salty and is used an ingredient in some foods, especially pickles to give a salty taste while not increasing the food's sodium content.
- **Canola Oil**– toxic; genetically engineered from rapeseed oil; processed at extremely high temperatures; depletes body stores of vitamin E; contains trans-fats; caused kidney, heart, thryroid and adrenal problems in lab animals; depresses the immune system; blocks enzyme function; no studies done on humans for safety.
- **Carrageenan**– comes from seaweed, undegraded has not caused cancer in animals. Degraded carrageenan has caused cancer in rats. Product labels do not distinguish between degraded and undegraded carrageenan. Those with intestinal problems such as Chron's, IBS and colitis should avoid.
- **Corn Syrup, High Fructose Corn Syrup**– highly refined processed sweetener associated with blood sugar problems, fatty liver and obesity. Causes mineral and B-vitamin deficiencies.
- **Ethyl Acetate**– nervous system depressant; prolonged inhalation can cause kidney, liver damage.
- **Invert sugar**– a 50-50 mixture of two sugars, dextrose and fructose, is sweeter and more soluble than sucrose (table sugar). Invert sugar forms when sucrose is split in two by an enzyme or acid. It provides "empty calories," contributes to tooth decay, and should be avoided.
- **Monosodium Glutamate (MSG), Free Glutamates**– may cause brain damage, esp. in children; always found in the following: autolyzed yeast, calcium caseinate, glutamate, glutamic acid, hydrolyzed corn gluten, hydrolyzed protein, hydrolyzed soy protein, monopotassium glutamate, monosodium glutamate, pea protein, plant protein extract, sodium caseinate, textured protein, yeast extract, yeast food and yeast nutrient. May be in the following: barley malt, boullion broth, carrageenan, citric acid, enzymes, anything enzyme modified, anything fermented, flavors and flavorings, malt extract, malt flavoring, maltodextrin, natural flavors and flavorings, natural chicken flavoring, natural beef flavoring, soy protein, soy protein concentrate, and foods that proclaim NO MSG, NO Added MSG or NO MSG Added. Monosodium glutamate is used to induce obesity in laboratory animals. Quite possibly induces obesity in humans.
- **Guar Gum**– may cause nausea, stomach upset or bloating. Guar gum, a natural gum, is an edible thickening agent extracted from the guar bean. The largest market for guar gum is in the food industry, where guar gum is used as a thickener and binder of free water in sauces, salad dressings, ice creams, instant noodles, pet foods, processed meats, bread improvers and beverages to name some. Guar gum has very similar properties to locust bean gum, which is extracted from the seeds of the carob tree.
- **Hydrogenated and Partially hydrogenated oils**– extremely unhealthy and chemically manufactured type of oil. Causes cancer, heart disease, high

cholesterol, diabetes, and weight gain.

- **Locust Bean Gum, Xanthan Gum**– may cause stomach upset, extracted by solvent extraction which may leave a toxic residue; may contain allowable amounts of lead, arsenic, and heavy metals.
- **Modified Food Starch**– processed with chemicals of questionable safety. Modified starches are used in processed foods to improve their consistency and keep the solids suspended. Starch and modified starches sometimes replace large percentages of more nutritious ingredients, such as fruit.
- **Mono & Diglycerides**– hydrogenated oils in disguise. Makes bread softer and prevents staling, improves the stability of margarine, makes caramels less sticky, and prevents the oil in peanut butter from separating out.
- **Nitrates and Nitrites**– form powerful cancer-causing agents in the stomach, considered dangerous by the FDA but not banned because they prevent botulism. Found most often in cured and smoked meats such as hot dogs, bologna, salami, smoked turkey, ham, bacon and sausage.
- **Nutrasweet, Aspartame**– may cause central nervous system disturbances, brain lesions and menstrual difficulties. Headaches are a common symptom. Metabolic breakdown products are formaldehyde and methanol--two known carcinogens. In combination with MSG causes multiple sclerosis symptoms.
- **Natural Flavors**– may be chemically extracted and processed and in combination with other food additives not required to be listed on ingredient labels. May contain MSG.
- **Phosphates, Phosphoric Acid**– can inhibit mineral absorption, especially calcium. Excess consumption can cause kidney damage, osteoporosis. Phosphoric acid is a main ingredient of carbonated soft drinks.
- **Potassium bicarbonate** (also known as potassium hydrogen carbonate or potassium acid carbonate)–is a colorless, odorless, slightly basic, salty substance. The compound is used as a source of carbon dioxide for leavening in baking, extinguishing fire in powder fire extinguishers, acting as a reagent, and a strong buffer in medications. The US FDA recognizes potassium bicarbonate as "generally recognized as safe". It is used as a base in foods to regulate pH.
- **Saccharin, Sweet 'n Low**– delisted as a carcinogen in 1997, however studies still show that saccharin causes cancer.
- **Silica, Silicon Dioxide, Silicates**– may be associated with kidney problems. Many forms of life contain silica structures including microorganisms such as diatoms, plants such as horsetail, and animals such as hexactinellid sponges. It is present in the cell walls of various plants (including edible ones) to strengthen their structural integrity. Silica is also used as a food additive, primarily as a flow agent in powdered foods, or to absorb water.
- **Sodium Benzoate**– can cause skin rashes, gastrointestinal upset, hyperactivity in children, neurological disorders; has caused birth defects in lab animals; moderately toxic if swallowed; those with asthma or liver problems should avoid.
- **Sodium Propionate**– may trigger headaches, behavioral changes, blood

pressure, kidney disturbances, water retention.

- **Soy Isolates**– contains toxins that cannot be completely removed with processing, enzyme inhibitors that block enzymes needed for digestion, phytates that inhibit mineral absorption; promotes clumping of red blood cells, kidney stones; depresses thyroid function; weakens immune system; fermented soy products have less toxins.
- **Soybean Oil**– contaminated with hexane from chemical extraction at high temperatures; may be genetically modified.
- **Sucralose, Splenda**– chlorinated sugar linked to shrinkage of thymus gland, enlarged liver and kidneys, miscarriage, and diarrhea in lab animals. Contrary to manufacturer's claims, sucralose is absorbed and metabolized by the body 11-27% according the to the FDA and 40% according to the Japanese Food Sanitation Council; contains small amounts of dangerous contaminants, such as heavy metals, methanol, arsenic, chlorinated disaccharides and chlorinated monosaccharides; no independent studies or long term studies of the effects on humans; those with chlorine allergies may suffer severe reactions.

A HOT DOG AND POPCORN AT THE MOVIES COULD TAKE YOUR BREATH AWAY

Taking a breather from cured meats and popcorn could save your lungs and your life. A 2007 study conducted by Columbia University Medical Center suggests that eating cured meats such as hot dogs, smoked turkey, ham, bologna, bacon, or salami may double your risk for lung disease. Concurrent news showed that the pervasive lingering aroma of artificially butter-flavored popcorn can literally kill you.

Researchers found that people who ate cured meat products at least 14 times a month were 78 percent more likely to develop chronic obstructive pulmonary disease (COPD) than people who did not eat these meats, even after the researchers sought to account for many other risk factors including smoking, overall diet, and age.[8]

COPD is a medical condition that includes chronic bronchitis and emphysema, which interfere with normal breathing. COPD is also the fourth-leading cause of death in the United States.

In food preparation, **curing** refers to various preservation and flavoring processes, especially of meat or fish, by the addition of a combination of salt, sugar, and either "**nitrate**" or "**nitrite**." Many curing processes also involve smoking. Nitrates not only help kill bacteria, but also produce a characteristic flavor, and give meat a pink or red color.

Nitrate, in the form of either sodium nitrate or potassium nitrate, breaks down in the meat into nitrite. Herein the problem lies: the nitrite further breaks down in the meat into another compound called nitric oxide. Nitric oxide binds to iron in the blood, preventing the iron from being utilized in the body.

Iron is a key component in substances that carry oxygen to the cells and hold it there, such as hemoglobin and myoglobin. This is especially important for the cells in lung tissue. Without adequate hemoglobin and myoglobin, the lungs are deprived of adequate oxygen, which damages lung tissue by cracking elastin and stiffening collagen.

THE FOLLOWING ADDITIVES
HAVE NO KNOWN TOXICITY

- **Annatto–** derivative of the achiote trees of tropical regions of the Americas, used to produce a red food coloring. Annatto is produced from the reddish pulp which surrounds the seed of the achiote. It is used in cheese (Cheddar and Red Leicester), margarine, butter, rice, smoked fish and custard powder. Annatto is commonly found in Latin America and Caribbean cuisines as both a coloring agent and for flavoring. Central and South American Natives used the seeds to make a body paint, and as a lipstick. For this reason, the achiote is sometimes called the *lipstick-tree*. In Venezuela, annatto (called locally 'onoto') is used in the preparation of hallacas, perico, and other traditional dishes.
- **Arrowroot–** natural thickener, derived from the root of a south american plant. It has no known toxicity. It can be used in cooking in place of corn starch (a processed refined carbohydrate).

Another toxic chemical has been linked to a rare and life-threatening form of fixed obstructive lung disease, medically termed as **bronchiolitis obliterans**. This disease is commonly known as "popcorn workers lung," because many workers at microwave-popcorn factories who are exposed to the chemical have developed the disease, which destroys the lungs. A transplant is the only cure.

Since 2001, academic studies have shown links between the disease and a chemical used in artificial butter flavor called **Diacetyl**. Repeatedly inhaling significant doses of heated diacetyl, a vapor that, if inhaled, can cause the small airways in the lungs to become swollen and scarred. Eventually, the scarring of airways can create a condition where it is possible to inhale deeply, but very difficult to exhale without extreme discomfort.[9]

Even less is known about the health effects of eating diacetyl in butter-flavored popcorn, or breathing the fumes after the bag is microwaved. In September 2007 the New York Times ran a story about a 53-year old Colorado man whose fondness for microwave buttered popcorn may have caused him to develop the disease. Initially diagnosed with generalized lung inflammation, the Colorado man's doctor eventually discovered that he ate at least two bags of microwave buttered popcorn per day for more than a decade. He often made it a point to inhale the butter-flavored steam that came out of the bags when he first opened them.[10]

Diacetyl is used to add a buttery flavor to many brands of microwave popcorn. Chronic exposure to heated diacetyl in food production and flavoring plants that utilize synthetic butter has been linked with hundreds of cases of lung damage. Flavoring manufacturers have paid out more than $100 million as a result of lawsuits by people sick with popcorn workers lung over the past five years. One death from the disease has been confirmed.

You may want to think twice the next time you are tempted to indulge in the typical movie fare of a hot dog and popcorn. The evidence continues to mount that processed foods and additives create health hazards. Real whole foods do not.

- **Beta Carotene–** Vitamin A - Beta-carotene is used as an artificial coloring and a nutrient supplement. The body converts it to Vitamin A, which is part of the light-detection mechanism of the eye and which helps maintain the normal condition of mucous membranes. Large amounts of beta-carotene in the form of dietary supplements increased the risk of lung cancer in smokers and did not reduce the risk in non-smokers. Smokers should certainly not take beta-carotene supplements, but the small amounts used as food additives are safe.
- **Coconut Oil, Palm Kernel Oil–** helps the body metabolize fatty acids; substitute for butter; use for frying and baking; use only non-hydrogenated.
- **Oligofructose (also called Fructooligosaccharide or FOS)–** is a soluble fiber found in a variety of common plants, fruits, and vegetables. Although it may be extracted from any of these sources, the most common source used in supplements is derived from chicory root, due to its naturally high FOS concentration. This ingredient is commonly used as an "artificial" sweetener since FOS is sweet to the taste, but the body cannot utilize its calorie content.
- **Inulin–** is a fructooligosaccharide derived from Chicory roots and other natural sources of inulin. As a prebiotic, Inulin stimulates the growth of friendly and healthy intestinal bacteria which supports good colon health. Since it also has a very low glycemic index, it is suitable for many people who are on restricted diets. Its taste is comparable to sugar. Inulin is often blended with the powdered forms of Stevia.
- **Stevia–** natural herbal sweetener, 100-200 times sweeter than sugar but does not affect blood sugar levels. Can be used by those with candida, diabetes, and hypoglycemia.[7]

As you can see, there aren't many additives that are safe, so you are best off buying as few packaged foods as possible!

Just because a packaged food is sold in a natural food market doesn't mean that it will be free of harmful additives. I have read the ingredient lists on plenty of foods in the natural food markets and have put them right back on the shelf. Cereals, crackers, cookies, sauces, salad dressings and other packaged foods can still contain maltodextrin, hydrogenated oils, sugars, and MSG. So the question as to whether Newman's O's are really better for you than Oreos, comes from your ability to interpret the ingredient list.

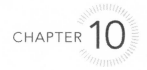

Alkalinity and the Most Important Foods for Good Health

In the summer of 1997, five years after my weight loss, I was suddenly struck ill with some ghastly symptoms I had never experienced before in my life: crampy abdominal pain, nausea, bloody diarrhea, loss of appetite, fever and fatigue. After several trips to the doctor, with no diagnosis and no relief, I finally ended up in the emergency room, severely dehydrated and "out of it." After two days in the hospital and lots of tests later, I was diagnosed with ulcerative colitis – an inflammatory disease of the large intestine, otherwise known as the "gut."

Ulcerative colitis is considered an autoimmune disease (your body begins attacking itself). There are four theories as to the cause, and there is apparently no known cure. One of the theories suggests that the disease is preceded by a virus or infection, another theory is that food sensitivities are responsible.

Needless to say, I was confused. I thought that abstaining from flour and sugar and other processed foods was going to make me immune to illness and disease, and yet here I was, weak and caught off guard by a seemingly incurable disease. My hospital stay lasted eight days, and when I was sent home I was told to eat a low fiber diet (of white flour and white flour products), and to take medications that quickly added pounds to my body. While in the hospital, I was given an IV with a sugar solution in it, and I spent the next two weeks fighting off cravings for sugar (this experience convinced me that sugar really is an addictive substance).

I took the medication until my symptoms subsided, but ignored all the dietary recommendations. Once again, I began to research the natural remedies and traditional foods for healing the colon. My research opened my eyes once again to a new aspect of health—the importance of a balanced body chemistry and a clean and well-functioning digestive system. I have been free of any colitis symptoms for many years.

DIGESTIVE WELLNESS

Good nutrition is not just a question of *what* we eat, but how efficiently the food is digested and utilized by our body. Most people don't think much about digestion unless it isn't working well. I didn't, until I was debilitated by ulcerative colitis. According to Elizabeth Lipsky, we don't really need to think about it, because it works automatically. In her book *Digestive Wellness*, Lipsky writes "The function of digestion is to break down foods into basic components for the cells to use for energy, as building materials, and catalysts. The uninterrupted flow of these nutrients into our system is critical to our long-term health. When we eat poorly or our digestion becomes blocked and sluggish, we compromise the ability of all our cells to work efficiently and healthfully. While it may seem obvious to some that what we eat affects the health of our digestive systems and our bodies, it is a revolutionary concept to many."

Of all the things I learned from the Edgar Cayce teachings, the one thing that stood out the most had to do with proper food combinations to ensure that food gets digested properly, nutrients get absorbed, and waste gets eliminated. Many contemporaries have espoused some of these food-combining rules. I also follow some of the Fat Flush Food Combinations, which can be found in Ann Louise Gittleman's book *The Fat Flush Plan*.

Plan-D incorporates these principles as they have worked for me and many of my clients. Remember, Cayce was recommending these food-combining principles in the early 1900's, long before any of the more contemporary books on healthy digestion became popular.

As a diet counselor, I have witness the improved health of my clients who have adopted these rules. Weight loss comes easier, with little to no bloating, gas, constipation, or diarrhea.

PLAN-D HEALTHY FOOD COMBINATIONS

- DO NOT EAT VEGETABLES AND FRUITS TOGETHER. The complex carbohydrates in vegetables require different enzymes for digestion than the sugars in fruits. If fruits and vegetables are eaten together, there is competition in the stomach for digestive enzymes. Usually the vegetables win, and the fruit goes partially undigested, leading to fermentation in the small intestine.
- DO NOT EAT MEAT WITH FRUIT. Sugars and animal proteins don't combine well.
- DO NOT DRINK LIQUIDS WITH MEALS. Water is good for many things, but not with meals. Liquids dilute digestive enzymes and have a numbing effect on the cells that secrete stomach acid.
- DO NOT ADD MILK OR CREAM TO COFFEE OR TEA. This was a very interesting gem given by Edgar Cayce. He said that when coffee or tea are mixed with milk or cream outside of the body (as in your coffee mug) it creates an indigestible curd—like leather in your system!
- EAT ONLY ONE PROTEIN AT A MEAL. This means no steak and lobster dinners, or chicken and fish combinations. When more than one type of protein is eaten together, digestion is impaired and toxicity results.

- EGGS ARE THE EXCEPTION TO THE PROTEIN RULE. Eggs are considered neutral and can be added to the above mentioned proteins. They go particularly well with dairy products (like frittatas) and add to the protein value of bean dishes. Eggs can be combined with sprouted-grain products.
- ANIMAL PROTEINS SUCH AS DAIRY, MEATS, FISH AND POULTRY DO NOT COMBINE WELL WITH GLUTEN-GRAINS (E.G. WHEAT, RYE, OATS, AND BARLEY). This means no bread with meat, no pasta with meat. However, animal proteins do combine well with baked potatoes, sweet potatoes, corn, or peas as long as you also include leafy greens in the meal.
- IN GENERAL, VEGETABLES COMBINE WELL WITH PROTEINS AND SHOULD ALWAYS BE EATEN TOGETHER.
- STARCHES COMBINE WELL WITH VEGETABLES AND SHOULD ALWAYS BE EATEN TOGETHER.
- YOGURT CAN BE COMBINED WITH FRUIT OR WHEY. Edgar Cayce recommended this helpful combination.
- NO CITRUS FRUITS WITH CEREALS OR MILK. Like the cream in coffee, the combination becomes acid and does not digest.

YOUR BODY'S PH: ACID-ALKALINE BALANCE

The first time I ever heard the term pH was on a TV commercial for Herbal Essence shampoo. Farrah Fawcett was tossing around her beautiful long hair, and they said the shampoo was pH balanced for beautiful hair. So I thought pH had something to do with hair. My first year college chemistry course cleared up that confusion.

In order for our bodies to be healthy and remain free of disease, we must maintain proper body chemistry. The body chemistry is determined mostly by what we eat and drink but is also determined by what we think and what we feel. All fluids, including body fluids, have a measurable degree of acidity or alkalinity. The scale used to measure these acid or alkaline levels is called the pH scale, which runs from 0 to 14. Values below 7 represent increasing acidity. Values above 7 represent increasing alkalinity. A value of 7, which is in the middle of the scale, is considered neutral (it is neither acidic of alkaline).

For optimal health, the human body should be kept in a slightly alkaline state. The blood should be at or near a pH of 7.4. The body works hard to maintain this pH, despite what we eat. Maintaining this alkalinity is so essential to our survival that the body mobilizes its special buffering system to neutralize excess acidity whenever the scale tips. A vital link in this complex buffering system is the body's *alkaline reserve*. The body draws on alkaline mineral elements to help restore alkalinity in the system. However, the minerals in the alkaline reserve must be replenished regularly through food.

All foods, after they are metabolized, leave either acid- or alkaline-forming mineral elements in the body. The alkaline forming foods are those which supply calcium, sodium, magnesium, potassium, iron, and manganese. The acid forming foods are those which supply copper, bromine, fluorine, chlorine, iodine, phosphorus, sulfur, and silicon.

Most fruits and vegetables are alkaline-forming, whereas meats, grains, and most fats and dairy products are acid-forming.

Most people who suffer from unbalanced pH are acidic. This condition that is known as acidosis, forces the body to borrow minerals—including calcium, sodium, potassium and magnesium—from vital organs and bones to buffer (neutralize) the acid and to safely remove it from the body. Because of this strain, the body can suffer severe and prolonged damage due to high acidity—a condition that may go undetected for years.

Mild acidosis can cause such problems as:

- Cardiovascular damage, including the constriction of blood vessels and the reduction of oxygen.
- Weight gain, obesity and diabetes.
- Bladder and kidney conditions, including kidney stones.
- Immune deficiency.
- Acceleration of free radical damage, possibly contributing to cancerous mutations.
- Hormone concerns.
- Premature aging.
- Osteoporosis; weak, brittle bones, hip fractures and bone spurs.
- Joint pain, aching muscles and lactic acid buildup.
- Low energy and chronic fatigue.
- Slow digestion and elimination.
- Yeast/fungal overgrowth.

The reason acidosis is more common in our society is mostly due to the typical American diet, which is far too high in acid-producing animal products like meat, eggs and dairy, and far too low in alkaline-producing foods like fresh vegetables. Additionally, we eat acid-producing processed foods like white flour and sugar and drink acid-producing beverages like coffee and soft drinks.

We use too many drugs, which are acid-forming; and, we use artificial chemical sweeteners like saccharin (Sweet 'n Low), aspartame (NutraSweet and Equal), or sucralose (Splenda) which are extremely acid-forming. One of the best things we can do to correct an overly acid body is to clean up the diet and lifestyle.

PH AND BONE LOSS:

A study conducted at the University of California, San Francisco, on 9,000 women showed that those who have chronic acidosis are at greater risk for bone loss than those who have normal pH levels. The scientists who carried out this experiment believe that many of the hip fractures prevalent among middle-aged women are connected to high acidity caused by a diet rich in animal foods and low in vegetables. This is because the body borrows calcium from the bones in order to balance pH.
— *American Journal of Clinical Nutrition*

Your body is able to assimilate minerals and nutrients properly only when its pH is balanced. It is therefore possible for you to be taking healthy nutrients and yet be unable to absorb or use them. If you are not getting the results you expected from your nutritional or herbal program, look for an acid alkaline imbalance. Even the right herbal program may not work if your body's pH is out of balance.

MAINTAINING PROPER PH BALANCE

The body should be kept in an alkaline state, that is the body fluids should be kept alkaline for optimal metabolic function. For this reason, your diet should consist mainly of alkaline forming foods—fruits and vegetables. The goal for your daily food intake is to eat 80% alkaline forming foods and 20% acid forming foods. Don't worry about trying to figure it out; Plan-D is designed to help you achieve this.

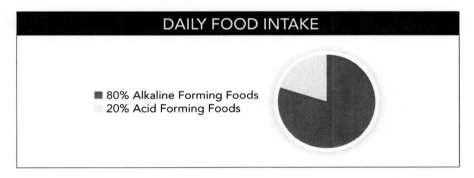

DAILY FOOD INTAKE

■ 80% Alkaline Forming Foods
  20% Acid Forming Foods

The chart on 128 outlines which foods are the most acid forming and which foods are the most alkaline forming.

Note that a food's acid or alkaline-forming tendency in the body has nothing to do with the actual pH of the food itself. For example, lemons are very acidic, however the end-products they produce after digestion and assimilation are very alkaline so lemons are alkaline-forming in the body. Likewise, meat will test alkaline before digestion but it leaves very acidic residue in the body so, like nearly all animal products, meat is very acid-forming.

Most Alkaline	Alkaline	Lowest Alkaline	FOOD CATEGORY	Lowest Acid	Acid	Most Acid
Stevia	Maple Syrup, Rice Syrup	Raw Honey, Raw Sugar (Rapadura)	SWEETENERS	Processed Honey, Molasses	White Sugar, Brown Sugar	NutraSweet, Equal, Aspartame, Sweet 'N Low
Lemons, Watermelon, Limes, Grapefruit, Mangoes, Papayas	Dates, Figs, Melons, Grapes, Papaya, Kiwi, Blueberries, Apples, Pears, Raisins	Oranges, Bananas, Cherries, Pineapple, Peaches, Avocados	FRUITS	Plums, Processed Fruit Juices	Sour Cherries, Rhubarb	Blackberries, Cranberries, Prunes
Asparagus, Onions, Vegetable Juices, Parsley, Raw Spinach, Broccoli, Garlic	Okra, Squash, Green Beans, Beets, Celery, Lettuce, Zucchini, Sweet Potato, Carob	Carrots, Tomatoes, Fresh Corn, Mushrooms, Cabbage, Peas, Potato Skins, Olives, Soybeans, Tofu	BEANS VEGETABLES LEGUMES	Cooked Spinach, Kidney Beans, String Beans	Potatoes (without skins), Pinto Beans, Navy Beans, Lima Beans	Processed Chocolate
	Almonds, Coconuts	Chestnuts	NUTS SEEDS	Pumpkin Seeds, Sunflower Seeds	Pecans, Cashews	Peanuts, Walnuts
Olive Oil, Apple Cider Vinegar	Flax Seed Oil, Coconut Oil	Fish Oil	OILS & VINEGARS	Corn Oil	Canola Oil, Soybean Oil	Hydrogenated Oils
		Amaranth, Millet, Wild Rice, Quinoa	GRAINS CEREALS	Sprouted Wheat Bread, Spelt, Brown Rice	White Rice, Corn, Buckwheat, Oats, Rye	Wheat, White Flour, Pastries, Pasta
	Raw Chocolate (Cacao)		MEATS	Venison, Cold Water Fish	Turkey, Chicken, Lamb	Beef, Pork, Shellfish
	Breast Milk, Coconut Milk, Almond Milk	Soy Milk, Goat Milk, Goat Cheese, Whey	EGGS DAIRY	Eggs, Butter, Yogurt, Buttermilk, Cottage Cheese	Raw Milk, Rice Milk	Cheese, Homogenized Milk, Ice Cream
Herb Teas, Lemon Water	Green Tea	Ginger Tea	BEVERAGES	Black Tea	Coffee	Beer, Soft Drinks

One of the most alkaline-forming foods that helps maintain a proper pH level in the body, and helps keep the body's metabolism revved up is apple cider vinegar. Plan-D includes the use of **raw unfiltered apple cider vinegar** to make the ***Vitality Vinegar Tonic*** as a key component of the plan. Apple cider vinegar contains all of the alkaline-forming minerals, especially potassium. Specific advantages of apple cider vinegar are detailed in the next chapter.

Although maintaining an alkaline balance is extremely important, you shouldn't go overboard in your efforts to alkalize. Plan-D has been designed to help you achieve the proper alkalinity, but of course it will ultimately be up to you to make the right food choices. Edgar Cayce said that excessive alkalinity is worse than excessive acidity. The body requires a certain amount of high-quality protein and fat every day for cellular maintenance and metabolic function, so acid- forming foods can't be eliminated altogether.

VEGETABLES - THE MOST IMPORTANT ALKALINE FOODS YOU SHOULD BE EATING EVERY DAY

Vegetables are the most alkaline forming foods you can eat, therefore they should play a starring role in your daily meals. The amount of vegetables you eat each day is directly proportional to the level of health you will experience and the amount of weight you will lose.

For optimal health and weight loss, you should consume four or more 1-cup servings of vegetables each day. At least two of those servings should come from dark green leafy types such as spinach, broccoli, cabbage, Brussels sprouts, chard, kale, bok-choy, collards, romaine and other dark green lettuces.

Also, include a "rainbow" of other brightly colored vegetables including red, orange, yellow, green, and purple. It is those biologically active substances in plants, the *phytochemicals* that give them their color, flavor, and natural disease resistance abilities.

Vegetables provide the broadest range of nutrients of any food classification and give us the highest amount of life force energy. They are brimming with vitamins, minerals, complex carbohydrates, protein and small amounts of essential fatty acids.

Vegetables are the single most important food to include in your diet if you want to lose weight. Studies published in *Nutrition Review* and the World Health Organization report *Diet, Nutrition and the Prevention of Chronic Disease*, conclude that the more plant foods you eat, the more weight you lose. According to these studies, "energy density" is the key concept to understanding the efficacy of plant foods in regard to weight loss.

Most plant foods are high in water and fiber, but comparatively low in energy, or calories. Thus they create a feeling of fullness without delivering the hefty load of calories delivered by foods higher in fat.

A typical lunch or dinner meal should include at least 1 ½ to 2 full cups of vegetables. Make sure that you include a variety of them with each meal – for instance, have at least 3 different vegetables to make sure that you are getting a variety of colors and nutrients. For instance, steam some broccoli, carrots, and snow peas and then take a portion of the medley to make up 1 ½ to 2 cups to include with your meal.

The best way to consume vegetables is in their fresh raw form; therefore *at least half of your vegetables should be eaten raw, as in a salad or slaw.* Salad can be any combination of raw vegetables; it does not have to include lettuce.

In Plan-D, the vegetable family has been divided into two categories—**non-starchy vegetables** and **starchy vegetables**. The non-starchy vegetables are further divided into two sub-categories—***dark green leafy vegetables*** and ***rainbow (colorful) vegetables***.

Each day, you may eat an unlimited amount of non-starchy vegetables, however you must eat a minimum of 4 cups in order to balance your alkalinity. At least two of those 4 cups should be dark green leafy vegetables. Dark green leafy vegetables have the most chlorophyll (the highest type of life-force energy).

They include spinach, kale, romaine lettuce, leaf lettuce, spring mix, mustard greens, collard greens, bok-choy and Swiss chard. They are good sources of many vitamins and minerals your body needs to stay healthy, like vitamin A, vitamin C, and calcium. In fact, you can get your daily requirement of calcium from eating plenty of dark green leafy vegetables as you can dairy products. Unlike dairy products however, green leafy vegetables are also great sources of fiber. The darker the leaves, the more nutrients the vegetable usually has. Iceburg lettuce does not count as a dark green leafy vegetable. You should *avoid iceburg lettuce as much as possible, as it has very little nutritional value* or life-force energy.

Here's some quick and easy ways to eat dark green leafy veggies:

- **Make a salad:** Leafy greens like spinach, romaine and arugula taste great when mixed in a salad with different kinds of veggies, such as tomatoes, cucumbers, carrots, celery, and radishes.
- **Wrap it up:** Make a wrap with tuna, chicken, or turkey and add spinach, spring mix, arugula, and other veggies for some extra flavor.
- **Add to soup:** Try mixing some leafy greens with your favorite soup.
- **Roll them into a meatloaf:** Add chopped spinach or other greens into the center of a meatloaf and then bake. This is called "Meatloaf Florentine". See the recipe on page 254.
- **Sauté or Stir-fry.** Lightly sauté leafy greens in coconut oil or add chopped leafy greens to your stir-fry. Chicken or tofu stir-fried with coconut oil and your favorite leafy greens is delicious!
- **Steam:** For something new, steam some collard greens, kale, or spinach. Add water to a pot and place a steamer basket with the vegetables into it. Next, bring the water to a simmer, cover with a lid, and wait a few minutes until your vegetables are slightly soft. The best way to retain nutrients in your steamed vegetables is to cook them in a special type of vegetable parchment paper called ***Patapar Paper.*** This was a unique method recommended by Edgar Cayce. This special paper is not the parchment paper found in grocery stores. The only place I know to purchase it is from an on-line source (see below.)

THE BEST WAY TO RETAIN NUTRIENTS IN YOUR VEGETABLES

Cooking with Patapar Paper can help you to find a new source of natural vitamins – right in your kitchen. Edgar Cayce found food sources of nutrients far superior to supplementation. He advised cooking with vegetable parchment as a way of preserving these food values.

Because of the oxidation which occurs when foods come in contact with the air, conventional cooking destroys some 50% of a vegetable's vitamin content and most of the vitamin C, which is essential to vitamin balance. Food salts (minerals in organic structure), which are building blocks for vitamins in the body are also adversely affected.

Not only does cooking foods in parchment prevent oxidation by excluding air from the cooking process, but is also preserves their natural flavors, making you a gourmet cook. The constant temperature of boiling water and the vacuum-like conditions within the bundle yield a consistent and uniform product every time. Starch and cellulose are "predigested," allowing nutrients to be released. Vegetables are cooked in their own juices, as Cayce advised, to keep these valuable nutrients from escaping.

One package of Patapar Paper is probably the best deal in town and won't break your budget. For only $5.00 to $6.00 you get a package of six durable 24-inch x 24-inch sheets. You can cut them to make smaller sheets. Sheets are tied with a string or twist tie and then placed in a pot of boiling water or in a steamer basket.

Vegetable parchment is safe, economical, versatile and easy to use. It has no taste or odor and is nontoxic. It is airtight, watertight (when precautions are taken to avoid punctures), and when wet, pliable. **With proper care, one sheet can be reused over 50 times!** You can't beat that for $5.00!

Cooking with Patapar Paper reduces kitchen work to a minimum, as there is no grease and no scrubbing afterwards. The tied bundle immersed in water makes a perfect double boiler, and many lightweight bundles can be placed within a single pot. With sufficient water in the pot at a slow boil, no attention is required while the food is cooking, since the liquid within the bundle cannot boil away.

PATAPAR PAPER COOKING INSTRUCTIONS

1) Fill cooking pot 1/3 full of water, place on stove and set burner for fast boil. Or use a steamer basket over boiling water.
2) Wet Patapar Paper, shake off excess water, and drape the paper over a bowl.
3) Pour in cut vegetables (without water) or grains (with measured water). Make more than one bundle if necessary to prevent overloading.
4) Lift up corners to center the contents and tie tightly with a string or a twist tie, tying low enough to prevent leakage.
5) Place bundles(s) in steamer basket, return to boil and set burner for slow boil. Set timer, allowing for differences between faster and slower cooking items.
6) When time has elapsed; turn off burner, remove cover, and allow bundles to cook a minute. Then place vegetables packages in a colander which has been placed inside a bowl, place grain packages directly in a bowl. Untie the bundle,

lift slowly by one corner and gently shake out the contents.

7) To avoid punctures, rinse sheet(s) immediately after emptying (gentle rub or brush lightly as needed), and hang to dry. Store when dry.

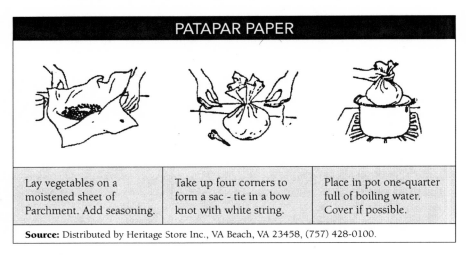

Lay vegetables on a moistened sheet of Parchment. Add seasoning.	Take up four corners to form a sac - tie in a bow knot with white string.	Place in pot one-quarter full of boiling water. Cover if possible.

Source: Distributed by Heritage Store Inc., VA Beach, VA 23458, (757) 428-0100.

NOTE: For maximum nutrition it is, of course, important to consume the vegetable juices that collect inside the parchment bundle. The juice can be poured off and drunk as a "vitamin cocktail," mashed in with root vegetables or squash, added to soup, or stew, or used in making homemade baby food. According to Edgar Cayce, it is best if vegetables are cooked separately in their own juices before combining them. Seasonings can be added after cooking.

Patapar Paper can be purchased on-line at: www.baar.com

CALCIUM:
Why We're Deficient and How to Replace What We've Lost

We are all becoming increasingly aware of the need for calcium in our diets as a necessary mineral for our long-term health. While Dr. Phil McGraw boasts a milk mustache in advertisements implying that the calcium from milk helps promote weight loss, we are never told which foods leach calcium from the body or that the absorption of calcium is dependent upon many other dietary and lifestyle factors. In this article I will explain how calcium is absorbed into the body, what conditions lead to leaching of calcium from the body, and how we can get enough calcium essential for proper metabolism, weight loss, and good health.

We need and use more calcium than any other mineral in the body. In fact there are 179 different known uses for calcium in the human body. It controls muscle contraction and relaxation, is responsible for impulse nerve transmission, and for the transfer of information between our brain cells.

Calcium controls osmosis and diffusion through the cell membranes, and also the passing of information within the cell. It controls the rhythm of the heart, the formation of enzymes and hormones, and also the DNA formation in chromosomes. Calcium is used in blood clotting, urine filtration, and in the formation and maintenance of the bones and teeth. In addition, and perhaps most importantly, calcium is the main buffer used to neutralize acids and to maintain the proper pH throughout the body.

The first thing we need to understand about calcium is its bioavailability—that is how much of the calcium that we eat is actually in a form that is absorbable that we can use. In order for calcium from our food or supplements to become bioavailable, it needs to be broken down, or digested, into its ionic form (Ca^{2+}) before it can be used by the body for any of the functions listed above. Calcium is one of the more difficult minerals for the body to digest and absorb because it depends on several other conditions to be in place. First, calcium needs an acid environment in the stomach to fully digest and dissolve (ionize) calcium from food or supplements. Drinking liquids with meals dilutes the enzymes and stomach acids that are crucial for maintaining this environment.

Another unfortunate challenge is that people over the age of 60 produce only ¼ of the stomach acid they did when they were 20. Additionally, 40 percent of postmenopausal women lack sufficient stomach acid for proper ionization of calcium.

Once calcium has dissolved, its absorption into the body is *totally dependent on the presence of vitamin D* in the intestine. Vitamin D, unfortunately, is not present in most of our food, so our body is dependent on the action of sunlight on our skin to synthesize vitamin D. Without intestinal vitamin D being present, most of the ionized calcium will pass through the body unused. Staying indoors and out of the sun, or lathering up with sunscreen when out in the sun, prevents the calcium in our diets from being ionized into a useable form. The reason we are told that Vitamin D is important for strong bones, is its key role in aiding the absorption of calcium, which is the main component of our bones.

The use of alkaline forming antacids like Tums (calcium carbonate) and H-2 blockers like Zantac, Tagamet, Pepcid AC, etc., alter the pH of the stomach by neutralizing stomach acid needed for ionization of calcium. So you can see that conditions in the stomach and adequate exposure of sunlight play a vital role in our ability to absorb calcium.

Calcium absorption also depends on the presence of the amino acid lysine, and many other trace minerals, including magnesium and boron. The necessary ratios of these trace minerals are not present in most calcium supplements and are severely lacking in processed foods.

Inability to absorb enough calcium is only part of our problem. We also need to keep our body chemistry properly balanced. The Standard American Diet (SAD) consisting of high amounts of red meats, refined sugars and grains, sodas, fried foods, and prescription drugs create acidic conditions in the body that contribute to increased bone loss due to leaching of calcium from the bones.

While our stomachs need to maintain a certain level of acidity in order to digest food, the rest of our body (blood) chemistry needs to be the opposite. Scientists have found that healthy people have body fluids that are slightly alkaline, 7.1 to 7.5 pH. Scientists and doctors have also found that over 150 degenerative diseases are linked to acidity, including cancer, diabetes, arthritis, heart disease, gall and kidney stones, and many more. All diseases thrive in an acidic, oxygen poor environment.

Keep in mind that a drop in every point on the pH scale is 10 times more acidic than the previous number. For example, from 7 to 6 is 10 times, and from 7 to 5 is 100 times, etc. From 7 to 2 is 100,000 times more acidic.

Sodas, especially diet sodas, may be the largest contributor to calcium loss. Colas have a pH of approximately 2.5. Almost no soda has a pH higher than 3.0. Diet sodas are the worst as they have the highest acid content. Diet sodas actually cause you to gain weight, not lose weight, because they create acidic body chemistry, altering your metabolism, leading to a slower metabolic rate.

Almost everything we do, including our lifestyles and our diets push us into the acidic range: proteins, carbohydrates, and unhealthy fats are all digested down to acids. Even metabolic functions and exercise create some acids (lactic acid). Body fluids range between 4.5 and 7.5 pH (Your blood must maintain an alkaline range of 7.35 to 7.45 pH). So even our natural functions produce acids, and if we do not get the proper minerals in the proper forms, our bodies will begin to degenerate. When you drink soda, the deterioration will be much faster.

Over the long term the effects of colas and other acid forming foods are devastating to the body. For instance, it would take 32 glasses of alkaline water at a pH of 9 to neutralize the acid from one 12 oz. soda. When you drink a soda, the body will use up reserves of its own stored alkaline buffers, mainly calcium from the bones and DNA, to raise the body's pH to a livable level of alkalinity. Acidic blood levels cause death! There are enough acids in one soda to kill you if you didn't possess a mechanism to neutralize them.

If you have enough calcium and other minerals, your body can stop the process. But when you use up the supply of available minerals to neutralize the acids, at that point you may get a very serious degenerative disease. Every soda that you drink will contribute to this acidity. Minerals are needed in our diets to stop the deterioration process. Unfortunately, most of the food that we eat no longer contains the minerals that we need, due to poor soil content. This may be the reason for all the degenerative diseases that are so prevalent today. Most degenerative diseases we call "Old-Age Diseases" like memory loss, osteoporosis, arthritis, diabetes, hypertension, and many more are actually life style diseases caused by acidosis, the lack of supplements, what acids we ingest, what nutrients we don't ingest, or toxins we don't properly eliminate.

What can we do to replenish our bodies with calcium and maintain proper body pH? The simplest thing we can do is stop eating processed foods, drink plenty of water, and begin to eat more calcium containing foods. This means that we need to eat 6-8 servings of vegetables and 2-3 servings of fruit each day. It is important to eat real foods that contain calcium, because they have the other trace minerals needed for absorption. Vegetable choices should consist of dark green leafy types such as collard greens, kale, cabbage, and broccoli, for their high calcium content. Other food sources for calcium are almonds, asparagus, blackstrap molasses, buttermilk, carob, cheese, figs, filberts, goat's milk, kelp, mustard greens, oats, prunes, sesame seeds, tofu, turnip greens, watercress, whey, and yogurt. Food sources of lysine include cheese, eggs, fish, lima beans, milk, potatoes, organic meats, and protein powders.

For those with diminished stomach acid, add 2 teaspoons of raw unfiltered apple cider vinegar to a glass of water and drink it 30 minutes before meals. The acetic acid in the vinegar acts like stomach acid and improves digestion. Apple cider vinegar can also be sprinkled on vegetables or combined with olive oil to make tangy vinaigrette.

As far as calcium supplements are concerned, we benefit the most from coral calcium in a powdered form that can be added to water and drank. Coral calcium is the only form of calcium that is already 98% ionized before putting it into your stomach, therefore it needs no stomach acid to be ionized and is easily absorbed into your body. Most other calcium supplements provide only 30-50% of the calcium they contain.

As mentioned before, calcium cannot be absorbed and utilized in our bodies without certain trace minerals, including magnesium, boron *and many others*, also being present. The full complement of these trace minerals is not found in most calcium supplementation tablets and are lacking to a great degree in the typical American diet. These trace minerals are important not only to facilitate the absorption of calcium (as in magnesium) but they are also needed by the body as well for the millions of biochemical reactions that are taking place in the body every day. Coral Calcium contains essential trace minerals from the sea that synergistically aid the immediate utilization of ionic calcium by our bodies.

Not all coral calcium is the same. If it is in the capsule or caplet form it may damage the digestive process. The ionic calcium that can be added to water is the best form to use.

You can take control of your own health by staying away from processed foods including sodas and white flour and sugar. If you do, you will prevent and even reverse calcium deficiency. As an added benefit, you will enjoy a permanently healthier and lighter you.

Calcium deficiency, which is also known as hypocalcaemia, is responsible for approximately 150 different degenerative diseases and conditions, as well as other problems that can be harmful or dangerous to the body. Here's just a partial list. Anything look familiar?

Arthritis	Colitis	Hiatal Hernia
Heart Palpitations	Heart Disease	Low Back Pain
Hypertension (High Blood Pressure)	Acid Reflux	Allergies
Loss of Mental Functions	Gout	Arrhythmia
Indigestion	Muscle Cramps	Cancer
Rickets	Eczema	Bone Spurs
Kidney and Gall stones	High Cholesterol	Asthma
Fibromyalgia	Insomnia	
Recessed gums	Headache	And about 125 others

CHAPTER 11

Plan-D
Superfoods

Let Thy Food Be Thy Medicine, and Thy Medicine Be Thy Food.
—Hippocrates

The reason Plan-D can positively affect so many different health conditions is because it is based on eating the healthiest foods available. It aims to properly support alkaline body chemistry, which in essence heals on a cellular level. This chapter details the health benefits of some of Plan-D's key foods. These are the foods that helped me lose weight and gain health, and they are the foods you should be incorporating into your meals on a regular, if not daily basis.

RAW UNFILTERED ORGANIC APPLE CIDER VINEGAR
I cannot overstate the importance of alkalizing your body. The body cannot heal itself in an acidic state, therefore chronic acidity makes it very difficult to sustain health. Adding insult to injury, unfortunately prescription drugs—the drugs that are intended to make us well—all create acidity.

However, you can compensate with the most effective food weapon known to properly alkalize your body—Apple Cider Vinegar. Apple cider vinegar has been highly regarded throughout history. Hippocrates, the venerated Greek healer and father of modern medicine, used apple cider vinegar for its many healing and cleansing properties. Apple cider vinegar is made from pressing fresh apples; therefore, it is not surprising that the vinegar contains as many health benefits as the apple itself. Apples are one of the richest sources of potassium, an important mineral for keeping the arteries of the body soft, flexible, and resilient, and for fighting off bacteria and viruses.

Although acidic on the outside of the body, the minerals in apple cider vinegar (calcium and potassium), when metabolized, leave an alkaline residue in the body. So strong is apple cider vinegar's alkalizing power, it is known for lowering cholesterol, relieving arthritis, dissolving kidney stones, and assisting in weight loss.

The best apple cider vinegar comes from pressed apples matured in wooden barrels. Raw unfiltered apple cider vinegar is the same cloudy, light-brownish color as unfiltered apple juice. When held up to the light, you should see floating particles of a cobweb-like substance that is called the "mother." This amazing Mother of Vinegar is naturally formed from the pectin and apple residues and appears as strand-like chains of connected protein molecules. The more raw and unfiltered the cider vinegar, the more "mother" shows in the bottle.

Raw, unfiltered, organic apple cider vinegar is different from refined and distilled vinegars found in most grocery stores. Those vinegars are the refined sugar and flour equivalents of the vinegar world. They have been filtered to remove the "mother" and pasteurized; therefore the nutrients have been removed or destroyed. Any vinegar that is clear and has no "mother" has no nutritional value.

Among its many health benefits, apple cider vinegar has been proven to help in reducing weight. In the early 1950's, D.C. Jarvis, a Vermont country doctor, published a book describing how he used apple cider vinegar to successfully treat a number of common ailments as well as chronic conditions such as high blood pressure, arthritis, and overweight.

Dr. Jarvis proved that adding apple cider vinegar to the daily diet leads to gradual weight loss. There is good science behind why this is true. Apples are a good source of pectin—a soluble fiber similar to the fiber that is in oat bran. Apple cider vinegar contains the same amount of pectin as apples. In addition to improving insulin sensitivity, soluble fiber can help you feel more full and more satisfied, and reduce the number of calories your body will absorb.

Plan-D incorporates a **Vitality Vinegar Tonic** developed by health Pioneer Dr. Paul C. Bragg, to help cleanse and alkalize our bodies. Dr. Bragg was a strong advocate of the use of apple cider vinegar, especially with honey, as a healing beverage. Bragg's family made their own apple cider vinegar from the apples they grew and used it as a staple in their diet. His father drank a combination of cider vinegar and honey to relieve the fatigue of long hours working on a farm. While recovering from tuberculosis as a teenager, Bragg rediscovered this healthful elixir and credited his renewed vigor and strength to it. Dr. Bragg and his daughter Dr. Patricia Bragg have written several books on the healing powers of apple cider vinegar, as well as on the topics of fasting, raw foods, and other subjects relating to health, diet, and fitness.[1]

The Braggs recommend adding 1 to 2 teaspoons of raw unfiltered organic apple cider vinegar to a glass of pure water and drinking it before meals three times per day. You may sweeten it with a small amount of honey or stevia if necessary. If it is too difficult to drink the *Vitality Vinegar Tonic* before each meal, you can drink one in the morning before breakfast, one before retiring at night, and one at another time during the day when it is convenient. Apple cider vinegar can also be sprinkled on vegetables and used to make tangy vinaigrette salad dressings.

EXTRA VIRGIN COCONUT OIL

Coconut oil has been mistakenly accused of raising cholesterol and causing heart diseases. We now know that it is one of the healthiest oils we can eat, but as I have mentioned before, the "fat lies" die hard. Coconut oil got its bad rap based on a study of a single cow. The study showed that this one cow did not flourish on a coconut oil diet. The results made perfect sense, since no one, not even a cow, could have coconut oil as the only source of fat in the diet. The essential fats were completely absent from this poor cow's diet, and to twist the results even further, the coconut oil that was fed to the cow was hydrogenated, thereby making it a trans-fat (seems to me this study should have been used to prove that trans fats are killers).[2]

Nevertheless, coconut oil was labeled as a cholesterol-raising culprit and was the baby that got thrown out with the bath water when all saturated fats were banished as "artery clogging" fats. More recent studies have shown that coconut is more of a miracle oil than we ever realized. First of all, it does not raise cholesterol, but in fact it lowers it. In the April 2008 issue of *Vegetarian Times Magazine*, Mary Margaret Chappell discusses the advantages of adding coconut oil to the diet. She points out that "Research now shows that the medium-chain fatty acids in coconut oil do not raise cholesterol or fat levels in the bloodstream and may actually help prevent chronic diseases." [3]

Further in the article, Gerard Mullin, M.D., Director of Integrative Nutrition Services at John Hopkins Hospital is referenced as addressing the value of coconut oil and its promise that it promotes a better balance of LDL and HDL cholesterols. He states, "I give coconut oil a thumbs-up. It tastes rich and people are finding it's not such a bad thing after all."[4]

We know that saturated fat is good for us, and coconut oil is one of the best sources of saturated fat because it comes from a plant source. It contains a high amount of lauric acid, the main component found in mother's milk, which is responsible for strengthening the immune system and protecting against viral and bacterial infections. Studies show it has many healing properties, including its effectiveness with treating HIV.

The way it protects against viruses and bacteria is amazing. Many viruses are enveloped by a protective membrane composed of fats. Current research indicates that the medium chain fatty acids in coconut oil destroy viruses and bacteria by dissolving the fatty envelope surrounding them, essentially causing them to disintegrate.[5] Coconut oil has also been shown to prevent cancer, osteoporosis, and diabetes.

The ability of coconut oil to promote weight loss is miraculous. It is considered the only "low fat" fat. All other fats contain 9 calories per gram, whereas coconut oil contains only 6.8 calories per gram. The reason for this is its molecular structure. Because it's a medium-chain fat, coconut oil acts more like a carbohydrate in that it gets burned for energy right away and does not easily store in the body as fat. This in effect increases metabolism and provides a special burst of energy. Because of its ability to speed up metabolism, coconut oil is my oil of choice for weight loss.

You may notice that nearly all of the Plan-D recipes call for coconut oil or coconut milk, which in the traditional method of fat and calorie counting would yield high grams of fat per serving. However, you need to understand that the fat from coconut oil does not make you fat nor does it make you gain weight.

In one study in which coconut oil was used at part of a high fat diet, researchers found not only that coconut oil did not increase body fat, but that the coconut oil-enriched diet actually produced a decrease in white fat stores. In another study, when genetically obese mice were given a diet high in either safflower oil or coconut oil and their number of fat cells was measured, those given coconut oil were found to have produced far fewer fat cells than those given safflower oil.[6]

The Plan-D recipes call for coconut oil for sautéing, stir-frying, and baking because of its remarkable stability and resistance to oxidation. As you now know, when oils are heated and used for frying, they become rancid and introduce harmful free radicals into the body when eaten. Coconut oil is the amazing exception, once again due to its medium-chain structure. It has a very high temperature threshold, which makes it an excellent oil for cooking. It can take heat up to about 350 degrees without breaking down the way other fats do. I use it exclusively for any type of pan-frying because it isn't absorbed into fried food like other vegetable oils, so it doesn't contribute extra calories to fried food. It also browns foods beautifully!

You might think that using coconut oil will make all of your food taste like coconuts. On the contrary, the coconut flavor you are most familiar with is an artificial flavor that is sweetened with refined sugar. Coconut oil tastes somewhat buttery and is extremely satisfying. The best way to incorporate coconut into your diet is to use the oil for cooking or adding to foods. Other ways to enjoy the oil from coconut is to use coconut milk, fresh coconut, or dried coconut.

OMEGA-3 FATS: FISH OIL, FLAXSEED OIL, AND FLAX SEEDS

As discussed in chapter 6, most Americans are deficient in omega-3 fats. For this reason, fish oil, flaxseed oil, and flax seeds are Plan-D superfoods. Taking fish oil supplements and adding flaxseed oil and flax seeds to your meals will ensure that you are getting the proper amount of omega-3 fats every day.

Our bodies need these fats for proper protection of our cell membranes and to help metabolize other fats in our diet. Like the fat contained in coconut oil, omega-3 fats raise metabolism and lower triglycerides levels. They also help the body burn fat more efficiently.

Fish oil contains two very important omega-3 essential fats—EPA (eicosapentaenoic acid) and DHA (docosahexaenoic acid). We need both of these fats, and only fish oil contains BOTH of them in a readily useable form. These two fatty acids have slightly different functions; EPA in combination with DHA is best for heart health, while DHA alone is best for the brain and the eyes.

Flaxseed oil also contains omega-3s, but it does not contain EPA and DHA in a readily useable form. In order to get both EPA and DHA from flaxseed oil, the body must first convert the alpha-linoleic acid (ALA) in flaxseed oil into EPA and DHA, a process that is long and complicated and may not be successful in everyone. The ALA in flax oil uses an enzyme in the body called delta-6 desaturase (D6D). However, D6D is made inoperative by high levels of insulin (from eating sugar or simple starches), alcohol, pollutants, or high levels of omega-6s from vegetable oils, fried foods, trans fats, and emotional stress. D6D also becomes less available as we age. Most importantly, there is a common inherited gene that causes a lifelong

D6D deficiency.[7]

This is why flaxseed oil should not be your only source of omega-3s. Fish oil is really the best source, unless you are a strict vegetarian. It is important to remember that we also need to make sure that we get enough saturated fat in our diet to ensure proper usage of EPA and DHA.

I recommend a combination of both fish oil and flaxseed oil, because high lignan flax oil has other health benefits. The lignans are the plant fibers from the flax seeds which protect against breast cancer, colon cancer, and prostate cancer. According the USDA, flax seeds contain 27 identifiable anticancer agents.

Many people like to use the flax seeds instead of the oil. The fat in the seed is well protected by its seed coat and doesn't easily turn rancid. In fact, the seed coat is so tough that if you don't grind the seeds, they will pass right through you unchanged, which means you don't get the benefit of their oils. You can grind the seeds in a coffee grinder, but you should use them right away, as their healthy oils will tend to go rancid quickly if left exposed to light and air for long periods of time.

Omega-3 fats have an amazing ability to provide satiety. You will feel full for a sustained period of time after adding one tablespoon of oil at a meal because the omega-3 fats cause the stomach to retain food for a longer period of time as compared to fat-free or low fat foods. In Plan-D, flax oil can be blended into yogurt, smoothies, salad dressings, and even maple syrup.

Both fish oil and flaxseed oil are very sensitive to light and heat; therefore, *they should never be heated or used for cooking.* Fish oil comes in gel caps or liquid oil and should be pharmaceutical grade, meaning all toxins and impurities have been removed. Flaxseed oil also comes in gel caps or liquid oil. Labels should read that it is high lignan and expeller pressed. It should be contained in a dark bottle, sealed tightly, and kept refrigerated at all times. The bottle should have an expiration date of no longer than four months from the date of pressing to ensure freshness and nutritional potency. To extend freshness you may freeze unopened bottles of flaxseed oil prior to use. Do not buy flaxseed oil that is on the store shelf at room temperature in a glass or plastic bottle. Flaxseed oil kept at room temperature is not of high quality and may possibly go rancid.

Fish oil is usually kept on the shelf in the store, but should be refrigerated after opening. The liquid forms of these oils are the best absorbed into the body, however gel caps are also acceptable. Gel caps do not need to be refrigerated, so they are great for traveling.

ORGANIC BUTTER

One of the "fat" lies is that butter is bad for you. But that would be a surprise to many people around the globe who have used butter for its life-sustaining properties for millennia. Dr. Price found that butter was a staple food for many supremely healthy people, because it contains many nutrients that protect humans from many diseases.

Butter can especially protect against heart disease (yes, that's right, I'm busting the fat lies wide open!) It contains vitamin A, which is needed for the health of the thyroid and adrenal gland, both of which play a role in the proper functioning of the heart. Butter is America's best and most easily absorbed source of vitamin A. Vitamins A and E, and the mineral selenium, all contained in butter, are strong antioxidants that protect us against free radical damage.[8]

Additionally, butter is a good source of iodine, a nutrient many people are deficient in. Iodine protects the thyroid gland, thereby helping to regulate metabolism. Butter has many other health benefits, from improving the immune system and preventing cancer, to assisting the body in the absorption of calcium and building strong bones. All the nutrients in butter make it an essential food, capable of supplying many of our daily nutrient needs.[9]

You will find only the use of butter and never that of margarine type products in Plan-D recipes. So, be prepared to enjoy the taste and benefits of one of nature's most enduring natural products—butter!

OLIVE OIL

Everyone knows how good olive oil is, so I don't need to espouse its virtues. Aside from coconut oil, olive oil is one of the most digestible of all the fats. Olive oil contributes to the prevention of heart disease and cancer, and has been used as a remedy for a wide variety of ailments.

You may use olive oil liberally for its monounsaturated fat, but don't heat it too much as you will destroy all of it's health-giving qualities. In fact, the reason extra-virgin olive oil is the best, and the reason why it's called "first cold pressed," is because it isn't heated above 150 degrees during the pressing process. To make sure you use olive oil properly, none of the Plan-D Recipes use it for cooking. It is recommended that it be used more for salad dressings.

One thing you may note about olive oil is that it will turn hard if you put it in the refrigerator. This is because, like most fruit, olives have waxes on their epidermis (epicarp) to protect them from insects, desiccation and the elements. These natural waxes are what allow an apple to be shined, and they are also why olive oil solidifies when its temperature is lowered. There is nothing wrong with this.

Often times a manufacturer will "winterize" their oil—meaning it is chilled and filtered to remove the waxes. A standard test to determine if olive oil has been sufficiently winterized is to put it in an ice water bath (32 degrees Fahrenheit) for 5 hours. No clouding or crystals should occur.

It has been my experience that most olive oils that you purchase in a grocery store have not been winterized. Oil that has not been winterized will clump and form needle-like crystals at refrigerator temperatures as the fats and waxes in the oil congeal. Some olive varieties form waxes that produce long thin crystals, others form waxes that congeal into rosettes, slimy clumps, clouds, a swirl of egg-white-like material, or white sediment that the consumer may fear represents spoilage. These visual imperfections may form outside the refrigerator during the winter when the oil is exposed to cold temperatures during transport, hence the term "winterize". Chilling or freezing olive oil does no harm and the oil will return to its normal consistency when warmed.

Olive oil will solidify at 36°F, but it will return to a liquid state as soon as the temperature rises. If your olive oil salad dressing has turned hard in the refrigerator, and you want to use it quickly, I suggest putting the bottle containing the dressing in a bowl of warm water for a few minutes to warm the oil so that it will return to its liquid state.

AVOCADOS

Not only are avocados delicious (they are my absolute favorite) but they are also chock full of nutrients. They're loaded with vitamin A (the potent antioxidant), have plenty of B vitamins, including folate, lutein (a phytochemical important for the eyes), magnesium, and 60 percent more potassium than bananas. One medium size avocado contains a whopping 15 grams of fiber, making it one of the most fiber-rich fruits on the planet.

Avocados are high in fat, but you don't need to be afraid of it, it's the good kind of heart healthy monounsaturated fat, which helps to lower bad (LDL) cholesterol. Avocados have four times more beta-sitosterol, a phytochemical that reduces the amount of cholesterol absorbed from food. So the combination of beta-sitosterol and monounsaturated fat makes the avocado an excellent cholesterol buster.

According to a study in Brisbane, Australia, eating avocados daily for three weeks improved blood cholesterol levels in middle-aged women better than a low-fat diet did. The avocado diet reduced total cholesterol 8 percent compared with 5 percent for the low-fat diet. Most important, avocados improved the good HDL-cholesterol ratio by 15 percent.

The daily amount of avocado ranged from ½ avocado for small women to 1 ½ for large women. The expected outcome was that by eating avocados, heart patients could cut their risk of heart attack by 10 to 20 percent and death rates by 4 to 8 percent in three to five years.[10]

Beta-sitosterol has an apparent ability to block the bad LDL cholesterol absorption from the intestine, resulting in lower blood cholesterol levels. The Australian study not only reported that eating either half or a whole avocado per day for a month succeeded in lowering cholesterol levels, but at the same time most people in the study lost weight![11]

ALMONDS

Almonds are a highly nutritious food. In addition to being an excellent source of dietary fiber, they supply important amino acids and several minerals, notably calcium, magnesium, potassium, and phosphorus. Almonds contain vitamin E, a powerful antioxidant, which is present in significant amounts and protects the other oils in the diet from spoiling. The B-complex vitamins, as well as carotene, which are converted to vitamin A in the body, are also found in almonds.

Like avocados, almonds are also rich in monounsaturated oils. This high oil content ensures maximum availability of the fat-soluble vitamin E, which is present in significant amounts. The powerful antioxidant properties of this vitamin further protects the oils from going rancid. The B-complex vitamins, as well as carotene, which is converted to vitamin A in the body, are also found in almonds. The almond also contains more phosphorus and iron in a combination easily absorbed into the body than any other nut. Current research confirming the immune boosting properties of each of these nutrients lend support to one of Edgar Cayce's bold assertions that "those who would eat two or three almonds each day need never fear cancer."[12]

I always carry a small bag of almonds with me to keep in my purse or in the car (they won't melt), for snacking. They are a great source of protein too.

It is very important to almonds and any other nuts *in their raw form.* Heating and roasting nuts destroys their health-promoting natural oils, the same as heating vegetable oil has a detrimental effect on health.

Almond butter and almond milk are two great ways to enjoy almonds. See the recipe for almond milk on page **217.**

OAT BRAN

Oat bran is the edible, outermost layer of the whole oat kernel. I chose it as the main ingredient in my flourless muffins for its many health benefits. Oat bran's most virtuous and versatile component is its soluble fiber. In January 1997, the FDA passed a unique ruling that allowed oat bran to be registered as the first cholesterol-reducing food, for its ability to bind to blood cholesterol and effectively flush it from the body.

Because oat bran is high in fiber, it promotes weight loss by reducing cravings, stabilizing blood sugar levels, and by providing a prolonged feeling of fullness along with a steady boost of energy. It is considered an excellent food for diabetics because the fiber causes dietary sugar to be absorbed more gradually and increases tissue sensitivity to insulin. In fact, studies show that people with type 1 diabetes who incorporate oat bran into their balanced diets reduce their insulin requirements.

The fiber in oat bran helps regulate bowel function and can alleviate constipation—a health problem that many overweight people suffer from which can lead to a number of bowel diseases, including colon cancer. The soluble fiber in oat bran activates white blood cells, which in effect strengthens the immune system and may prevent some cancers.

Oat bran can be eaten raw or cooked. Prepared as a hot cereal like oatmeal, it serves as a nice breakfast food. I also use it in place of breadcrumbs in recipes. And of course, you can make muffins with it.

WILD CAUGHT SALMON

Salmon is an incredibly healthful fish full of essential omega-3 fatty acids, but you need to make sure that you are eating wild caught salmon instead of farm-raised salmon. Wild salmon roam freely in the ocean and eat little crustaceans called krill, a big part of their natural diet. Krill contain a powerful antioxidant carotenoid called astaxanthin, which is the source of the crustacean's red color, and the subsequent pink color of the salmon who eat them.

Farm-raised salmon live a very different life from its wild cousin. They are raised in small pens, leaving very little room for the fish to move about freely. They're fed grains, an unnatural diet for fish, and antibiotics to prevent diseases that can result from living in such close quarters. Farmed salmon have more antibiotics administered by weight than any other form of livestock. The natural color of farmed salmon is an unappetizing gray, so they're fed colorings (chemically synthesized forms of astaxanthin), so that they turn pink to make them more palatable for our plates. On the packaging of all farm-raised salmon you will see the statement "Farm raised, color added." What's more, according to the independent Environmental Working Group, farmed salmon contained high levels of contaminants called PCBs (polychlorinated biphenyls) when the organization tested farmed salmon purchased in U.S. grocery stores.

Wild salmon is one of the best sources of omega-3 fatty acids, however because of the make-up of their feed, farmed salmon contain higher levels of omega-6 fats and lower levels of omega-3s.

Most farmed salmon is called "Atlantic Salmon", while wild salmon are called "Alaskan, Sockeye, or Chum." As a general rule, you should strive to eat only wild caught fish of any kind, as opposed to farm raised.

ORGANIC EGGS

Organic eggs contain nearly all known nutrients except for vitamin C and are a nearly perfect form of protein. They are good sources of the fat-soluble vitamins A and D, plus they contain essential fatty acids. While many people have been afraid to eat eggs due to their high cholesterol levels, recent studies suggest that eggs contain several nutrients that promote heart health and actually lower the risk of heart disease.

The best thing about eggs is their ability to assist in weight loss. Eggs are rich in lecithin, a compound that helps to cleanse and detoxify the liver. Cleansing the liver results in effortless weight loss. As with other animal products, you should eat organic eggs. Hard-boiled eggs make great snacks, and they travel well too!

ORGANIC YOGURT

Yogurt is a fermented dairy product made by adding bacterial cultures to milk. These "Live and Active" cultures carry on the conversion of the milk's lactose sugar into lactic acid. This clever process gives yogurt is unique tart and sour flavor and unique pudding-like texture. The texture is the reason the Turks gave it the name *yoghurmak*, meaning "to thicken." The lactic acid bacteria that are traditionally used to make yogurt—*Lactobacillus bulgarius, Lactobacillus acidophilus, Bifidobacterium lactis,* and *Streptococcus thermophilus*—are also responsible for many of yogurt's health benefits.

Yogurt containing live and active cultures has been demonstrated to improve intestinal health by suppressing harmful bacteria in the intestine. Yogurt also lowers cholesterol. In a recent study of older adults, intake of about 1 cup of yogurt with live cultures per day for one year prevented an increase in blood total and low-density lipoprotein (LDL) cholesterol levels.[13]

Several other studies have suggested that the consumption of high levels of cultured milk products, such as yogurt and buttermilk, may reduce the risk of colon cancer. The anticancer effects of these foods extend well beyond the colon, however. Various probiotic species have demonstrated immune-enhancing and antitumor effects, but they also play a critical role in the detoxification of many cancer-causing substances, including hormones, meat carcinogens, and environmental toxins.[14]

When buying yogurt, the more natural the product is, the more beneficial it will be to your health. Plain Organic yogurt is best, as it will have the lowest amount of naturally occurring sugars (from lactose) and the highest amount of live and active cultures.

Yogurt-lovers should take notice: there are products in the marketplace that take advantage of yogurt's healthful image. Beware of yogurts containing artificial colors, flavorings, or sweeteners such as aspartame or sucralose (Splenda), modified food starch, and added sugars such as high fructose corn syrup. Vanilla and other flavored yogurts and yogurts with fruit already mixed in are usually inferior yogurts in terms of nutritional value and levels of live and active cultures.

FLOURLESS BREAD (SPROUTED WHOLE GRAIN BREAD)

This is another one of those "too good to be true" foods. Giving up flour and sugar doesn't mean giving up bread. There is a process, called sprouting, which releases the vital nutrients stored in whole grains and makes delicious breads that are richer in protein and vitamins than breads baked from dry grains ground into flour. The bread contains significantly higher concentrations of nutrients. The sprouting process causes a natural change that makes the protein and carbohydrates in the grains easier for the body to digest and use. The baking process preserves the nutrients and retains the natural fiber and bran found in the whole grains.

Most of the flourless breads available are made with a combination of organic sprouted grains. These breads are ideal for weight loss because they are filling, regulate blood sugar levels, and do not cause cravings. Believe me, you will not want to overeat on this bread! Use it anywhere you would use other types of bread.

STEVIA

Stevia is a natural sweetener derived from a plant in the daisy family that was originally found growing in the rainforests of South America. The leaves of the stevia plant, known as "sweet leaf," have been used for over 1500 years by the Guarani Indians of Paraguay as a healing tonic.

In addition to its natural sweetening qualities, stevia has many health benefits. There have been over 500 scientific studies performed on stevia since it was first discovered in 1899. The results of the studies reveal that stevia has the following positive effects on human health when added to the daily diet:

Stevia is effective in regulating and normalizing blood sugar levels in people who suffer from diabetes and hypoglycemia.

Stevia aids the weight loss process because it contains no calories and may, therefore, be used in recipes that satisfy the sweet tooth and balance the diet, eliminating feelings of deprivation or lack of variety. A small amount of stevia goes a long way and will help to reduce cravings for sweets and fatty foods.

Stevia inhibits the growth of oral bacteria. This may explain why regular users of mouthwashes and toothpastes containing stevia are less susceptible to colds and flu. Studies also show improvement with bleeding gum problems.

Stevia can be applied externally to the skin to rapidly heal wounds and cuts, and to clear up eczema, dermatitis, and acne.

Stevia contains inulin, a natural fiber that stimulates the growth of helpful intestinal bifidobacteria. This may explain why stevia improves digestion and soothes an upset stomach.

Stevia is my sweetener of choice. I recommend using it to sweeten teas, yogurt, oatmeal, smoothies, and anything else you like!

AGAVE NECTAR (ALSO CALLED AGAVE SYRUP)

Agave nectar is a natural sweetener that comes from the Agave Plants. It can be used to sweeten any type of beverage or food. Agave nectar has a low glycemic level and is a delicious and safe alternative to table sugar. It will not over stimulate the production of insulin. Unlike the crystalline form of fructose, which is refined primarily from corn, Agave Nectar is sweet in its natural form. This nectar does not contain processing chemicals. Even better, because it is sweeter than table sugar, less is needed in your recipes and meals. It can be most useful for people who are diabetic, have insulin resistance (Type II, non-insulin dependant) or are simply watching their carbohydrate intake.

The Agave Nectar contents aid the functioning of the gall bladder, helping to break down and metabolize dietary fats. Its contents also work against the blocking of arteries and veins due to high cholesterol levels.

The oligosaccharides found in agave nectar serve as food for intestinal microflora, otherwise known as friendly bacteria. Clinical studies have shown that oligosaccharides can increase the number of these friendly bacteria in the colon while simultaneously reducing the population of harmful bacteria. For this reason, agave would be ideal to add to yogurt.

Agave can be used for the same purposes as stevia. You will find agave in many of the Plan-D recipes.

CHAPTER 12

Processed-Free Vitamins

Less than a century ago, the existence of vitamins and their role in human nutrition were virtually unknown. Today, whole shops are dedicated to an ever-growing industry that has been built around them. Extensive research confirms that we definitely need an adequate amount of vitamins and minerals for optimal health, but can the vast world of synthetic vitamins really be a true substitute for the type of health we receive from eating whole natural foods?

Before I discuss the importance of vitamins and minerals, I want to give you a little background on Recommended Daily Allowances (RDAs). A little over forty years ago, there was a fleet of sailors who developed a disease called scurvy while out at sea. Scurvy is a disease caused by a deficiency of vitamin C. Because these sailors had no access to citrus fruits or other foods containing vitamin C, they got very sick. When they returned to shore, they were given oranges and limes to eat. It was documented how many oranges and limes it took to reverse the symptoms of scurvy. This minimum amount became the recommended daily allowance for vitamin C. However, this amount was only the minimum amount *to not get scurvy*— it was not the amount to keep a person functioning optimally.

Shortly thereafter, the rest of the RDAs were instituted by the U.S. Food and Nutrition Board as a standard for the daily amounts of vitamins and minerals needed by a healthy person. The amounts, however, only provide us with the bare minimum required to ward off deficiency diseases such as scurvy, beriberi (a vitamin B1 deficiency), rickets (a vitamin D and calcium deficiency), and night blindness (a vitamin A deficiency). What these amounts do not account for are the amounts needed to maintain maximum health, rather than borderline health.

OPTIMAL DAILY ALLOWANCE

In order to be optimally healthy, we need to ensure that our vitamin and mineral intake is optimum. Scientific studies have shown that doses higher than the RDAs help our bodies work better. The RDAs therefore, are not very useful for determining what our intake of vitamins and minerals should be. When it comes to discussing vitamins and minerals, I prefer to speak more in terms of *optimal daily allowances* (ODAs). These are the amounts needed for vibrant good health. In today's world, we do need to take supplements to make sure that we get the optimal daily allowance of vitamins and minerals. However, our first source of these important nutrients should be our foods, therefore our supplements should also come from our foods.

THE ROLE OF VITAMINS AND MINERALS

Vitamins are required by our bodies to perform a variety of functions. Chemically, they are divided into two groups—those that are fat soluble (A, D, E, and K) and those that are water soluble (the B vitamins and vitamin C). If we take in more fat soluble vitamins than our bodies need, they are stored in our fatty tissues and can be used later if our intake decreases, therefore, we don't need to eat them every day. However, the water soluble vitamins cannot be stored and are excreted in the urine daily, therefore they must be continually supplied by our food.

Vitamins are unable to do their job without an adequate supply of minerals in the body. Minerals also perform many biochemical functions, and are essential components of the skeletal system and other body tissues. Our bodies require vitamins and minerals for the following functions:

- Regulate metabolism
- Assist with release of energy during digestive processes
- Assist enzymes with chemical reactions that facilitate bodily functions
- Assist body in fighting off diseases,
- Help boost immune system responses
- Help maintain balanced moods
- Assist the body to assimilate benefits from exercise and macronutrients (fats, carbohydrates, proteins). [1]

Because of their important functions, we need to make sure we have enough vitamins and minerals. In our chemically polluted and stress-filled world, our nutritional requirements have been increasing, but the number of calories we require has been *decreasing,* as our activity level as a society has declined. This means we are faced with the need to get *more* nutrients from *less* food. At the same time, due to the cooking and processing of foods, which destroy most nutrients, getting even the Recommended Daily Allowance of vitamins and minerals from our modern diet has become difficult, if not impossible to achieve.

Additionally, because the nutrients in the soil that our food is grown in have been depleted over time, the food itself does not contain the amount of nutrients that it used to. For example, the apple your great grandfather ate had more nutrients in it than the apple you eat today, even if the apple comes from the same tree. That is because the soil that the tree is growing in has been depleted over time and the apple that it bears contains less nutrients as a result. And although the food itself has fewer nutrients in it in today's world, our bodies still have the same requirements for nutrients that our great grandfathers did in order to be optimally healthy. Consequently, in order to obtain the optimal amount of many nutrients, it is necessary to take them in supplement form. However, taking supplements should never be a replacement for eating real whole foods. We need both, but we have to be careful about what type of supplement we take.

SYNTHETIC VERSUS NATURAL WHOLE FOOD SUPPLEMENTS

Vitamin supplements can be divided into two groups: *synthetic* and *natural* (also called whole food supplements). Most over the counter vitamin supplements like One-A-Day, Centrum, Kirkland, and many others are synthetic—meaning they are made in a laboratory from isolated chemicals that mirror their counterparts found in nature but are not from real food. Natural vitamin and mineral supplements *are* derived from real food sources, specifically vegetables, fruits, herbs, and seaweeds.

What is the difference between synthetic and natural vitamins and minerals? There is a world of difference between synthetic vitamins that are in pill form versus vitamins that are contained within nature's foods. Although the chemical differences between a vitamin found in food and one created in a laboratory is slight, synthetic supplements contain the isolated vitamins only, while natural supplements also contain all of the other nutrients in foods not yet discovered, such as antioxidants and phytochemicals that help the vitamins do their jobs. Natural vitamins also retain the necessary enzymes that are specific to the foods they are derived from, which assist the body in utilizing the vitamins and minerals properly.

Another difference is that synthetic vitamins may also include coal tars, artificial coloring, preservatives and stabilizers such as maltodextrin, stearates and dioxides, sugars, and starch, as well as other additives. You should beware of such harmful elements.

Natural whole food supplements are made by condensing or compressing real whole foods and then evaporating off the water. The actual process is achieved by placing vegetables and fruits in a large blender and then dehydrating the mixture to evaporate the water at very low temperatures. The low temperature is crucial so as not to destroy the enzymes and cofactors contained in the foods. The enzymes are very important synergists that are required for digesting and assimilating vitamins and minerals. The remaining dried "powders" are then placed in capsules or combined with vegetable cellulose to form solid tablets.

If you are deficient in a particular nutrient, the synthetic chemical source will work to an extent, but you will not get the benefits of the vitamin as found in whole foods. Synthetic vitamins just do not work like foods, and foods are what our bodies were designed to use for healing, prevention and energy. There is no substitute, and no matter how you look at it, synthetic vitamins are an invention of scientists, so they are prone to cause side effects, be incomplete and lack what we need to overcome or prevent health problems.

For years synthetic vitamins have been sold and marketed as the "magic bullet" for all health conditions. The problem is that vitamins, when not still contained in their original food (oranges, bananas, spinach, broccoli, etc.) are merely chemicals. Our bodies do not recognize synthetic vitamins as nutrients, because they don't work the same way as whole foods. Dr. Vic Shayne provides insight into the limitation of synthetic vitamins. In his article, <u>Why Vitamin Pills are Not Enough</u>, he explains why synthetic supplements cannot be substituted for healthy, whole foods:

- Foods contain not just vitamins, but the co-factors (synergists) and helper nutrients that allow vitamins to work
- Foods are never found in high potency, so you won't suffer any toxic side effects that have been proven to exist with all vitamin pills.
- Vitamins are just a small part of what our bodies require for health and healing. It is very often that it is the other food properties that help us while the vitamins are secondary.
- Vitamin pills need other nutrients in order to work. 2

For these reasons, and more, synthetic vitamin pills, despite their use and overuse, are lacking the properties of real nutrition, which can only come from eating nature's real, whole, raw foods. The ONLY supplement that someone should take, therefore, is a whole food formula WITHOUT any isolated (singular vitamin). In order to know whether your vitamin and mineral supplement comes from whole foods, you have to carefully read the labels. Instead of just names of vitamins and minerals on a label, you should be looking for the names of foods and herbs on the label, such as kale, dandelion, kelp, ginger, cinnamon, apples, carrots and broccoli.

It is a very common misconception that we need to take high dosages of vitamins to keep us healthy. Remember, real whole foods are never found in high potency, so don't be fooled by high milligrams, high potency, standardization or any other such terms that just do not apply to real foods from nature.

If you take an isolated vitamin supplement to resolve a suspected deficiency, remember that in order for vitamins to be efficient they must work in conjunction with particular minerals, and vice versa. The taking of individual vitamins alone will not necessarily resolve the deficiency. There must be a balance between the vitamins and minerals for the vitamins to work as desired.

To help you understand the required interaction between vitamins and minerals refer to the chart below. This shows which minerals need to be present in combination with specific vitamins to resolve vitamin deficiencies.

MINERALS REQUIRED FOR VITAMIN ASSIMILATION	
VITAMIN DEFICIENCY	**SUPPLEMENTS NEEDED FOR ASSIMILATION**
Vitamin A	Choline, essential fatty acids, zinc, vitamins C, D, and E
Vitamin B Complex	Calcium, vitamins C and E
Vitamin B_1 (thiamine)	Manganese, vitamin B complex, vitamins C and E
Vitamin B_2 (riboflavin)	Vitamin B complex, vitamin C

Vitamin B$_3$ (niacin)	Vitamin B complex, vitamin C
Pantothenic acid (B$_5$)	Vitamin B complex, vitamins A, C, and E
Vitamin B$_6$ (pyridoxine)	Vitamin B complex, vitamin C, and potassium
Biotin	Folic acid, vitamin B complex, pantothenic acid (vitamin B$_5$), vitamin B$_{12}$, vitamin C
Choline	Vitamin B complex, vitamin B$_{12}$, folic acid, inositol
Inositol	Vitamin B complex, vitamin C
Para-aminobenzoic acid (PABA)	Vitamin B complex, folic acid, vitamin C
Vitamin C	Bioflavonoids, calcium, magnesium
Vitamin D	Calcium, choline, essential fatty acids, phosphorus, vitamin A and C
Vitamin E	Essential fatty acids, manganese, selenium, vitamin A, vitamin B$_1$ (thiamine), inositol, vitamin C
Essential fatty acids	Vitamins A, C, D, and E
MINERAL DEFICIENCY	**SUPPLEMENTS NEEDED FOR ASSIMILATION**
Calcium	Boron, essential fatty acids, lysine, magnesium, manganese, phosphorus, vitamins A, C, D, and E
Copper	Cobalt, folic acid, iron, zinc,
Iodine	Iron, manganese, and phosphorus
Magnesium	Calcium, phosphorus, potassium, vitamin B$_6$ (pyridoxine), vitamins C and D
Manganese	Calcium, iron, vitamin B complex, vitamin E
Phosphorus	Calcium, iron, manganese, sodium, phosphorus, vitamin B$_6$ (pyridoxine)
Silicon	Iron and phosphorus
Sodium	Calcium, potassium, sulfur, vitamin D
Sulfur	Potassium, vitamin B$_1$ (thiamine), pantothenic acid (B$_5$), biotin
Zinc	Calcium, copper, phosphorus, vitamin B$_6$ (pyridoxine)

Source: Balch, Phyllis and James Balch, M.D. Prescription for Nutritional Healing.

HOW TO CORRECTLY TAKE A MULTIVITAMIN
When you take supplements, the ultimate goal is for your body to efficiently absorb and utilize them. For that to occur, a supplement needs to be protein-bound. Natural,

whole food supplements are protein-bound. Furthermore, to help facilitate vitamin and mineral efficiency, supplements should always be taken with food. Vitamins A, D, E and K are only soluble in fat, meaning they can only be absorbed into the body when oil or fat is present in the meal. All other vitamins are water soluble, meaning they can be dissolved by any food containing water. Because multivitamins are very concentrated, they need a full or nearly full stomach to get adequate absorption into the body through the digestive process. Take a multivitamin in the middle of or at the end of a meal, NOT at the beginning of a meal and not with just a snack.

Just like you need to eat more than once a day in order to get vitamins from your food, you should take your vitamin supplements in divided doses—one with the morning meal and one with the evening meal. It is important to take your second dosage with the evening meal because your body needs the vitamins for regeneration at night.

Finally, vitamin supplements are supposed to be just that—supplements. They are not intended to replace what you would get from eating the actual food. *There is no vitamin pill or supplement that can make up for a diet that is lacking in variety and nutrients.* Following Plan-D ensures that you get a variety of food as well as the proper amount of vitamins and minerals from whole food supplement.

RECOMMENDED DAILY ALLOWANCE (RDA) VERSUS OPTIMAL DAILY INTAKE (ODI)

	RDA [2004]	ODI [2006]
FAT SOLUBLE VITAMINS		
Vitamin A	4,000 - 5,000 IU	5,000 - 10,000 IU
Vitamin D	200 - 400 IU	400 IU
Vitamin E (d-alpha tocopherol)	15 IU	200 IU
Vitamin K	Has no RDA	100 - 500 mcg
WATER SOLUBLE VITAMINS		
Carotenoids containing Beta-carotene	1,000 – 4,000 IU	5,000 - 25,000 IU
Vitamin B1 (thiamine)	1 – 1.4 mg	50 - 100 mg
Vitamin B2 (riboflavin)	1.6 mg	15 - 50 mg
Vitamin B3 (niacin)	13 – 18 mg	15 - 50 mg
(niacinamide)	13 – 18 mg	50 - 100 mg
Pantothenic acid (vitamin B5)	4 – 7 mg	50 - 100 mg
Vitamin B6 (pyridoxine)	2 – 2.2 mg	50 - 100 mg
Vitamin B12 (cobalamin)	3 mcg	200 - 400 mcg
Biotin (part of the B vitamin family)	100 200 mcg	400 - 800 mcg

	RDA [2004]	ODI [2006]
Choline (also part of the B vitamin family)	Has no RDA	50 - 200 mg
Folic Acid (vitamin B9, also called folate)	400 mcg	400 - 800 mcg
Vitamin C with mineral ascorbates (Ester C)		1,000 - 3,000 mg
Para-aminobenzoic acid (PABA, part of the B vitamin family)	Has no RDA	10 - 50 mg
Bioflavonoids, mixed (vitamin P)	10 – 25 mg	200 - 500 mg
MINERALS		
Boron	Has no RDA	3 - 6 mg
Calcium	1,000 – 1,300 mg	1.500 – 2,000 mg
Chromium	Has no RDA	150 - 400 mcg
Copper	0.7 – 1.3 mg	2 - 3 mg
Iodine (kelp is a good source)	150 mcg	100 - 225 mcg
Iron	8 - 18 mg	18 - 30 mg
Magnesium	310 - 420 mg	750-1,000 mg
Manganese	Has no RDA	3 - 10 mg
Molybdenum	45 - 50 mcg	30 - 100 mcg
Potassium	4700 mg	99 - 500 mg
Selenium	55 – 70 mcg	100 - 200 mcg
Vanadium	Has no RDA	200 – 1,000 mcg
Zinc	8 – 11 mg	30 - 50 mg

Sources:

1. Balch J & Balch, P. *Prescription for Nutritional Healing, 4th Edition* (New York: Avery Publishing Group, 2006), 9.
2. *Dietary Reference Intakes (DRIs): Recommended Intakes for Individuals, Elements,* Food and Nutrition Board, Institute of Medicine, National Academies, http://www.iom.edu/Object.File/Master/21/372/0.pdf , National Academy of Sciences, 2004.

CHAPTER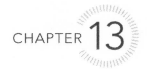

Swing Your Arms and Bounce

"Walking is man's best medicine."
—*Hippocrates*

The most important aspect of gaining health is choosing healthy foods. However, in order for true healing to occur, we have to balance our healthy food choices with moderate physical activity. Throughout history, humans have been movers and shakers. The longest-lived peoples in human history moved their bodies at an active moderate pace nearly every day of their lives. They walked, jumped, stretched, plowed, gardened, herded and hunted animals, balanced heavy objects on their heads and backs, and built structures. Some cultures also engage in daily activities that discipline and tone the body, such as Thai Chi and yoga.

Calorie burning aside, the value of exercise is more extensive than you ever imagined. Our bodies were designed to move—not sit around for hours and hours on "end" (rear-end, that is)— and there is a very good reason for that. The quality of our health is entirely dependent upon how we move. Most of us know about our circulatory system, which circulates blood throughout our body and relies on our heart as the "pump" to make this action happen. Also within our body is a relatively unknown *secondary circulatory system* underneath the skin, called the *lymphatic system*, which rids the body of toxins, bacteria, heavy metals, dead cells, cholesterol, trapped protein, and fat globules. The lymphatic system is basically the garbage disposal of the body.

THE RIVER OF LIFE

Like the cardiovascular system, the lymphatic system is made up of channels, or vessels, valves, and filters (lymph nodes). Unlike the circulatory system however, the lymphatic system has no "pump." Instead, the fluid that moves through the lymphatic system (called "lymph") relies on us to "move our bodies" in order to stimulate the healthy flow of lymph. Muscle action, deep breathing, and gravitational pressure from exercise are what keep the lymph flowing freely. In other words, "exercise" is the only pump for the lymphatic system.

In 2001, a well-respected cardiologist from Philadelphia, Gerald M. Lemole, M.D. wrote a book called *The Healing Diet*, which describes the link between the health of the lymphatic system and the overall health of the body. Once a skeptic about the power of lifestyle changes, he is now a strong believer in the philosophy of the venerated Greek healer Hippocrates—that walking (exercise) is man's best medicine. In his book, Dr. Lemole calls the lymphatic system "our river of life."

According to Dr. Lemole, when the lymphatic system is flowing freely, our body works fine. When it becomes sluggish, or backs up, we gain weight, get sick, or both. The lymphatic system slows down and becomes sluggish when we are inactive, and especially when we sit for long periods of time. The consequences of a sluggish lymphatic system can be serious, even life threatening. In addition to being part of the body's plumbing and repair system, the lymphatics are an essential part of our immune system. In addition to filtering out toxic materials, the lymph nodes also produce substances that fight off invading viruses and bacteria and destroy abnormal cells that developed within the body, such as cancer cells.

"Exercise is the most powerful conditioner of the lymphatic system," says Dr. Lemole. Conditioning and purifying the lymphatic system is essential for ridding the body of fat, especially the unsightly cellulite that builds up on our thighs and buttox. Therefore, Plan-D emphasizes the types of exercise that will condition and cleanse the lymphatic system—bouncing and swinging your arms while walking briskly.

SWING YOUR ARMS

According to Jordan Rubin, author of *The Maker's Diet*, the oldest physical activity of the human race can be expressed in one word—*walking*. A brisk two-mile walk (with long strides and vigorous arm movements) every day increases enzyme and metabolic activity and may increase calorie burning for up to twelve hours afterward![1]

Dr. Lemole says walking should be your first option for the purposes of keeping the lymphatic system healthy. As you remember, I *walked* my way to a 100 pound weight loss. Walking was my main form of exercise, for 30 to 60 minutes each day at least five days each week. I encourage you to do the same. Walk briskly, dramatically swinging your arms along with your pace. Allowing your arms to hang limply at your sides does not keep the lymphatic system moving.

Begin your walk with a warm-up period of normal pace walking for about 5 minutes. Then begin to walk briskly. If you are just beginning a walking program, start out with 20-minute brisk walks, and work your way up to 30 to 60 minutes as your body responds to your daily activity. You may walk outside in the sunshine (the preferred method), or you may walk indoors on a treadmill. The distance you walk is not as important as the length of time. As long as you are walking, you will benefit from the exercise in many ways.

Dr. Lemole may be the first doctor to truly explain the reason why exercise has proved to be such a powerful remedy for lowering cholesterol and major reductions in heart disease. According to Dr. Lemole, clearing the lymphatic system can substantially reduce the risk of atherosclerosis, or blockage of the arteries. A study he performed on primates demonstrated that clearing the lymphatic system allows the body to more efficiently clear excess cholesterol out of the arteries. The excess cholesterol is carried through the lymphatics to the veins and then to the liver, where it can be broken down and discarded. Furthermore, according to the results of two separate U.S. studies, brisk walking does the same job of lowering LDL (bad cholesterol) as cholesterol-lowering drugs, and more besides. Exercise not only significantly reduces LDL, but also increases levels of HDL (good cholesterol). Researchers found that brisk walking over 12 miles a week will lower LDL, but only sustained moderate exercise, such as jogging 20 miles a week, will raise HDL.[2]

The pace of brisk walking is different for each person. I like the recommendation of obesity specialist Gus Prosch Jr., M.D. for determining how fast one should walk. "Imagine that you are wearing thin clothing and that the temperature outside is below freezing, the wind is blowing hard, and it is raining and you have to go to the bathroom very badly and you are a mile from home. How fast would you walk to get there? Now, that's brisk walking!"

BOUNCE YOUR WAY TO HEALTH

A few years ago I attended a weight loss convention where one of the featured speakers shared he had lost 200 pounds in 18 months. He claimed that the only exercise he engaged in during his weight loss was jumping on a trampoline. He humorously revealed that he "wore out" five mini- trampolines by the time he reached his goal weight.

His story made sense to me, because the action of bouncing, or more recently known as rebounding, gives the lymphatic system a complete cellular cleansing. Dr. Prosch was a big proponent of rebounding, or using a mini-trampoline, claiming that it may be one of the best forms of exercise for cleansing the lymphatic system. In his article titled *Twelve Vital Nutritional And Health Topics* he writes " this form of exercise is different from other physical activities because it puts gravity to work in your favor. By subjecting each of the sixty trillion cells in your body to greater gravitation pull, waste products are squeezed out and nutritional elements and oxygen are drawn into the cells. The cells function more efficiently and the metabolism increases to its maximum. As the lymphatic vessels have one-way valves in them, and the lymph flows only one way (towards the heart) when one jumps up on the rebounder, the lymph is thrown up also and cannot go back down the vessels because of the one-way valves. This acts as a suction pump to pull out and suck out the lymph and return it back to the circulation where it is supposed to be."[3]

The exercise of rebounding has many other health benefits. In her book *The Fat Flush Plan*, author Ann Louise Gittleman espouses the benefits of rebounding:

> Use of a mini-trampoline (or rebounder) has proven to be an efficient form of exercise with virtually no harmful side effects. Your cardiovascular fitness will excel, and you will be toning your body at the same time. It

fires up cellular metabolism, energizing every cell with fresh oxygen and nutrients. The low impact (such as the light pressure on the thighs) stimulates waste drainage, easing waste material out of the lymphatic system. In approximately two weeks, you should notice that your legs, buttox, and ankles are becoming toned and those orange peel-like cellulite deposits are smoothing out.[4]

You can purchase a mini-trampoline at any sports store, some department stores, or on-line. They typically stand about 8 inches off the ground and are anywhere from 36 to 40 inches in diameter. They cost anywhere from $30 to $150, depending on the size and type.

Gittleman recommends bouncing every day for five minutes. Dr. Prosch suggested a more detailed rebounding routine. He recommended the following method for rebounding:

> Jog on the rebounder for two minutes, then jump with both feet on the rebounder for two minutes and repeat this process over and over for twenty minutes in all. If you get dizzy at first, this is because the toxins are being pulled out of the spaces between your cells too rapidly. You should slow down or stop for a few minutes before continuing, if this should happen.[5]

If you feel unsteady on the rebounder, place a high back chair next to the rebounder and hold on to it while you are bouncing.

One great thing about rebounding is that anyone can do it, regardless of age or physical challenges. Even those who can't walk can still benefit from the effects of rebounding by sitting on the rebounder while someone else bounces on it. Just the motion of bouncing stimulates the lymphatic system.

DEEP BREATHING

Deep breathing also improves the function of the lymphatic system. The lymph collected throughout the body drains into the blood through two ducts situated at the base of the neck, the main one being the thoratic duct. Breathing drives this action.

You should breathe deeply through your nose and exhale through your mouth. Do this 10 times in a row, then return to normal breathing. Do this several times throughout the day. Because of its action on the lymphatic system, deep breathing is also a great stress reliever.

EXERCISE IN THE MORNING

Traditional physiological science has proven that exercising in the morning is the best way to improve overall metabolism. After having slept all night, the lymphatic system is at its lowest rate; therefore moving the body first thing in the morning stimulates the flow of lymph and keeps your metabolism burning all day.

Edgar Cayce also stressed the importance of keeping the lymphatic system clean and flowing freely. He too recommended a daily program of brisk walking in the morning "when the dew is on the ground, for it is using the energies that enable the body to produce better eliminations of toxic forces." Apparently, there is a higher vibrational energy in the morning hours. The oxygen and ozone in the fresh, outdoor air keep the blood flow balanced through the lungs, heart, liver, and kidneys.[6]

If you can't exercise in the morning, do not use that as an excuse not to exercise! Exercise at any time of the day is better than no exercise at all. And although walking and rebounding are the main Plan-D recommendations, you should also engage in other forms of physical activity to help stimulate your lymphatic system. Yoga, Pilates, bicycling, swimming, hiking, resistance training, and other sports are all excellent forms of exercise and should be enjoyed as a part of your healthy lifestyle.

CHAPTER 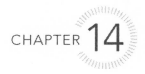14

PLAN-D:
A PLAN FOR BALANCED EATING AND LIVING

Balance is key to achieving and maintaining your health. The balance that comes from eating high life-force energy foods, getting enough sunshine, exercise and rest paves the way for a healthy positive attitude and a spiritual connection to life. Plan-D focuses on restoring balance in your physical body, thereby restoring your body's natural size, weight, and optimal health. Balanced eating provides the body with the necessary fiber and nutrients to cleanse the liver, alkalize body fluids, stabilize blood sugar levels and eliminate cravings.

A BALANCED AND CLEANSING WAY OF LIVING

The word *diet* comes from the Greek word *dieta,* which means "discipline" or "way of living." The Latin root of the word means "a day's journey." Plan-D is designed to cleanse and nourish your body on a daily basis. Plan-D does not include any refined sugars, refined carbohydrates or harmful oils. Unhealthy foods and poor eating habits may have robbed your body of the ability to support health and/or weight loss by creating chemical imbalances, food allergies or food addictions. As long as you continue to eat foods that contain refined carbohydrates, your body chemistry will remain unbalanced.

Plan-D emphasizes the following essential components to nourish, cleanse and support your body:

- Portion sizes and quality of food consumed
- Fiber in the form of vegetables, fruits, legumes, whole grains, nuts, and seeds
- Lemon water
- Vitality Vinegar Tonic
- Pure Water

- Health Promoting Oils
- Metabolism boosting spices and herbs
- High-quality multiple vitamin and mineral formula
- Positive mental attitude
- Exercise and relaxation
- Journaling
- Avoid refined and processed foods

PORTION SIZE AND FOOD QUALITY

Plan-D is a path to overall wellness. You are encouraged to focus on eating for long-term health rather than short-term weight loss or quick-fix health remedies. Obsessive counting of calories, carbohydrates and fat grams is discouraged because the traditional method of doing so does not take into account the nutrient density of the food or the metabolic properties of food. For example, 100 calories from an apple is not the same as 100 calories from a candy bar or a cookie. The apple contains fiber, nutrients, and enzymes, as well as cleanses the body. The candy bar contains no fiber, no nutrients and no enzymes; in fact it robs the body of nutrients, upsets body chemistry, makes you feel hungry an hour later, and makes you fat.

Additionally, foods high in fiber have been shown to enhance blood sugar control and assist in the reduction of absorption of between 30 and 180 calories per day. While healthy omega-3 oils and coconut oil do contain a high amount of calories, they actually increase our body's ability to burn fats more efficiently, thereby increasing our metabolism. Some foods, such as celery and lettuce, have what are called "negative calories", meaning that our bodies expend more energy (calories) to digest the foods than the foods themselves contain. For these reasons, the traditional formula of calories in, calories out is an oversimplified and inaccurate way of achieving optimal health.

Nature supplies food for us in its purest state, and nature has always intended that we eat it in that form. When you improve the quality of the foods you eat and eat them in the proper quantities, there is no need to count calories. In fact, you will find that following the portion guidelines outlined in this chapter will yield a daily calorie level that is within a healthy range.

To help you figure out portions, a detailed list of foods and their portion sizes is provided on pages **174-183.** In general, the following guidelines can be used to help you gauge healthy portion sizes:

- A 1 cup portion is about the size of a baseball
- A half-cup portion is about the size of half a baseball
- A 3-ounce portion of cooked meat, fish, or poultry is about the size of a computer mouse or a deck of cards
- One ounce of cheese looks like three stacked dice or a stick of string cheese
- One ounce of nuts is about a handful

A note about calories, carbohydrates, fat, etc: Approaching food as "a way of eating for life" helps you put the joy back into eating while supporting health and fitness. You are encouraged to make food choices based on balance, variety and portion size. Plan-D emphasizes eating a wide variety of vegetables, fruits, whole grains, legumes, nuts, seeds, oils, and protein foods. In this way, you can focus on healthy, satisfying meals without undue emphasis on nutritional details that may distract you from the big picture of pleasurable eating in a way that supports health and weight management as part of a healthy lifestyle.

FIBER IN THE FORM OF VEGETABLES, FRUITS, WHOLE GRAINS AND SEEDS

Plan-D is high in both soluble and insoluble fiber. Fiber is important for regulating blood sugar levels and normalizing bowel function. It helps prevent colon cancer, hemorrhoids, obesity, and many other disorders. Fiber has been found to be helpful in facilitating weight loss since it promotes satiety and reduces cravings.

Soluble Fiber

The "soluble" in soluble fiber means that it dissolves in water (though it cannot be digested by humans). Soluble fiber is the type that binds with certain substances that would normally result in the production of cholesterol, and eliminates them from the body. In this way, soluble fiber helps lower blood cholesterol levels and reduces the risk of heart disease. Soluble fiber also prevents and relieves BOTH *diarrhea and constipation*. Nothing else in the world will do this for you! The soluble fiber in Plan-D comes from whole oats and oat bran, apples, apple cider vinegar, brown rice, barley, quinoa, corn, potatoes, carrots, yams, sweet potatoes, turnips, rutabagas, parsnips, beets, squash, mushrooms, chestnuts, avocados, bananas, mangoes, papayas, flaxseeds, and psyllium husks.

Insoluble Fiber

While soluble fiber dissolves in water, insoluble fiber, referred to in the past as "roughage," passes through your intestines largely intact. Both types of fiber are found mainly in plant sources such as vegetables, fruits, whole grains, nuts, seeds, and legumes. A good goal for dietary fiber intake is **25-35 grams per day**, with an approximate ratio of **65-75% insoluble fiber** and **25-35% soluble fiber**. If you consume the Plan-D recommended daily servings of these foods, you do not need to worry about keeping track of the amount or types of fiber. When you eat the proper amount of vegetables, fruits, nuts, seeds, and whole grains you will get an adequate amount of fiber.

Vegetables, beans and whole grains are some of the best sources of both types of fiber. One cup of cooked carrots has almost the same amount of fiber as 3 slices of whole wheat bread or 2 cups of oatmeal. A half-cup of kidney beans contains 7.3 grams of fiber. Many foods such as oats, oat bran, psyllium husk and flaxseeds are rich in both insoluble and soluble fiber.

Fiber Supplements

If you feel you need additional fiber, a fiber supplement may be helpful. The best natural fiber sources are *psyllium husk and ground flaxseeds* because they are rich in water-soluble fibers. When taken with water before meals, these fiber sources bind to the water in the stomach to form a gelatinous mass that makes a person feel full and can help prevent overeating. Fiber also helps block the absorption of calories from carbohydrates, which in turn stabilizes blood sugar levels and facilitates healthy weight loss. A healthy combination of ground Flax Seeds, Sunflower Seeds, and Almonds, called *FSA* for short, makes a great fiber supplement that can be sprinkled into smoothies, yogurt, salads, or added to other foods. See page 209 for the recipe.

LEMON WATER

Upon rising, before you consume anything else, drink an 8-ounce glass of warm water with fresh lemon juice. The purpose of this drink is to cleanse your liver (your body's main fat burning organ) and to stimulate your metabolism into action.

HOW TO PREPARE: Add the juice of ½ a fresh lemon to 8 ounces of warm water. Water should be the temperature of a cup of tea. Use only fresh lemon juice; bottled lemon juices contain a preservative, which will defeat the purpose of the cleansing lemon water. *The warm lemon water counts toward 8-ounces of your daily water intake.*

HINT: To save time on squeezing lemons daily, you may freeze a batch by squeezing enough lemon juice to fill an ice cube tray. Each morning you can put your "lemon juice cube" into your warm water, allow it to melt, stir and drink.

VITALITY VINEGAR TONIC

The power of the Vitality Vinegar Tonic comes from its main ingredient—raw unfiltered organic apple cider vinegar. Apple cider vinegar is a secret weapon that has been used for generations for everything from alleviating arthritis, dissolving kidney stones, and assisting in weight loss. Raw unfiltered apple cider vinegar added to water assists in the reduction of excess weight by improving digestion, adding soluble fiber to the diet to stabilize blood sugar levels and blocks absorption of calories, and creating a feeling of satiety. The main action of apple cider vinegar is to assist in alkalizing your body chemistry. In combination with proper food choices, the Vitality Vinegar Tonic ensures that you achieve a proper body pH.

HOW TO PREPARE: Add 2 teaspoons of raw unfiltered apple cider vinegar to an 8-ounce glass of water at room temperature. If the tonic is too tart for your taste, a half-teaspoon of raw honey or agave nectar, or a few drops of stevia may be added. Drink this tonic three times daily, preferably 20 minutes before each meal. If you cannot drink this before meals, drink one in the morning, one in the evening, and one at some other time during the day when it is convenient. *The three 8-ounce glasses of Vitality Vinegar Tonic counts toward 24 ounces of your daily water intake.*

HINT: You can prepare a large volume of Vitality Vinegar Tonic by filling a 1-gallon container with water and adding ¾ cup raw apple cider vinegar. You can then serve your daily aliquots of the tonic from the larger container. The one-gallon container will last for 5 to 6 days. DO NOT REFRIGERATE, the vinegar will preserve the water and allow you to keep the water at room temperature.

PURE WATER

Your body's metabolism will become depressed if you don't drink enough water each day. When your metabolism slows down, food has a tendency to turn into fat and you become much more fatigued. Plan-D incorporates a minimum of 64 ounces of water each day—including the 8 ounces of morning lemon water and 24 ounces of Vitality Vinegar Tonics before meals. Water is also vital for cleansing the colon, absorbing and transporting nutrients, and flushing out waste products, including fat and toxins.

Since we all have different body sizes, we all require different amounts of water. To determine how much water your body needs, divide your current weight by two. The resulting number is the number of ounces of water you need to drink daily.

> For example, if you weigh 150 pounds:
> **Current weight in pounds ÷ 2 = ounces of water per day you need to drink**
> 150 lbs. ÷ 2 = 75 ounces of water per day

You may notice that this amount of water exceeds the typical recommendation of 64 ounces per day for adults. Unless you weigh 128 pounds, 64 ounces of water will not be adequate for proper hydration. If you are an adult and weigh less than 128 pounds, 64 ounces is recommended as the minimum amount of water. If you live in a dry climate or if you are extremely athletic, you will probably need more than half your body weight in ounces of water. If you are following Plan-D to lose weight, you will need to adjust your water intake according to your reduced weight!

YOUR TOTAL DAILY WATER INTAKE: Forty ounces of your daily requirement will come from a combination of the morning lemon water and the Vitality Vinegar Tonics. You would then add enough pure water to make your optimal daily water requirement.

If for example you weigh 150 pounds, your required 75 ounces of water will include 8 ounces of warm lemon water, 24 ounces of Vitality Vinegar Tonic, and 43 ounces of pure water.

NOTE: If you are not currently drinking your optimal amount of water per day, you must add water gradually. Your body can only absorb so much water at one time; therefore, you should add 8 ounces more water per day for one week. The next week add another 8 ounces of water per day. Do this each week until you reach your optimal amount of water per day.

For example, if you are currently only drinking 32 ounces of water each day, but you need to work your way up to 75 ounces per day, you will need to do it gradually week by week:

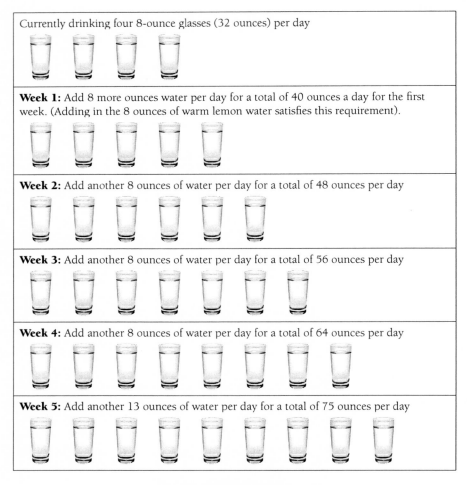

Currently drinking four 8-ounce glasses (32 ounces) per day

Week 1: Add 8 more ounces water per day for a total of 40 ounces a day for the first week. (Adding in the 8 ounces of warm lemon water satisfies this requirement).

Week 2: Add another 8 ounces of water per day for a total of 48 ounces per day

Week 3: Add another 8 ounces of water per day for a total of 56 ounces per day

Week 4: Add another 8 ounces of water per day for a total of 64 ounces per day

Week 5: Add another 13 ounces of water per day for a total of 75 ounces per day

HEALTH PROMOTING OILS

As discussed in Chapter 6, it is absolutely essential to include the right types of fats and oils in your daily meals. You will enjoy a variety of health-promoting fats and oils such as coconut oil, butter, omega-3 oil, olive oil, avocados, nuts, and seeds.

METABOLISM-BOOSTING HERBS AND SPICES

Adding these spices to your food entices your taste buds, raises your body temperature and boosts your metabolism for efficient calorie burning. Studies have shown that some of these seasonings triple the body's ability to burn calories for fuel rather than store them as fat.

DAILY INTAKE: To your taste.

CHOOSE FROM: Cayenne, dried mustard, cinnamon, ginger, dill, garlic, anise, fennel, cloves, bay leaves, coriander, parsley, cilantro, apple cider vinegar, and cumin.

HIGH QUALITY MULTI-VITAMIN

A multiple vitamin supplements your meals to ensure that optimal daily intakes of vitamins and minerals are achieved.

Only vitamins that come from a whole-food source should be taken. Synthetic vitamins are lacking in essential cofactors necessary for proper absorption. See chapter 12 for details about whole food vitamins versus synthetic vitamins.

How To Take A Multivitamin: Because multivitamins are very concentrated, they need a full or nearly full stomach to get adequate absorption into the body through the digestive process. Take your multivitamin in the middle of or at the end of a meal, NOT at the beginning of a meal and not with just a snack. A snack will not provide enough food in the stomach for adequate absorption of the vitamins and minerals.

Take multivitamins in divided doses, one with the morning meal and one with the evening meal. For instance, if the recommended daily dosage of your multivitamin is 4 capsules, you should take 2 capsules with the morning meal and 2 capsules with the evening meal. It is important to take your second dosage with the evening meal because your body needs the vitamins for regeneration at night while you are sleeping.

A POSITIVE MENTAL ATTITUDE

The key to physical healing is having a positive attitude and a strong belief that you will be successful in achieving your health goals.

A positive mental attitude results from a life dedicated to self-improvement. With a personal commitment to following *Plan-D* to the best of your ability today, you don't have to be overly concerned about yesterday or tomorrow. As I have mentioned several times before, it is not recommended or implied that you should approach this plan with black and white thinking or a lofty goal for perfection. If you temporarily fall back into old unhealthy food patterns, you can gently bring yourself back to center the next day, or even with the next bite. *NEVER BEAT YOURSELF UP OR THINK YOU HAVE TO START OVER.*

You are encouraged to strive for progress, not perfection. Imagine leaving your house to go out for a walk. You get three blocks away from home, and you trip on a crack in the sidewalk and fall to the ground. What do you do? Do you stay down for years and blame the crack in the sidewalk for your slip? Do you get up and go all the way back home and start your walk over, negating the three blocks of progress you had already made? Or, do you adopt a positive attitude, pick yourself up, dust yourself off, and continue on your committed path with the understanding that "slips happen" and it is your healthy response to those slips that empower you to continue on from where you are? I recommend the latter. It is this healthy positive attitude that has allowed me to keep my weight off for nearly 17 years. I have had my share of "slips", but I have never allowed them to completely derail me from my committed path, and neither should you.

"Starting over" thinking is one of the most damaging thought forms in any attempt to improve one's health and it has no place in Plan-D. No one is perfect. Without changes in attitude, most people are unable to maintain a healthy lifestyle.

EXERCISE AND RELAXATION

Regular exercise is absolutely critical to any effective health program. As discussed in chapter 13, walking and rebounding are excellent forms of movement that will keep your body fit and your lymphatic system flowing freely. However, any activity that you enjoy is recommended.

In addition to moving your body, allowing it to relax and regenerate is equally important. Relaxation is a process vital to good health. Quiet time, breathing exercises, or meditation, even for a minute will bring strength, whether walking, standing still, or resting. Taking a long hot bath or sitting in a hot tub is another way to relax your body and your mind. Put on some light music, light a candle, and soak for 20-30 minutes.

Make time every day to do something restful and enjoyable.

JOURNALING

As I mentioned in my story, writing became an invaluable tool that allowed me to overcome my emotional attachments to unhealthy foods. Writing in a journal can be a new form of comfort food without the calories, or as enlightening as a session with a psychologist without the hourly fee. Keeping a journal is more than an outlet for creativity. It's a meditative, stress-relieving experience as potent as any pill. Writing things down is a way of coping with life. It's a way of communing with yourself. A journal is a place of emotional freedom, a place where you can be completely honest.

Writing is a powerful tool that allows us to access feelings that we may not always be aware of until we start writing about them. The practice of writing in a journal on a regular basis helps us to see patterns in our behaviors and thinking. Writing also strengthens and trains our minds to look for our motivations for wanting to eat when we're not hungry.

A journal can be used in any of the following ways:

- Write at least one page in a journal every day, preferably in the morning. Writing in the morning helps to ground us in our intentions for the coming day.
- Write out feelings rather than acting on them or avoiding them. Describe your feelings when you feel a lot of anything, even if you can't put names to your feelings.
- Use your journal to write down what you eat every day. This encourages honesty and accountability. I have included a daily checklist on page **185** to help you keep track of your food intake.
- Write about decisions you have to make. List pros and cons of your choices. This will help clear your thinking process.
- Ask yourself questions that will help you change your thinking and behaviors. In her book *The Right Questions*, author Debbie Ford presented a set of 10 essential questions to guide us to an extraordinary life. I found many of the questions can apply directly to situations where food and life choices are involved. For example, in any situation, you can ask yourself the following

questions and then write your answers and feelings in a journal:

- Will this choice bring me closer to my goals or take me away from my goals?
- Will this choice bring me long-term fulfillment or will it bring me short-term gratification?
- Will this choice add to my life force or will rob me of my energy?
- Will I use this situation as a growth opportunity or will I use it to beat myself up?
- Does this choice empower me or does it dis-empower me?
- Is this an act of self-love or an act of self-sabotage?
- Am I acting out of commitment or am I acting out of emotion?[1]

Keeping a journal is easy. You can use a softbound composition notebook, loose-leaf paper, or a hardbound book with blank pages. It doesn't matter what you write on, it just matters that you write!

AVOID REFINED AND PROCESSED FOODS

The success of Plan-D depends as much on what you don't eat as on what you do. **Reduce or eliminate the following:**

- **Excessive Caffeine:** This means those sugary coffee drinks and caffeinated colas. Caffeine is a non-nutritive substance that has been found to elicit cravings. Just two cups of coffee will make your body secrete 80% more adrenaline than normal. Adrenaline increases insulin secretion, which in turn lowers blood sugar levels and triggers feelings of hunger, which you may identify as cravings. Secondly, caffeine is a liver stressor, which will inhibit your body's ability to effectively burn fat.
- **Carbonated Drinks:** Sodas, especially diet sodas, are potentially the largest contributor to calcium loss leading to a host of degenerative diseases. Diet sodas are the worst as they leave a high acid residue in the body. In fact, diet sodas actually cause you to gain weight, not lose weight, because they create acidic body chemistry, altering your metabolism, leading to a slower metabolic rate.
- **Refined "White" Foods:** As mentioned before, you will not achieve optimal health if you continue to eat refined and processed foods; therefore they are not included in Plan-D. In general, you should avoid the following white foods:
  - Refined White Sugar
  - Refined White Flour
  - White Rice
  - Artificial Sweeteners
- **Trans-Fats (Partially Hydrogenated or Hydrogenated Oils):** Read every food ingredient list and avoid anything with these deadly oils. Fast food joints and restaurants use them liberally. Beware!

- **Processed Soy Foods:** Products made from soy in its unfermented state should be avoided. These would include soy burgers, soy hot dogs, soy crumbles, soy yogurt, soymilk, and isolated soy proteins that are added to many foods to increase protein content. Soy protein isolates are found in most protein bars and many canned and frozen dinner type foods. Unfermented soy foods are said to inhibit our bodies from absorbing calcium, protein, magnesium, zinc and iron because they are quite high in phytic acid. Phytate is a salt that makes calcium, zinc, iron and other nutrients insoluble so that the body does not absorb them properly. The fermentation process (for tofu, tempeh, miso, soy sauce, and tamari sauce) reduces the phytates in soybeans, so only those unfermented forms of soy are OK to include in Plan-D. Most whole foods nutritionists agree that certain derivatives of soy, such as soybean oil, hydrolyzed vegetable protein, hydrolyzed soy protein, and soy protein isolates should be avoided.
- **Pork and Shellfish:** With the exception of some occasional crisp bacon, as the Cayce readings recommend, pork and pork products, and shellfish are not recommended on Plan-D for several reasons. First, pigs and shellfish are the scavengers and garbage collectors of their environments. They are unclean and the most polluted and toxic beings on the planet. Eating these creatures increases our own risk of ill health and toxicity. If you do occasionally indulge in some crisp bacon, make sure it comes from an organic source (or at least antibiotic-free), and is uncured without added nitrates, nitrites, or chemical preservatives.

PLAN-D DAILY SUMMARY	
Food Type	Amount Per Day
Non-Starchy Vegetables Dark Leafy Greens Rainbow Vegetables	 Unlimited, 2 portions minimum Unlimited, 2 portions minimum
Legumes	2 portions
Beneficial Carbohydrates Starchy Vegetables Whole Grains	4 portions
Fruits	3 portions
High Quality Proteins	8 portions
Health Promoting Fats and Oils Coconut Oil and Coconut Products Omega-3 Oils Other Oils, Nuts and Seeds	 2 to 4 portions 2 to 4 portions 4 portions
High Quality Multiple Vitamin	Divided Dose—one in the morning, one in the evening with a meal
Warm Lemon Water	One 8-ounce glass upon arising
Vitality Vinegar Tonic	Three times daily, 20 minutes before meals
Adequate Water	Body Weight (lbs.) ÷ 2 - 32 = number of ounces of pure water per day
Exercise	30-60 minutes or more

PLAN-D DAILY SPECIFICS

DARK GREEN LEAFY VEGETABLES
Daily Amount: Unlimited (minimum of 2 portions per day)
Portion Size: 1 cup raw, cooked, or raw juiced

Arugula	Beet greens
Bok-choy	Butterhead lettuce
Cabbage, all types	Chard, all types
Chinese Cabbage (Napa Cabbage)	Collard greens
Dandelion greens	Endive
Escarole	Frisse
Green loose-leaf lettuce	Kale
Mustard greens	Raddichio
Red loose-leaf lettuce	Romaine
Spinach	Spring mix
Turnip greens	Watercress

RAINBOW VEGETABLES
Daily Amount: Unlimited (minimum of 2 portions per day)
Portion Size: 1 cup raw, cooked, or raw juiced

Artichokes	Alfalfa Sprouts	Asparagus
Bamboo shoots	Bean sprouts	Beets
Bell peppers	Broccoli	Brussels sprouts
Carrots	Cauliflower	Celery
Chives	Cucumbers	Daikon
Eggplant	Jicama	Kohlrabi
Leeks	Mexican Gray Squash	Mushrooms
Okra	Onions, all types	Parsley
Radishes	Rutabagas	Rhubarb
Sauerkraut	Scallions	Shallots
String Beans, green and yellow	Snap Peas	Snow Peas
Sorrel	Sprouts, all types	Summer Squashes
Tomatoes	Turnips	Water Chestnuts
Yellow Crookneck Squash	Yellow Straightneck Squash	Zucchini

LEGUMES

Daily Amount: 2 portions per day
Portion size: Each of the following equals 1 portion

LEGUMES	PORTION SIZE (COOKED)
Adzuki beans	½ cup
Black beans	½ cup
Black-eyed peas	½ cup
Cannelini beans (white Kidney beans)	½ cup
Garbanzo beans	½ cup
Hummus	½ cup
Kidney beans	½ cup
Lentils, all types	½ cup
Lima beans	½ cup
Navy beans	½ cup
Pinto beans	½ cup
Split peas	½ cup
White beans	½ cup

BENEFICIAL CARBOHYDRATES:
STARCHY VEGETABLES AND WHOLE GRAINS

Daily Amount: 4 portions per day
Portion size: Each of the following equals 1 portion

STARCHY VEGETABLES:	PORTION SIZE (COOKED)
Green Peas	½ cup
Acorn Squash	½ cup
Banana Squash	½ cup
Butternut Squash	½ cup
Hubbard Squash	½ cup
Parsnips	½ cup
Pumpkin	½ cup
Spaghetti Squash	½ cup
Potatoes	½ cup measured if boiled, mashed, or fried 4 ounces weighed out if baked
Sweet Potatoes	½ cup measured if boiled, mashed, or fried 4 ounces weighed out if baked
Yams	½ cup measured if boiled, mashed, or fried 4 ounces weighed out if baked

WHOLE GRAINS:	PORTION SIZE (COOKED)
Amaranth	½ cup
Barley	½ cup
Brown rice	½ cup
Buckwheat	½ cup
Bulgur	½ cup
Corn kernels	½ cup
Corn on the Cob	½ cob
Cornmeal, whole grain with germ	2 tablespoons, dry
Kamut	½ cup
Millet	½ cup
Oats	½ cup
Polenta, cooked	½ cup
Quinoa	½ cup
Red Rice	½ cup
Rye	½ cup
Spelt	½ cup
Wild rice	½ cup
Whole Wheat	½ cup

WHOLE GRAIN BREADS:	PORTION SIZE
Sprouted Grain Bread	1 slice
Sprouted Grain English Muffin	½ muffin
Sprouted Grain Bagel	½ bagel
Sprouted Grain Burger Bun	½ bun
Sprouted Grain Hot Dog Bun	½ bun
Sprouted Grain Tortilla	1 tortilla
Corn Tortilla (6-inch)	2 tortillas
Baked Blue Corn Tortilla Chips	1 ounce, about 18 chips
Plan-D Flourless Muffins	1 muffin
Whole Grain Pancakes	two 4-inch pancakes
100% Whole Spelt Bread	1 slice
100 % Whole Wheat Bread	1 slice
Gluten-Free Breads	1 slice

WHOLE GRAIN PASTAS:	PORTION SIZE (COOKED)
Ezekiel Sprouted Grain pasta	½ cup cooked
Brown Rice pasta	½ cup cooked
Corn pasta	½ cup cooked
Quinoa pasta	½ cup cooked
Whole Spelt pasta	½ cup cooked
Whole Wheat Orzo	½ cup cooked
Whole Wheat pasta	½ cup cooked

WHOLE GRAIN CRACKERS:	PORTION SIZE
Ak-Mak 100% whole wheat cracker	5 sections
Brown Rice Cakes, unsalted	2 rice cakes
Mary's Gone Crackers (gluten-free organic whole grain and seed crackers)	Check package for portion size
Rye-Vita 100% Rye Crackers	2 crackers

WHOLE GRAIN CEREALS, BRAN, GERM	PORTION SIZE (COOKED)
Ezekiel Sprouted Grain Cereal	½ cup
Granola (low sugar content)	½ cup
Kasha	¼ cup uncooked, about ½ cup cooked
Oat Bran	¼ cup uncooked, about ½ cup cooked
Oatmeal	¼ cup uncooked, about ½ cup cooked
Puffed cereal, unsweetened	1 cup
Shredded Wheat Cereal	Shredded Wheat Cereal
Uncle Sam's Cereal	3/4 cup
Wheat Bran	¼ cup uncooked
Wheat Germ	¼ cup
Whole Grain Hot Cereals, unsweetened	¼ cup uncooked, about ½ cup cooked
Other whole grain unsweetened cereal	¾ cup or check package for serving size

MISCELLANEOUS	
Rice Milk, unsweetened	1 cup

FRUITS
Daily Amount: 3 portions
Portion Size: Each of the following equals 1 portion:

FRUIT	PORTION SIZE
Apples	1 large
Applesauce, unsweetened	1 cup
Apricots, fresh	4 medium
Apricots, dried	8 halves
Bananas	1 medium
Berries	
Blackberries	1 cup
Blueberries	1 cup
Cranberries	1 cup
Raspberries	1 cup
Strawberries	1 ½ cup
Cherries	20 large
Dates	4 whole
Figs, fresh	2 whole
Figs, dried	2 whole
Grapefruit	1 medium
Grapes, all types	20
Kiwi fruit	2 small
Mango	1 small
Melons	
Cantaloupe	½ small
Honeydew	¼ medium
Watermelon	2 cups cubed
Nectarine	2 small
Oranges	1 large
Papaya	1 ½ cups
Peach	2 medium
Pear	1 medium
Persimmon	2 medium
Pineapple	1 cup cubed
Plums	4 medium

Prunes	4 medium
Prune Juice	½ cup
Raisins	4 tablespoons
Tangelos	1 large
Tangerines	2 medium
Frozen Fruit, natural unsweetened	1 cup
Dried Fruit, unsweetened, no sulfites	¼ cup
Fruit Juice, fresh	1 cup (8 ounces)
100% Fruit Jams and Preserves	1 tablespoon
Honey, raw	1 tablespoon
Agave nectar	2 tablespoons
Maple Syrup, pure	1 tablespoon

HIGH QUALITY PROTEIN

Daily Amount: Up to 8 portions per day total
Portion Size: Each of the following equals 1 portion:

FOOD	PORTION SIZE
FISH (WILD CAUGHT IS BEST)	
Cod	1 ounce cooked
Grouper	1 ounce cooked
Haddock	1 ounce cooked
Halibut	1 ounce cooked
Herring	1 ounce cooked
Mahi mahi	1 ounce cooked
Mackerel	1 ounce cooked
Orange Roughy	1 ounce cooked
Sardines (canned in water or olive oil only)	1 ounce
Salmon, fresh	1 ounce cooked
Salmon, canned boneless skinless	1 ounce
Salmon, canned with bones and skin	1 ounce
Sea Bass	1 ounce cooked
Snapper	1 ounce cooked
Sole	1 ounce cooked
Tilapia	1 ounce cooked

Trout	1 ounce cooked
Whitefish	1 ounce cooked
Tuna, fresh	1 ounce cooked
Tuna, canned in water only	1 ounce

POULTRY

Chicken	1 ounce cooked
Cornish game hen	1 ounce cooked
Duck	1 ounce cooked
Turkey	1 ounce cooked
Chicken or Turkey Bacon (no nitrates or nitrites)	1 ounce cooked
Chicken or Turkey Sausage (no pork casings, no nitrates or nitrites)	1 ounce cooked
Chicken or Turkey Deli Meats and Hot Dogs (no synthetic additives, nitrates or nitrites)	1 ounce cooked

MEAT (ALL LEAN TYPES)

Beef	1 ounce cooked
Buffalo	1 ounce cooked
Lamb	1 ounce cooked
Liver (must be organic)	1 ounce cooked
Veal	1 ounce cooked
Venison	1 ounce cooked
Beef Deli Meats and Hot Dogs (no synthetic additives, no pork casings, no nitrates or nitrites)	1 ounce cooked

EGGS

EGGS	1 egg

DAIRY

Milk	1 cup
Yogurt	1 cup
Goat Yogurt	1 cup
Kefir	1 cup
Cottage Cheese	½ cup
Ricotta cheese	½ cup

Goat Cheese, soft	1 ounce
All other soft cheeses (bleu cheese, feta, etc.)	1 ounce
Hard Cheeses (Cheddar, Jack, Mozzarella, etc.)	1 ounce

FERMENTED SOY FOODS	
Tofu	½ cup
Tempeh	½ cup

PROTEIN POWDERS	
Whey Protein Powder (lactose free with negligible carbohydrates—unsweetened or stevia sweetened brands only)	1 scoop (about 25 grams protein)
Goat Whey Protein Powder (lactose free with negligible carbohydrates—unsweetened or stevia sweetened brands only)	2 scoops (about 33 grams protein)
Hemp Protein Powder— unsweetened or stevia sweetened brands only	4 tablespoons (about 15 grams protein)
Brown Rice Protein Powder - unsweetened or stevia sweetened brands only	2 tablespoons (about 15 grams protein)

MISCELLANEOUS	
Almond Milk, unsweetened	1 cup
Hemp Milk, unsweetened	1 cup

HEALTH PROMOTING FATS AND OILS:

EXTRA VIRGIN COCONUT OIL AND COCONUT PRODUCTS
Daily Amount: 2 to 4 portions per day, at least 2 portions should come from extra virgin coconut oil.
Portion Size: The portion size varies depending on the type of coconut product. Refer to the below list for portion sizes
Note: Coconut oil is best used for cooking, however it can also be added into smoothies, soups, oatmeal and other hot cereals, and as a spread in place of butter.

Food	Portion Size
Extra Virgin Coconut Oil (Best used for cooking)	1 tablespoon
Coconut Milk, fresh or canned, unsweetened	1/3 cup
Fresh Coconut Meat	2 ounces
Coconut Cream, unsweetened	1 tablespoon
Dried coconut, unsweetened	2 tablespoons

OMEGA-3
Daily Amount: 2 to 3 portions per day.
Portion Size: The portion size varies depending on the type of oil. Refer to the below list for portion sizes.
Note: Always take omega-3 oils with a meal. DO NOT TAKE MORE THAN TWO PORTIONS AT THE SAME MEAL.

You must divide the portions equally and take them at different times throughout the day. These oils are extremely sensitive to heat and light, therefore they should never be heated or used for cooking. Keep them in dark bottles in the refrigerator.

Omega-3 Fats	Portion Size
High Lignan Flaxseed Oil	1 tablespoon
Hempseed Oil	1 tablespoon
Fish Oil	1 teaspoon
Cod Liver Oil	1 teaspoon

OTHER BENEFICIAL FATS AND OILS
Daily Amount: Up to 4 portions daily
Portion Size: The portion size varies depending on the type of fat/oil. Refer to the below list for portion sizes.

Extra Virgin Olive Oil	1 teaspoon
Olives	5 olives
Avocado	1/4 avocado
Butter, organic	1 teaspoon
Peanut Oil, Expeller Pressed Unrefined	1 teaspoon
Safflower Mayonnaise	1 teaspoon
Sesame Oil, Expeller Pressed Unrefined	1 teaspoon

SEEDS

Flaxseeds	1 tablespoon
Hempseeds	1 tablespoon
Pumpkin Seeds, also called Pepitas	1 tablespoon
Sesame Seeds	1 tablespoon
Sunflower Seeds	1 tablespoon

NUTS

Almonds	1 ounce, about 23 almonds
Brazil Nuts	1 ounce, about 5 nuts

Cashews	1 ounce, about 18 nuts
Hazelnuts	1 ounce, about 20 nuts
Macadamia	1 ounce, about 10 nuts
Nut and Seed Butters, includes Sesame Tahini	1 tablespoon
Peanuts, dry roasted, unsalted	1 ounce, about 28 nuts
Pecans	1 ounce, about 19 pecan halves
Pistachios	1 ounce, about 47 nuts
Walnuts	1 ounce, about 10 walnut halves
FSA – a combination of ground flax seeds, sunflower seeds, and almonds (see recipe page 209	1 tablespoon

FAT BURNING HERBS AND SPICES

Daily Amount: There are no specific portions sizes for herbs and spices. Use them liberally in your cooking or added to foods. These herbs and spices are thermogenic, meaning they create heat in the body, raise metabolism and burn fat.

Allspice	Cardamom
Cayenne	Cinnamon
Coriander	Cumin
Dried mustard	Garlic
Ginger	

BEVERAGES

Teas may be sweetened with stevia or a small amount of agave nectar.

Dandelion root tea	Green tea
Milk thistle tea	Red rooibos tea
White tea	Yerba Mate
All naturally decaffeinated herbal teas	

SWEETENERS

Stevia (unlimited)

OTHER NATURAL SWEETENERS

A total of 1 tablespoon per day (combined) of the following:
Agave Nectar (2 teaspoons)
Raw Honey (1 teaspoon)
Pure Maple Syrup (1 Tablespoon)

CONDIMENTS AND SEASONINGS

Enjoy these condiments and seasonings added to foods and recipes:

Apple Cider Vinegar, Raw Unfiltered	Baking powder, non-aluminum	Baking soda
Brown Rice Vinegar	Celtic Sea Salt – use sparingly, not more than 1 teaspoon per day	Herbamare seasoning
Herbs, dried, all types	Herbs, fresh, all types	Mustard
Pure Extracts, vanilla, almond, mint, etc.	Salsa, fresh or jarred	Soy Sauce, reduced sodium
Spices, no added stabilizers (read labels carefully)	Taco Seasoning, see recipe page 240	Tomato sauce and paste, canned, no additives
Wheat-Free Tamari Sauce, reduced sodium	Miso	

WATER AND SUPPLEMENTS

Morning: Upon arising, drink one 8 ounce glass of warm water with the juice of ½ a lemon.

20 Minutes Before Meals: Drink one 8-ounce glass of Vitality Vinegar Tonic

Twice each day: Take a high quality food-based multiple vitamin and mineral supplement, with a meal.

Throughout the Day: Drink an adequate amount of pure water for a total of half your body weight in ounces of water.

IF YOU MUST...

Coffee: 1 or 2 cups daily, black or sweetened with a natural sweetener. No milk or cream.

Sugar: Rapadura or Sucanat unrefined organic whole cane sugar
(1 portion = 1 teaspoon)

Non-sprouted bread: 100% whole wheat or other whole grain bread (read labels carefully) 1 slice = 1 grain portion

Non-sprouted tortilla: 100% whole wheat or other whole grain tortilla (read labels carefully) – 1 tortilla = 1 grain portion

Popcorn: organic, popped in coconut oil, seasoned with sea salt – 3 cups = 1 grain portion

PLAN-D DAILY CHECKLIST

Morning Lemon Water ☐ 8 oz.	**Dark Leafy Green Vegetables–minimum of 2 cups daily** ☐ ½ cup ☐ ½ cup ☐ ½ cup ☐ ½ cup ☐ ½ cup ☐ ½ cup
Vitality Vinegar Tonic ☐ 8 oz. ☐ 8 oz. ☐ 8 oz.	**Rainbow Vegetables– minimum of 2 cups daily** ☐ ½ cup ☐ ½ cup ☐ ½ cup ☐ ½ cup ☐ ½ cup ☐ ½ cup
Coconut Oil/Coconut Products ☐ 1 portion ☐ 1 portion ☐ 1 portion ☐ 1 portion	**Legumes** ☐ 1 portion ☐ 1 portion
Omega-3 Oil ☐ 1 portion ☐ 1 portion ☐ 1 portion ☐ 1 portion	**Beneficial Carbohydrates: Whole Grains & Starchy Vegetables** ☐ 1 portion ☐ 1 portion ☐ 1 portion ☐ 1 portion
Beneficial Fats and Oils ☐ 1 portion ☐ 1 portion ☐ 1 portion ☐ 1 portion	**Fruits** ☐ 1 portion ☐ 1 portion ☐ 1 portion
Pure Water ☐ 8 oz. ☐ 8 oz. ☐ 8 oz. ☐ 8 oz. ☐ 8 oz. ☐ 8 oz. ☐ 8 oz. ☐ 8 oz. ☐ 8 oz. ☐ 8 oz. ☐ 8 oz. ☐ 8 oz. ☐ 8 oz. ☐ 8 oz. ☐ 8 oz. ☐ 8 oz.	**High Quality Protein** ☐ 1 portion ☐ 1 portion ☐ 1 portion ☐ 1 portion ☐ 1 portion ☐ 1 portion ☐ 1 portion ☐ 1 portion
High Quality Multiple Vitamin ☐ 1 dose, morning ☐ 1 dose, evening	**EXERCISE** ☐ 20 min ☐ 20 min ☐ 20 min ☐ 20 min

MEAL PLANNING AND SAMPLE MENUS

The following meal plans will help you design your Plan-D meals. Keep in mind that these plans are not set in stone; they are a guideline for you to follow. They are intended to help you understand how to create balanced meals. Find the meals and snacks you like and mix and match. The goal is to ultimately understand how to select and balance foods whether cooking at home or eating in a restaurant. Be sure to put your personal touch to the menus. You can alter them to suit your individual taste.

It's best to follow the portion guidelines as precisely as possible. A kitchen scale and a set of measuring cups and spoons are essential kitchen tools.

If you stay out of greasy fast food establishments and instead choose restaurants that offer a wide variety of options, you can always find something that will work for you when you go out to eat. Simply remember not to eat anything made with sugar or flour, or anything that has been deep-fried. This could be as easy as ordering something like salmon, turkey, a hamburger (without the bun), steak, roast beef slices, or of course, chicken—and then adding a side of veggies. Or order a large portion of veggies and a side of brown rice or starchy vegetable.

Each menu consists of three meals and two snacks. It is important not to exceed the portions sizes, as they are designed for balancing your blood sugar levels and releasing weight. If you are too hungry in between meals, you should eat more protein, fats, or non-starchy vegetables. DO NOT EAT MORE LEGUMES OR BENEFICIAL CARBOHYDRATES, unless you are a serious athlete or a person who expends a massive amount of energy and calories during the day.

TIPS FOR MAKING MEALS:

Buy already roasted chickens at a natural food store and use them for dinners or to add to salads.

Make a trip to the natural food store. There are many varieties of frozen vegetable medleys and frozen fish that would be easy for you to prepare. They also have brown rice that is pre-cooked in the freezer section. Look for a box that contains three pouches of pre-cooked organic brown rice. It will be very easy for you to eat brown rice if you do it this way. Stock up! Note: It is not recommended to microwave the rice. You can put the pouches in a steamer and heat them that way.

Hummus is a garbanzo bean dip that can be purchased at any grocery store, or you can make it yourself (see recipe on page **235**). Hummus contains no saturated fat, no cholesterol or sugars and is high in protein and fiber. Aside from being good for you, hummus also tastes great. It is a perfect food for processed-free living. There are many different companies that make hummus. Make sure to get one that is fresh with no preservatives.

Several companies make healthy jarred marinara sauce without sugar or other additives that is good for topping baked potatoes, cooked vegetables or pastas. Read ingredient lists carefully.

It is best to make your own salad dressings, as most commercially prepared dressings are loaded with undesirable oils or additives.

If you must buy a salad dressing, a good brand is Bragg's. They carry two varieties of vinaigrettes that contain apple cider vinegar, which is extremely helpful for weight loss, lowering cholesterol, and overall good health.

Most commercial canned soups are loaded with sodium and harmful chemical preservatives. Go to a natural food market and look for such brands as Health Valley or Amy's. Better yet, make your own large pot of soup and freeze the rest for enjoyment later.

Some good whole grain crackers are: Ak-Mak, Harvest Whole Wheats, Rye-Vita, Wasa, Mary's Gone Crackers, or tamari brown rice crackers. You may also purchase crackers made from flax seeds. Do not eat any other types of crackers.

Flourless sprouted grain breads and bread products can be purchased at natural food markets and some mainstream grocery stores. These flourless whole grain breads are extremely healthy for you. Some stores may also carry sprouted grain English muffins, bagels, burger buns, hot dog buns, pita bread, and tortillas. Because there are no preservatives in sprouted grain breads, they are perishable and will usually be found in a refrigerated unit or in the freezer section of the store. When you bring them home, you should keep them refrigerated or frozen. If you keep the bread frozen, you can take out as many slices as you need and pop them in the toaster to defrost.

Healthy frozen entrees are hard find, but natural food markets carry some acceptable frozen items. Amy's Organics is a line of organic vegetarian frozen entrees, with several gluten-free varieties. Organic Bistro is another acceptable frozen entrée that contains organic vegetables, grains, meats, and poultry. Sunshine Burgers are my favorite organic vegetarian patties made from organic brown rice, nuts, and seeds.

All of these frozen items are organic and free of preservatives. They come in one or two serving sizes, so it's easy to control portions.

DAILY NUTRITIONAL MUST-DO'S

- Drink a glass of warm water with the juice of ½ lemon first thing in the morning before breakfast.
- Drink a glass of Vinegar Vitality Tonic three times each day 20 minutes before meals, or whenever it's convenient
- Drink a minimum of 8 glasses of pure room temperature water per day. Water is essential to clear waste from the blood. Thirst is often mistaken for hunger.
- Do not drink liquids with meals.
- Eat a raw salad daily.
- Take omega-3 oil and vitamin supplements in divided doses.
- Use coconut oil for cooking, in recipes, or added to foods.
- Take the time to chew food well.

SAMPLE MENUS

DAY 1	
Breakfast	½ cup Slow Cooker Irish Style Steel Cut Oats, p. 213 (save leftovers for later this week) 1 Tablespoon coconut oil mixed in to cooked oats 1 cup berries of your choice 1 cup plain yogurt, sweetened with stevia and 1 Tablespoon FSA, p. 209, and 1 Tablespoon Flaxseed oil mixed in to yogurt
Snack	1 ounce raw walnuts, 1 peach
Lunch	1 cup Red Lentil Soup, p. 234 (save leftovers for later this week) 1 Tablespoon coconut oil mixed in to soup 1 Hard Boiled Egg 2 cups Spring Mix with 1 cup mixture of chopped rainbow veggies 2 Tablespoons Sweet Herb Vinaigrette, p. 236
Snack	2 kiwis, 1 Agave Granola Bar, p. 263 (save leftovers for later this week)
Dinner	4 ounces Pecan Crusted Tilapia, p. 257 3 cups Mixed Vegetable Curry, p. 243 Take fish oil supplement with dinner
DAY 2	
Breakfast	Dee's Favorite Breakfast, p. 206
Snack	1 banana, 12 almonds
Lunch	Southwestern Sweet Potato Wrap, p. 225 2 cups Mixed Baby Greens with 1 cup mixture of chopped rainbow veggies 2 Tablespoons Sweet Herb Vinaigrette, p. 236
Snack	1 ½ cup strawberries, 2 Allowable Sin, p. 268
Dinner	4 oz. Meatloaf Florentine, p. 254 1 cup Garlic Mashed Cauliflower. p. 242 2 cups steamed broccoli and asparagus Take fish oil supplement with dinner
DAY 3	
Breakfast	½ cup Slow Cooker Irish Style Steel Cut Oats, p. 213 1 Tablespoon coconut oil mixed in to cooked oats 1 cup berries of your choice 1 cup almond milk, p. 217, or other milk Take fish oil supplement with breakfast
Snack	1 cup yogurt, 1 peach
Lunch	Tantalizing Taco Salad, p. 229
Snack	2 oz. cooked chicken wrapped in large lettuce leaves 1 cup raw rainbow veggies with ¼ cup Roasted Garlic Hummus, p. 235

Dinner	1 cup Red Lentil Soup, p. 234 (leftovers) 1 Tablespoon coconut oil mixed in to soup 2 cups steamed mixed rainbow veggies 1 Tablespoon Flaxseed Oil drizzled on steamed veggies or take fish oil supplement with dinner
DAY 4	
Breakfast	Pumpkin Smoothie, p. 207
Snack	1 orange, 1 oz. walnuts
Lunch	Bean soft tacos: 2 corn tortillas, ½ cup pinto beans, diced red bell peppers, diced onions, ½ avocado, 1 ounce cheese, 2 Tablespoons salsa 2 cups Romaine lettuce, sliced cucumber, carrots, celery 2 Tablespoons Agave Lime Dressing, p. 237
Snack	1 slice Whole Grain Zucchini bread, p. 221, 1 peach
Dinner	4 oz. Roasted Lemon Herb Chicken, p. 250 4 oz. baked sweet potato 1 cup Ginger Beets and Fennel, p. 244 1 cup steamed zucchini, yellow squash and broccoli 1 Tablespoon Flaxseed Oil drizzled on steamed veggies or potato, or take fish oil supplement with dinner
DAY 5	
Breakfast	½ cup spinach and 1 cup mixture of diced bell peppers, onions, and any other veggies you like, sautéed in 1 Tablespoon coconut oil 2 eggs, scrambled, added to veggies 1 slice sprouted grain toast or English muffin, drizzled with 1 teaspoon Flaxseed oil or butter
Snack	1 orange, 1 oz. pecans
Lunch	1 cup Hardy Barley Salad, p. 230, over 2 cups Spring Mix ½ cup Roasted Garlic Hummus, p. 235
Snack	1 cup plain yogurt, sweetened with stevia 1 cup blueberries
Dinner	4 oz. Simply Baked Sesame Halibut, p. 255 ½ cup Minty Quinoa, p. 248 2 cups mixed veggies stir-fried in 1 Tablespoon coconut oil take fish oil supplement with dinner
DAY 6	
Breakfast	1 Plan-D Flourless Muffin, p. 218 1 cup plain yogurt sweetened with stevia, with 2 Tablespoons ground flaxseeds and 1 Tablespoon Flaxseed oil mixed in 1 banana
Snack	1 cup plain yogurt, sweetened with stevia 1 cup blueberries

Lunch	Veggie Sandwich: 2 slices sprouted grain bread, 1 ounce cheese, ¼ cup hummus, ½ avocado, sliced cucumber, tomato slices, sliced red onion, shredded carrots, handful of baby lettuces or Romaine lettuce 1 hard boiled egg
Snack	1 ½ cup strawberries, 2 Allowable Sin, p. 268
Dinner	Sensational Sweet and Sour Turkey Meatballs, p. 251 ½ cup cooked brown rice 2 cups mixed veggies stir-fried in 1 Tablespoon coconut oil take fish oil supplement with dinner
DAY 7	
Breakfast	½ cup Whole Grain Cereal with ½ cup Almond Milk, p. 217, or other milk 1 banana 1 cup plain yogurt sweetened with stevia, with 2 Tablespoons ground flaxseeds and 1 Tablespoon Flaxseed oil mixed in
Snack	1 oz. raw almonds, 1 peach
Lunch	Spinach Salad: 2 cups spinach with 1 hard boiled egg, 1 ounce of cooked turkey bacon, shredded carrots, diced cucumber, diced zucchini, cherry tomatoes, chopped celery, sliced onion, ¼ cup hummus. 1 Tablespoon Flaxseed oil 2 Tablespoons Sweet Herb Vinaigrette, p. 236
Snack	2 brown rice cakes with ½ mashed avocado
Dinner	Herb Crusted Salmon on Greens, p. 256 Mashed Sweet Potatoes with Coconut Milk, p. 247 2 cups Steamed mixed veggies take fish oil supplement with dinner

PLAN-D SHOPPING LIST

Vegetables
- Green leafy vegetables like spinach, romaine, spring mix, kale, or chard
- Alfalfa sprouts
- Carrots, celery, beets, green beans and eggplant
- Leeks, shallots and cruciferous vegetables such as broccoli, cauliflower, cabbage and Brussels sprouts
- Avocado
- Garlic and onions
- Fresh Ginger Root

Fruits
- Fresh Whole Lemons
- Apples, pears, and oranges
- Bananas, watermelon
- Pineapple

- Strawberries, blueberries, raspberries
- Peaches

Nuts/Seeds
- Raw Almonds
- Raw Walnuts
- Raw sunflower seeds
- Flax seeds (already ground or whole)

Oils
- Flax Oil (Barleans or Spectrum-High Lignan)
- Unrefined Coconut Oil (Spectrum or Jarrow)
- Extra-Virgin Olive Oil
- Fish Oil (Carlsons or Nordic Naturals)

Breads/Beans/Crackers/Rice/Grains
- Canned or dry beans or lentils
- Hummus
- Brown rice
- Oatmeal, oat bran, quinoa and quinoa pasta
- Uncle Sam Cereal, Puffed Kashi, or other sugar free cereals
- Ezekiel Bread products
- Ak-Mak Crackers
- Harvest Whole Wheat Crackers
- Raw Flax Seed Crisps

Miscellaneous
- Bragg's Apple Cider Vinegar
- Eggs (preferably free range omega-3 enriched)
- Whey Protein Powder
- Stevia (liquid extract or packets)
- Lärabar (a fruit and nut energy bar)
- Think Organic (a fruit and nut energy bar)
- Greens+ Energy Bar
- Herbal Teas and Green Tea
- Coconut Milk
- Almond Milk or Rice Milk
- Plain Yogurt

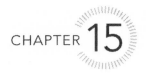

CHAPTER 15

Plan-D When Eating Out

When eating out or traveling, you've got to have a strategy or a plan ahead of time. If you fail to plan, you plan to fail. Don't leave your healthy eating commitment in the hands of others. You must take charge!

We live in a world that doesn't support healthy eating, so you've got to support yourself! My motto is always, **_BRING YOUR OWN_**. In most cases, the best way to make sure a healthy choice will be available is to bring it yourself. Follow this rule as often as possible and your chances of sticking with healthy choices are vastly improved.

SOCIAL EVENTS (POT LUCKS, WEDDINGS & CELEBRATIONS, DINNER PARTIES)

Always bring something to the potluck that is healthy for you and that others will enjoy eating. This way, you know your needs will be taken care of. If there are other dishes at the potluck that are healthy and that you enjoy, that's a great bonus!

When someone invites you for a meal at their home, ask what they'll be serving. If it doesn't suit your needs, ask for what you need or ask if you can bring something.

Despite what you may feel, it is not rude to exempt yourself from any food. There are many people who do not eat certain foods for various reasons, and you can be one of them!

RESTAURANTS AND FAST FOOD

One of the biggest challenges with eating out is avoiding the trans-fats. Basically most anything that is cooked in oil in a restaurant is cooked in unhealthy oil. There are some places that are better than others though. Olive and sesame oils are usually readily available in Italian, Greek, Spanish, Chinese, and Thai restaurants.

Seafood is always a great choice, and you can get salmon pretty much anywhere these days. Salmon and other fish should be grilled, broiled, poached, or baked in wine and seasoned with lots of garlic (specify fresh garlic, otherwise garlic salt will be used) and onions.

Some Japanese and Chinese dishes use peanut oil for stir-frying. This is acceptable.

A smart choice in Mexican restaurants is Fajitas (grilled meats and vegetables) with corn tortillas instead of flour. Guacamole, as long as there is no mayonnaise added to it, is also a great choice. Avocados contain a great source of healthy fat. Always ask for lemon wedges so you can squeeze the juice over veggies or salads. The lemon juice helps to cut the fats in the meal and assists in metabolism.

Hold back on mayonnaise because most commercially prepared mayonnaise products are made with partially hydrogenated soybean oil. That leaves out tuna, egg, shrimp, and chicken salads as well as cole slaw and potato salad.

When it comes to bread, muffins, crackers, and rolls, any made with refined white flour should be avoided. You will find that you just have to skip the bread basket in most restaurants because they just don't serve high enough quality bread. This would also be the case for pastas, which are almost always made from white flour.

Vegetables should be steamed without any seasonings or sauces.

Always order a green salad without dressing and ask for olive oil, lemon wedges, and balsamic vinegar on the side. This way you avoid the sugar that is usually in prepared vinaigrettes. You can add your own oil and vinegar and squeeze the lemon juice over the salad as well.

Ask how food is cooked so you can avoid the bad oils.

Ask for no croutons on salads (it always sucks when you forget to ask them to leave off the croutons and then you have to pick them out).

Ask for whole grain foods like brown rice and whole wheat breads (however, like I said, often times the restaurant's idea of whole wheat bread is not up to standards).

Your best bets for breakfast will be oatmeal or other whole grain cereal, eggs, fruit or veggies, cheese or cottage cheese, milk or plain yogurt. Eggs can be poached or boiled (hard or soft), or have them as an omelet with veggies.

Herbal teas are also good choices when eating out.

Here are some more tips for eating out:

- Plan ahead as much as possible.
- Go with a plan in mind (i.e., "wherever I go tonight, I'm going to have grilled fish, vegetables and a baked potato").
- Ask a lot of questions: How is the food prepared (i.e. grilled, fried, battered or breaded, etc.). Can I get extra vegetables? Can I substitute salad, vegetables or baked potato for French fries? Do you have brown rice instead of white?
- Always order salad dressing on the side and ask for no croutons.
- If others in your party don't mind, ask the server not to bring bread or chips to the table. If others in your party want the bread and chips, place the basket

away from you so that it's not within your easy reach.

- Always ask for whole wheat bread when menu items come on bread (i.e. sandwiches, burgers, toast, etc.) Sometimes I bring my own bread so I can switch it out.
- Always ask for real butter. Most restaurants use margarines in sauces and on toast.
- In Mexican restaurants, always ask for soft corn tortillas instead of white flour tortillas.
- Get whole beans instead of refried, and don't eat the rice, it's usually white rice that's been fried in vegetable oil.
- Avoid greasy fast food joints like burger places, taco stands, Chinese food, and fried chicken.

TRAVELING

By Car (this is easy, you can bring most of your own food)

Pack a small cooler with fresh fruit, cut up veggies, small cartons of milk, yogurts, cheese, tuna or egg salad. Pack a bag with dry foods such as Plan-D Flourless Muffins, dry cereal, Ak Mak crackers, Ezekiel bread, peanut or almond butter, raw nuts and seeds (or make your own trail mix). Bringing your own food reduces the need to eat fast food.

For long trips, bring enough food for most meals, and then stop at a sit down restaurant for the main meal.

By Plane (this is not as easy due to the poor quality of airport food, but still do-able)

My motto applies here: Bring Your Own as much as possible. I usually pack a small soft side cooler (lunch box size) to carry on the plane. I make up a lunch (or dinner) ahead of time and pack it to eat on the plane. Make sure you bring plastic cutlery and napkins. Beverages are usually free on the plane.

Early morning flights are easy. I bring yogurt and fruit and sometimes a muffin or cereal. These fit easily in my purse or carry on.

The same types of food that you take in the car can apply here also (crackers, nuts, fruit and veggies, etc.) When you have healthy snacks in your bag, you reduce the need to eat crappy food.

Some airports have great eating establishments, others don't. If you don't know the airport, you'd better be prepared!

STAYING IN OTHER'S HOMES

Bring Your Own. I can't stress it enough! I always bring a few things that I know may be difficult to get, such as whole grain cereals and crackers.

When you arrive, ask your host if you can make a trip to the grocery store to get a few things.

If meals will be shared, make sure you have input on what will be served.

Taking care of your healthy food needs when in social situations, in restaurants, and while traveling is vital to your success. This is the greatest act of self-care you can give to yourself. For most of us, relying on convenience and poor quality food to take care of our needs has been our downfall. Long term health and weight reduction means that you have to be prepared!

CHAPTER 16

Plan-D In Action:
STORIES OF SUCCESS

I was actually a skinny kid until I got out of high school. At that point I did start to gain some extra weight but was able to keep it under control with exercise and various fad diets. The real weight gain happened when as a young wife and new mother I stopped exercising and did not watch my food intake.

It was not until my son entered preschool that I started to exercise again and to eat a low-fat diet that I lost those extra 30 pounds. I even became a personal certified trainer. The problem I discovered, however, was that despite my exercising every day and cutting fats out of my diet, the weight crept back up on me.

As a certified personal trainer, I found it embarrassing that I could not lose those extra pounds of middle-age fat. Even though I continued to eat a low fat diet and conducted exercise classes every day, my body just would not give up those pounds. It bothered me to be advising my clients on weight loss when I continued to struggle with getting and keeping fit. It was really frustrating when I thought I was eating correctly.

In searching to find answers, I came across Dee's first book at one of the local natural food stores. Her plan made so much sense to me that I decided to sign up for her eight-week class. The classes were great! Dee taught me so much about nutrition and the science of food.

Following her plan, I started to eliminate all refined and processed foods from my diet while adding in more natural foods *including* healthy fats. I now always start my day with hot lemon juice water. Plus, with all of the veggies, fruits, grains, and healthy oils that I eat on her plan, I find that I never feel deprived. I cannot tell you how wonderful it was to be able to eat real oils again as I started making Dee's salad dressings.

I loved Dee's recipes so much. Not only have I happily lost and kept off those stubborn 25 extra pounds, my husband has lost 20 pounds by eating Dee's meals.

I feel so good and have more energy. My skin has gotten clearer, and my hair has a new shine and fullness to it that even my hairdresser commented on how healthy my hair is now.

It is so rewarding when my clients notice how trim I now look. I tell people that I was battling with fat every day and now I feel like I have won the war.

I want women experiencing the change of life who now have a weight problem to know that there is a right way to lose the weight. They can eat healthy without starving themselves.

—*Kathy Kopack, Scottsdale, Arizona*

When I was growing up my family owned their own restaurant, and as a young girl I helped out. I loved to eat the home-style foods, especially the desserts. Sweets were my downfall. As a result, I grew up weighing more than I should have.

Over the years, I yo-yo dieted using all of the popular diet programs but had only moderate success. Then several years ago, my weight really increased and I decided that I had to do something to get and stay healthy.

I had to confront the fact that my weight and health problems were about food choices and how I ate. About this same time, I attended a health seminar presented by Dee McCaffrey. She talked about her own weight history, and how she lost 100 pounds and kept it off for over 15 years.

Dee's plan made so much sense to me. I bought the book that day, read it, and immediately changed how I ate. I cleaned out my pantry of all processed food items. I then filled my refrigerator and cupboards with fresh fruits and vegetables, whole grains, lean proteins, vinegar, healthy fats like flaxseed and coconut oil. Following Dee's guidance, I started to drink lots of water with lemon juice added to it. Plus, I began to exercise at home on my own.

The results have been amazing. Within one year of following Plan-D I lost 84 pounds.

I am off all blood pressure medicine, and my health has improved so much that I can now walk up and down the stairs wherever I go. I sleep better at night and am not sluggish during the day. This is the first time in my life that I have such good results from a food plan.

The best is that I am not tempted to backslide because I now truly understand the negative effects of eating processed and refined foods on my body. I tell all of my friends and family that Plan-D is the only way to eat. I feel that I have a new lease on life!

—*Judy Sharpe, Peoria, Arizona*

I have always enjoyed food, and since my high school days have struggled with being overweight. Portion control and poor food choices were my downfall.

I have a real sweet tooth, and when I would find a food I liked, my tendency was to eat a lot of it all in one sitting. As I struggled over the years with my weight, I never understood how others could seem to eat so much and not gain weight. I dreamed of having a metabolism like my friend Bob who could eat like a horse and still stay skinny.

One Saturday I decided to check out a free introductory talk that Dee McCaffrey was giving about her nutrition plan. I was so intrigued by what she was sharing that I decided to attend her 8-week course.

When I attended Dee's food education classes I was amazed to find that if you eat a diet rich in natural foods and avoided processed foods, portion size would not be an issue. You could then eat as much natural food as you want. Dee even taught me that adding a brisk walk to my morning routine would keep my metabolism rate elevated during the day.

As I implemented these food lessons, I totally changed how I ate. It became easy to avoid processed food made with refined sugars and flours. Instead I added lots of vegetables, fruits, grains, and healthy oils like flaxseed to my food plan. I have even learned to satisfy my sweet tooth by enjoying naturally sweet fruits like mangos, apples, and papayas.

Learning to eat good, natural foods and adding exercise to my life was the answer. I found that I could have what Bob had!

The results were almost immediate. Within eight weeks, I went from 215 pounds to 180 pounds, and dropped two clothes sizes, all without feeling deprived. Today, not only do I feel better, I have more energy than I've had in a long time.

Dee was the first person to offer me nutritional advice that made sense. I know that this is a plan for life – and, it is a very good life.

—*John Bogumill, Chandler, Arizona*

Food has never been very important to me; in fact, I would just as soon ignore food as eat it. That is probably because for so many years everything I would eat would cause digestive problems. I grew up eating a very traditional diet of meats, potatoes, fats, breads, and red meat. My mom, who is in her nineties, still eats red meat everyday.

Throughout my adult life, I could never figure out a food plan that would sit well on my stomach. I just assumed that there was not a way to eat that would agree with me, and so I would eat as little as possible, or I would just skip meals altogether. As a result, I was always underweight for my height and build. I figured that this was the way my life was going to be and I toughed it out.

It was when a friend, who was being helped for migraine problems by Dee

McCaffrey, invited me to meet Dee that my life changed. After listening to my health story, Dee designed a food plan specific to my nutrition and digestion issues. But, it was not a one-time plan that cured me. Instead, Dee has worked with me over the past several years on a regular basis to modify and evaluate every aspect of the food plan she recommends.

It has been this process of fine tuning the types, quantities and combinations of foods that has helped us discover which foods my body tolerates and thrives on, and which foods I need to avoid. Following Dee's plan, I eliminated all dairy, wheat, refined sugars, and even fish from my diet. Instead, I've learned how to build my diet around whole grains like quinoa, lots of fresh vegetables, fruits, coconut milk, and natural sugars like honey or agave. I have also discovered that using protein powder in recipes, and to make smoothies, is the best way for me to absorb protein.

Today while I am still slender, I am at a healthy weight. Plus, before eating as Dee recommends, I was not only extremely underweight, I suffered from osteoporosis. After following Dee's nutrition guidelines for the past several years, the results of my most recent bone density scan showed that I have improved to the point of being back in normal range.

Now, I cook everything for myself, and have learned to plan ahead when going out to dinner or over to friend's homes. All my friends know that I will bring my own dinner, and are intrigued by the good foods I make for myself.

It has been great to see how watching me get healthy has impacted my family. I have a brother-in-law who has had some medical problems and I have inspired him to seek nutritional help. My niece even has sought help from Dee after seeing how my health improved.

Learning about nutrition from Dee was what I needed because nutrition was not taught in school when I was growing up. No one taught me about eating right. I was lucky to have met Dee. I have been so happy with the changes in my life, and I now feel so good. I have learned how to eat foods that work with my digestive system, and as a result have experienced renewed health.

She is very supportive, and I appreciate her on-going commitment to assist me in being healthy. Because of Dee, I have a new strategy for aging.

—*Ted Kreimier, Scottsdale, Arizona*

"Living in a fog" is the best way that I know to describe how I felt before I adopted Dee's eating plan. For years I was always so tired that I could barely drag myself through the day; it was a struggle just to stay awake. The doctors labeled it Chronic Fatigue Syndrome. Worse were the constant stomach pains and bloating with which I suffered that the doctors blamed on Irritable Bowl Syndrome.

Sure I tried various medicines, took recommended vitamins, and even took antidepressants prescribed by my doctor. While these medicines did help me feel better and be functional enough to pursue other help, they did not cure me. Unfortunately, I had the distressing side-affects of weight gain and feeling sluggish. It seemed that my body's metabolism kept slowing down. I would tell my husband that I felt so toxic.

Fortunately that is not the end of my story. The turning point came when my husband happened to catch a health segment being shown on one of our local TV stations that featured Dee McCaffrey. After hearing how a client of Dee's who followed her nutrition plan experienced a turn around in her health, my husband encouraged me to contact Dee.

I was at a point to try something different from all of the low calorie diets and medicines that I had been using. The problem I found with regular diets is that they are about cutting calories and not really about correct nutrition. Nothing I was doing was healing me.

When I had my first meeting with Dee, right off the bat she told me that I looked toxic! I knew then that I was on the correct track. Dee designed a plan that I followed to the letter. After completing a digestive cleanse, I totally changed how I ate by cutting from my food plan all gluten, dairy, processed foods, sugars, and anything artificial. Instead Dee designed a plant-based meal plan for me that was full of vegetables, grains, beans, lean protein, and fruits. I even got to add healthy oils like flaxseed and coconut oil, which was a revelation to me.

Almost immediately I felt the change – it was so amazing how my body responded to eating this new way. My body finally started to function normally for the first time in ten years as both my IBS problems and the chronic fatigue symptoms stopped. Not only was I no longer feeling sluggish and bloated, my extra thirty pounds of weight literally started to fall away. I was eating so much food and yet did not have to count calories.

I had to face the reality that I am a flour, refined sugar and food addict. Coming from an Italian family where meals included lots of pastas, breads, and desserts, I had made those my major food groups. Today, I make different choices, and for me, eating healthy is an all or nothing decision. I would tell readers of Dee's book that if you have tried other diets and food plans and nothing has worked, do try Plan-D – it is different and you will see results.

My friends and family began commenting on how much brighter I looked. My energy level improved to the point that I no longer went through the day groggy and it was no longer a struggle to stay awake. My husband and daughter tell me how much they like me this way, and have become my biggest support system. Today if they see me being tempted to eat bread, they almost rip it out of my hands. They support the new food choices that I make whether at home, at restaurants, or when we go on vacation. It does take more time to plan ahead, and commit to a mindset to not backslide, but for me it is so worth it.

—*Audry Britton, Glendale, Arizona*

I am a breast cancer survivor. Although over the years I had tried various weight loss programs, it was not until my cancer surgery in 2005 that I faced the realization that I was not eating as healthy as I should. I knew I had to improve the way I ate to lose weight and to stay healthy. My lucky day was when a friend referred me to Dee McCaffrey because meeting Dee was an answer to my prayers.

I enrolled in Dee's food education course, and was totally enthralled by the information Dee shared. I am the type of person who needs to learn the "why" behind things. Dee taught me the "why" of her food plan, and the relationship of her recommended foods on good health.

I immediately changed how I eat. Today I feel so much better about what I put into my body. I no longer have any desire for processed foods with its disgusting fats, salt, and sugars. Dee influenced me to join a workout exercise program. I feel great and love that my muscles are stronger and I have so much more energy.

Although I still need to lose a few additional pounds, over the past two years I have been able to maintain a steady weight, despite daily medications I have to take. I am very happy with this as following Plan-D for me is not just about weight loss. It is about how wonderful I feel every day.

I tell everyone that Dee is my guardian angel. I was blessed to have met her when I was ready to learn and willing to face the truth that my old food habits were slowly killing my body. Without Dee I would not have known how to change my food habits and where to get the right information. She came into my life at the point I needed her most, and she gave me a recipe for long-term health. I just wish that I could have met her twenty years earlier.

—*Elizabeth Theilin, Glendale, Arizona*

Developing high blood pressure was a wake-up call for me. I was so upset at being put on blood pressure medicine and knowing the potential negative effects on my kidneys that I resolved to find a way to get healthy and get off the medicine.

About this same time I came across an advertisement about Dee McCaffrey's sugar-free living plan. It sparked my interest and I decided to sign-up for her eight-week nutrition class.

For me, attending Dee's eight-week food education program was life changing. She helped me to fully embrace a new way of eating as she taught me how the food choices that I make impact my metabolism. In fact, her plan is the only one that I have tried that got my metabolism working right.

I found Dee's plan to be so sensible and easy to follow because the plan is explained and laid-out in layman's terms. I found that when I ate a diet comprised of at least 60% fruits, vegetables, whole grains, and beans, along with healthy oils as Dee recommended, my energy level increased and my blood pressure decreased.

I credit following Dee McCaffrey's food plan for my being able to naturally lower my high blood pressure. It felt wonderful when my doctor was able to get me off prescribed blood pressure medicines.

Within three months of eating this way and by eliminating all processed foods which contain refined sugars, flours and unhealthy fats, I not only lost 15 pounds, I found that I had more energy than I had had in years! I am 63 years old and still have the energy to work 16-18- hours per day.

I did not know what feeling good was until I adopted Dee's program. This is a plan that I take with me wherever I go including bringing my own salad dressing with me to restaurants. My new motto is, "cook my own; carry my own". Today, Dee's food plan is the kingpin for all of my food choices and food decisions.

—*Ted Alber, Tempe, Arizona*

I was referred to Dee McCaffrey for treatment of my arthritis by my own doctor, whose arthritis had been helped from following Dee's food plan. Although I was also 65 pounds overweight, I figured that the extra weight was just age-related. I was not looking to lose weight when I met Dee for consultation.

Within three days of adopting Dee's food plan, I noticed I had less joint pain as I walked to my mailbox. I continued to eliminate processed foods, refined sugars and wheat products, and increased my intake of vegetables, fruits, healthy oils, and lean protein as she recommended. Not only did my arthritis pain disappear, my extra weight literally melted away.

Within four months, I had lost 65 pounds. It has been one year now and my weight has remained steady at a wonderful 125 pounds.

I get up in the morning without aches and pains; my skin is better; my hair is shinier and healthier. Even my nasal allergy symptoms have been reduced to the point that I no longer have to take allergy medicine.

As my arthritis pains decreased, Dee worked with me to include yoga exercise into my daily routine. It is amazing how good I feel.

From working with Dee and following her plan, I now know that food is a fuel, not a reward. I understand the effect of food on my body's pH, and the need to eliminate refined sugars, meats that are tainted with antibiotics and hormones, and unhealthy fats for me to stay healthy.

Today my body works *so* well. This plan is simple to follow and so satisfying that I am not tempted to backslide. With all of the vegetables, fruits, healthy oils, and lean protein that I eat daily, I am never hungry.

Recently, I was flattered and delighted when a local television station included my story on one of their health segments. I was so happy to let others know about how well Dee's food plan works.

I rave about this food plan to my family and friends. I encourage everyone to give Plan-D a week and see how much better they will feel.

—*Colleen Politi, Glendale, Arizona, Caring Harps Music for Bedside*
www.caringharps.com

CHAPTER 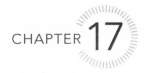 17

Plan-D Recipes

A SPECIAL NOTE TO DIABETICS

Some of the recipes in this book call for natural sweeteners that are not appropriate for diabetics to consume. Although raw unfiltered honey, pure maple syrup and Rapadura contain valuable enzymes and nutrients; the natural sugars contained in them can exacerbate a diabetic condition. The preferred sweeteners for anyone who is diabetic, and the ONLY sweeteners I recommend, are *stevia* and agave nectar. Stevia does not affect blood sugar levels and in fact has been shown to heal the pancreas in type 2 diabetics. Agave nectar is a very low glycemic sweetener, approved by the Glycemic Research Institute and is therefore safe for diabetic consumption. Even if you are not diabetic, you would do well to replace sugar with these healthy alternatives. Artificial sweeteners such as saccharine (Sweet 'n Low), Aspartame (Nutrasweet and Equal), Acesulfame Potassium (Acesulfame K), and Sucralose (Splenda) should be avoided due to their unnatural chemical properties, which have been linked to many health conditions and diseases.

A SPECIAL NOTE TO CELIACS

If you are intolerant to wheat and/or gluten, the majority of the recipes in this book are safe for you to consume. It is the philosophy of processed-free living to minimize exposure to wheat and gluten containing grains.

BRILLIANT BREAKFASTS

Dee's Favorite Breakfast

This meal packs a lot of nutrition into one small bowl!

Servings: 1 (serving size = 1 cup yogurt plus toppings and mix-ins)

Ingredients:
1 cup plain fat-free yogurt (preferably organic)
½ teaspoon cinnamon
1 teaspoon pure vanilla extract
3 drops liquid stevia extract
2 tablespoons ground flaxseeds or FSA (see page 209)
2 tablespoons raw oat bran
1 tablespoon dried unsweetened shredded coconut or coconut flakes
1 tablespoon sliced almonds
1 cup fresh fruit, such as blueberries, raspberries, kiwi fruit, sliced strawberries (or a medley of several different fruits)
1 portion Omega-3 oil

Instructions:
Combine yogurt, cinnamon, vanilla and stevia in small bowl. Stir and mix until you no longer see the color of the vanilla. Add flax seeds or FSA, oat bran, and oil. Mix well until all oil is absorbed. Top with dried coconut, sliced almonds, and fruit. Enjoy!

Nutrition per serving:
382 calories; 15 g Total Fat; 3 grams saturated fat; 17 g protein; 45 g carbohydrates; 8 grams dietary fiber; 0 mg cholesterol; 177 mg sodium.

Did you know?
All of the fat grams in this recipe come from the type of oil that makes your body burn more fat and help to lower cholesterol levels, so don't be alarmed by it's high fat content. The heart healthy omega-3 from flax oil and flax seeds, the metabolism-boosting saturated fat from coconut, and the cholesterol lowering monounsaturated fat from almonds are all Plan-D friendly. People who regularly include these types of oils in their diets safely lose weight and are healthier than those who don't!

Pumpkin Smoothie

Servings: 1

Ingredients:
1/3 cup coconut milk
2/3 cup water
3 drops liquid stevia extract
1 tablespoons ground flaxseeds or FSA (see page 209)
1 scoop (about 1/8 cup) Protein Powder (whey, goat, rice, or hemp)
1 tablespoon pumpkin pie spice
1/2 cup cooked pumpkin, canned or fresh
1 portion Omega-3 oil

Instructions:
Place all ingredients into a blender and blend until smooth and creamy. Drink immediately.

Nutrition per serving:
465 calories; 30 g Total Fat; 10 grams saturated fat; 29 g protein; 19 g carbohydrates; 4 grams dietary fiber; 0 mg cholesterol; 197 mg sodium.

Did you know?
You can make your own pumpkin pie spice by combining the following:

1 ½ teaspoons ground cinnamon
¾ teaspoon ground ginger
¼ teaspoon ground nutmeg
¼ teaspoon ground cloves

Nutritional Powerhouse Smoothie

Smoothies are highly nutritious and simple to prepare complete meals. They are also one of the easiest ways to incorporate the good healthy oils into your meal.

Servings: 1

Ingredients:
1/3 cup coconut milk
2/3 cup water
3 drops liquid stevia extract
1 tablespoons ground flaxseeds or FSA (see page 209)
1 scoop (about 1/8 cup) Protein Powder (whey, rice, or hemp)
1 tablespoon Green Powder
½ cup fresh or frozen blueberries or other fruits of your choosing
1 portion Omega-3 oil

Instructions:
Place all ingredients into a blender and blend until smooth and creamy. Drink immediately.

Nutrition per serving:
455 calories; 30 g Total Fat; 10 grams saturated fat; 28 g protein; 18 g carbohydrates; 3 grams dietary fiber; 0 mg cholesterol; 194 mg sodium.

Variations:
You can change the ingredients for different taste profiles. Add nuts and nut butters, carob powder, cacao powder, or yogurt.

FSA
(Flax Seeds, Sunflower Seeds, and Almonds)

This is a great fiber supplement. Sprinkle into yogurt, oatmeal, or onto salads!

Servings: 3 (serving size = 1 tablespoon)

Ingredients:
1 tablespoon raw whole flax seeds
1 tablespoon raw sunflower seeds
1 tablespoon raw almonds

Instructions:
Place 1 tablespoon each of sunflower seeds, almonds, and flaxseeds into a coffee grinder or seed mill. Grind until the mixture comes to a fine powdery consistency. Store in a tightly sealed container away from light.

Nutrition per serving:
48 calories; 4 g Total Fat; <1 gram saturated fat; 1.5 g protein; 1.5 g carbohydrates; 0.7 grams dietary fiber; 0 mg cholesterol; 0 mg sodium.

Bell Pepper, Basil and Spinach Crustless Quiche

Servings: 4

Ingredients:
8 eggs
½ cup green bell pepper, diced
½ cup red bell pepper, diced
½ cup fresh basil
1 cup fresh spinach
½ cup chopped onion
2 cloves garlic, minced
½ cup coconut milk
Salt and pepper to taste (optional)
1 tablespoon coconut oil, plus more for coating pan

Instructions:
Preheat oven to 375°F.

Place oil in a skillet over medium heat. Sauteé peppers, onions, and garlic until the peppers are soft, about 10 minutes. Add the spinach and basil and cook just until slightly wilted, about 1-2 minutes. Remove from heat.

Whisk eggs, coconut milk, salt and pepper if using, together in a large bowl, or place in a blender and blend until well mixed.

Coat a 9-inch pie pan (deep dish works best) or an oven safe skillet with coconut oil. Spread the cooked vegetables over the bottom of the dish or pan. Pour egg mixture over top of vegetables. Place dish or pan on center rack of oven and bake for 30-45 minutes, or until center of quiche is set. Let cool slightly then cut into four equal pieces.

Nutrition per serving:
227 calories; 15 g Total Fat; 7 gram saturated fat; 15 g protein; 7 g carbohydrates; 1 grams dietary fiber; 425 mg cholesterol; 170 mg sodium.

Did you know?
Making a crustless quiche is not much different than making a regular quiche. Actually it's easier, because you have one less thing to deal with. You always need some oil in the recipe to keep it from sticking to the pan, so we use coconut milk in the recipe and coconut oil for coating the pan.

You can add more veggies to this recipe, just remember to cook them first before adding to the quiche. If the veggies are not cooked first, your quiche may become too watery.

Easy Veggie Crust Variation: Bake some sweet potatoes. Then slice them and layer them on the bottom of the pie pan before topping with the veggies and eggs. This gives you a nice sweet potato "crust."

Banana Granola Pancakes

Servings: 4-5 (serving size = 2 pancakes)

Ingredients:
2 cups whole wheat flour
2 teaspoons baking powder
1 teaspoon baking soda
2 teaspoons cinnamon
½ teaspoon sea salt
2 cups unsweetened almond milk or other milk
1 egg
1 large ripe banana, mashed
¼ cup agave nectar
½ cup granola

Instructions:
Heat a griddle or large nonstick skillet over medium heat until hot.

In a medium mixing bowl, combine flour, cinnamon, baking powder, baking soda, and sea salt.

In a separate bowl, whisk the egg, milk, agave and mashed banana together. Add to the flour mixture and mix well to make batter. Add granola into the mixed batter.

Pour batter onto griddle ¼ cup at a time making sure the edges of each pancake don't touch. Cook until golden brown and bubbles appear on top of the pancakes. Flip and continue cooking until the other side is golden brown. Makes about 8 to 10 pancakes.

Nutrition per serving:
285 calories; 5 g Total Fat; <1 gram saturated fat; 13 g protein; 44 g carbohydrates; 8 grams dietary fiber; 60 mg cholesterol; 551 mg sodium.

Did you know?
Most granolas pack a high sugar content. This recipe used a granola that has 7 grams sugar per ½ cup serving.

Creamy Brown Rice Breakfast Pudding

Here's a yummy recipe to help you put that leftover brown rice to good use.

Servings: 6 (serving size = 1 cup)

Ingredients:
½ cup coconut milk
½ cup water
3 cups unsweetened almond milk
4 eggs
1 cup agave nectar
1 teaspoon pure vanilla extract
zest of 1 lemon
1 teaspoon ground cardamom
¼ teaspoon ground nutmeg
3 cups cooked brown rice
coconut oil for coating the cooking dish

Instructions:
Preheat oven to 350°F.

In a large bowl, whisk together the eggs, coconut milk, almond milk, agave nectar, vanilla, lemon zest, cardamom, and nutmeg. Stir in the brown rice.

Coat a casserole dish with coconut oil. Pour the mixture into the dish. Bake for 1 to 1 ½ hours. Let cool slightly and then serve warm.

Nutrition per serving:
222 calories; 9 g Total Fat; 4 gram saturated fat; 9 g protein; 26 g carbohydrates; <1 grams dietary fiber; 198 mg cholesterol; 167 mg sodium.

Did you know?
You can purchase pre-cooked organic brown rice from the frozen section of a natural food market.

Slow Cooker Irish Style Steel Cut Oats

Steel cut oats typically take 30 to 45 minutes to cook on the stovetop, and also require constant attention and stirring. Using a slow cooker takes away the hassle. If you set this recipe up before bedtime, you'll wake up to a hearty ready-to-eat breakfast!

Servings: 8 (serving size = 1/2 cup)

Ingredients:
1 cup coconut milk
3 ½ cups water
1 ¾ cups steel cut oats
½ teaspoon sea salt
¼ teaspoon allspice
coconut oil for coating the slow cooker

Instructions:
Coat a 4-quart slow cooker with coconut oil. Combine coconut milk, water, oats, sea salt, and allspice in the slow cooker. Cook on high for 2 to 4 hours or on low for 8 hours.

Nutrition per serving:
184 calories; 8 g Total Fat; 4 gram saturated fat; 5 g protein; 25 g carbohydrates; 4 grams dietary fiber; 0 mg cholesterol; 175 mg sodium.

Did you know?
Oats are high in soluble fiber, which binds to cholesterol and effectively flushes it from the body. Steel cut oats are simply the whole grain oat cut into small pieces, creating an oatmeal with a distinctive chewy texture. Steel cut oats are often called Irish or Scottish oats owing to the traditional use in those countries.

HEALTH PROMOTING BEVERAGES

Michael's Amazing Tonic™

My husband Michael likes to mix apple cider vinegar into apple juice and adds a little bit of flavored stevia. He's very liberal with the vinegar, so try adding more than this recipe calls for! The combination of the apple juice and vinegar creates a slightly fizzy sensation when mixed together.

Servings: 1 (serving size = 1 cup)

Ingredients:
1 cup unfiltered organic apple juice
2 teaspoons raw unfiltered apple cider vinegar
3 drops liquid stevia

Instructions:
Put all ingredients in glass. Stir and enjoy.

Nutrition per serving:
120 calories; 0 g Total Fat; 0 gram saturated fat; 0 g protein; 25 g carbohydrates; 1 grams dietary fiber; 0 mg cholesterol; 25 mg sodium.

Did you know?
A company called Sweet Leaf sells a variety of naturally flavored liquid stevia. Michael's favorite for his tonic is grape or orange!

Minty Maté Tea

The flavor of brewed maté tea is reminiscent of some varieties of green tea. Many consider the flavor to be very agreeable, but it is generally bitter if steeped in boiling water, so make it using hot but not boiling water.

Servings: 1 (serving size = 1 cup)

Ingredients:
1 peppermint tea bag
1 maté tea bag
hot but not boiling water

Instructions:
Put teabags in a mug. Add hot water. Let steep for 5 minutes. Add stevia or agave if desired. Enjoy!

Nutrition per serving:
0 calories; 0 g Total Fat; 0 gram saturated fat; 0 g protein; 0 g carbohydrates; 0 grams dietary fiber; 0 mg cholesterol; 0 mg sodium.

Did you know?
University of Illinois scientist Elvira de Mejia conducted a study that showed maté (mah' tay) tea drinkers had experienced a significant increase in the activity of an enzyme that promotes HDL (good) cholesterol while lowering LDL (bad) cholesterol. Maté tea has been used for centuries in South America as a medicinal tea.

Cranberry Pomegranate Fusion

Two antioxidant powerhouses, the juices of cranberries and pomegranates make a super healthy beverage.

Servings: 1 (serving size = 1 cup)

Ingredients:
1 cup water
2 tablespoons 100% cranberry juice
2 tablespoons 100% pomegranate juice

Instructions:
Add juices to the water in a glass and stir. Sweeten with stevia if desired.

Nutrition per serving:
28 calories; 0 g Total Fat; 0 gram saturated fat; 0 g protein; 7 g carbohydrates; 0 grams dietary fiber; 0 mg cholesterol; 5 mg sodium.

Did you know?
Pomegranate juice has about three times more antioxidants ounce for ounce than does red wine or green tea. Pomegranate juice has been shown to work well as a blood thinner. It also has been shown to reduce plaque in the arteries, and to raise "good" levels of cholesterol while helping lower "bad" cholesterol.
Aside from its high antioxidant content, cranberry juice inhibits the growth of mouth bacteria that causes plaque. As long as there is no sugar added to it, a healthy dose of cranberry juice ensures your teeth are fresh and clean all the time.

Raw Vanilla Almond Milk

This almond milk is delicious, easy to make and is far superior to commercially available almond milk, which often has added sugars and preservatives.

Servings: 4 to 6 (serving size = 1 cup)

Ingredients:
1 cup raw almonds, soaked in water overnight
3 cups water
1 teaspoon pure vanilla extract

Instructions:
Place the raw almonds in a bowl and add enough water to cover them. Place the bowl in the refrigerator and let the almonds soak overnight or for at least 6 hours.

When ready to make the almond milk, drain the almonds in a colander and rinse thoroughly. Place 3 cups water into a blender and add the soaked almonds. Blend until the mixture is smooth.

Strain the mixture through a cheesecloth, or strainer into a big bowl. Save the almond pulp in a container for use in smoothies.

Put the strained almond milk back into the blender and blend in the vanilla extract. This milk will last in the refrigerator for about 3-5 days.

Nutrition per serving:
40 calories; 3 g Total Fat; 0 gram saturated fat; 1 g protein; 2 g carbohydrates; 1 grams dietary fiber; 0 mg cholesterol; 2 mg sodium.

Did you know?
Almond milk is a perfect alternative for those who are lactose-intolerant, and can easily be exchanged for any other milk in recipes. It is rich in vitamin E, protein, and minerals such as zinc, magnesium, potassium, calcium, and iron.

MAGNIFICENT MUFFINS AND WHOLE GRAIN BREADS

Plan-D Flourless Muffins™

This is the homemade version of my famous flourless oat bran muffins sold in natural food markets throughout the Southwest. You can exchange the raisins and walnuts for other fruits and nuts, or try replacing the applesauce with mashed bananas or pumpkin puree for different varieties.

Servings: 12 (serving size = 1 muffin)

Dry Ingredients:
2 cups oat bran
2 1/8 teaspoons non-aluminum baking powder
1 tablespoon cinnamon
½ teaspoon nutmeg
½ teaspoon sea salt

Wet Ingredients:
1 cup unsweetened almond milk
½ cup unsweetened applesauce
2 egg whites
1 teaspoon vanilla extract
½ teaspoon liquid stevia

Third Set of Ingredients:
½ cup raisins
½ cup(s) walnut pieces
½ cup agave nectar or raw honey

Instructions:
Preheat oven to 400°F. Line muffin pans with paper muffin cups or coat with coconut oil.

Combine dry ingredients in a large mixing bowl and mix together thoroughly with a wire whisk. In a separate mixing bowl combine the wet ingredients with the wire whisk until the mixture becomes somewhat frothy. Slowly add the wet ingredients to dry ingredients and mix thoroughly with a spoon. Fold in the walnuts and raisins.

The last step is to add the agave nectar very slowly to the mixture while stirring. The batter should become lighter in texture.

Fill muffin cups and bake for 20 minutes or until the muffins are golden brown and a knife inserted into the center comes out clean. Let cool 10 minutes in the pan, and then transfer to a wire rack to cool completely.

Nutrition per serving:
126 calories; 5 g Total Fat; 0 gram saturated fat; 5 g protein; 17 g carbohydrates; 4 grams dietary fiber; 0 mg cholesterol; 180 mg sodium.

Whole Wheat Banana Bread

Whole-wheat wheat flour is not typically used in quick breads, but it really adds to the flavor and nutrition in this classic favorite.

Servings: 16 slices or muffins (serving size = 1 slice or 1 muffin)

Ingredients:
½ cup organic butter (1 stick), softened
2 tablespoons coconut oil, softened
½ cup Rapadura unrefined whole cane organic sugar
¼ cup agave nectar
2 eggs
3 large ripe bananas, mashed
2 tablespoons unsweetened applesauce
1 teaspoon vanilla extract
2 cups stone ground whole wheat flour
1 teaspoon baking soda
1 teaspoon sea salt
¼ cup ground flaxseeds

Instructions:
Preheat oven to 350°F. Coat a 9x5-inch loaf pan with coconut oil, or if making muffins, line muffin pans with paper muffin cups or coat with coconut oil.

In a large bowl, cream butter, coconut oil, and Rapadura sugar with an electric mixer. Add the eggs, bananas, applesauce, agave nectar, and vanilla. Beat well to thoroughly combine.

In a separate bowl, mix together the flour, baking soda, flaxseeds and salt.

Stir the banana mixture into the flour mixture and mix well. At this point the batter will be fairly thick. Pour the batter into the prepared loaf pan. If making muffins, fill each muffin cup about ¾ full.

Bake 1 hour for loaf or 20 to 30 minutes for muffins, or until a knife inserted in center comes out clean. Let cool in pan for 10 minutes then transfer to a wire rack to complete cooling.

Nutrition per serving:
185 calories; 9 g Total Fat; 5 gram saturated fat; 4 g protein; 21 g carbohydrates; 2 grams dietary fiber; 53 mg cholesterol; 260 mg sodium.

Did you know?
Rapadura™ is an unrefined organic whole cane sugar that can almost be considered a whole food. It is prepared by pressing the juice from the sugar cane stalk and then evaporating off the water. The remaining coarse, golden crystals retain a significant amount of the essential vitamins, minerals, and nutrients contained in the natural sugar cane.

Whole Grain Zucchini Bread

Here's another whole-grain version of a classic quick bread.

Servings: Makes 12 slices or 12 muffins (serving size = 1 slice or 1 muffin)

Ingredients:
2 eggs, beaten
1 cup agave nectar
½ cup butter, softened
2 tablespoons coconut oil, softened
2 tablespoons unsweetened applesauce
1 teaspoon vanilla extract
1 teaspoon almond extract
1 large ripe banana, mashed
2 cups whole-wheat pastry flour
1 cup whole spelt flour
1 tablespoon cinnamon
1 teaspoon non-aluminum baking powder
1 teaspoon baking soda
1 teaspoon sea salt
2 cups zucchini, grated

Instructions:
Preheat oven to 350°F. Coat a 9x5-inch loaf pan with coconut oil, or if making muffins, line muffin pans with paper muffin cups or coat with coconut oil.

In a large bowl, cream butter, eggs, agave nectar, coconut oil, applesauce, mashed banana, vanilla, and almond extract.

In a separate bowl, combine the whole-wheat pastry flour, whole spelt flour, cinnamon, baking powder, baking soda, and sea salt. Once thoroughly combined, add in the creamed ingredients and stir to mix thoroughly. Gently stir in the grated zucchini until evenly distributed. Pour into the prepared loaf pan. If making muffins, fill each muffin cup about halfway.

Bake 50 to 60 minutes for loaf or 20 to 30 minutes for muffins, or until a knife inserted in center comes out clean. Let cool in pan for 10 minutes then transfer to a wire rack to complete cooling.

Nutrition per serving:
228 calories; 12 g Total Fat; 7 gram saturated fat; 6 g protein; 24 g carbohydrates; 4 grams dietary fiber; 70 mg cholesterol; 375 mg sodium.

Gluten-Free Carrot Cake Muffins

Brown rice flour is a common ingredient used in gluten-free baking. Because there is no gluten, these muffins will not rise in the typical way that wheat flour muffins do, however they are wonderfully light and airy.

Servings: Makes 12 muffins (serving size = 1 muffin)

Ingredients:
1 ¾ cup brown rice flour
2 teaspoon baking soda
2 teaspoons cinnamon
½ teaspoon nutmeg
¼ teaspoon ground cloves
2 cups grated or finely chopped carrots
1 can (8 ounce) crushed pineapple (canned in its own juice), including juice
1 cup dried currants
½ cup unsweetened shredded coconut
3 large eggs
¾ cup agave nectar
½ cup coconut oil
½ cup chopped walnuts

Instructions:
Preheat oven to 325°F. Line muffin pans with paper muffin cups or coat with coconut oil.

Sift the flour, baking soda, cinnamon, nutmeg, and cloves into a large bowl. Resift and set aside.

In a second large bowl, combine the carrots, pineapple plus juice, currants, and shredded coconut. Set aside.

In a third bowl, beat the eggs with an electric mixer until very light. Add the agave nectar in a thin stream while beating. Beat until the mixture is very light and frothy. Add the oil in a thin stream while beating.

Pour the egg mixture into the carrot bowl. Stir to gently combine. Sift half the flour mixture over the bowl. Gently fold in. Repeat with remaining flour. Fold in walnuts.

Pour into prepared muffin cups. Bake for 30 minutes or until knife inserted in center comes out clean. Cool in the pan and then turn out onto wire racks to cool completely.

Nutrition per serving:
307 calories; 16 g Total Fat; 10 gram saturated fat; 6 g protein; 35 g carbohydrates; 1 grams dietary fiber; 74 mg cholesterol; 174 mg sodium.

Seasoned Spelt Pizza Dough

This recipe takes a little time, but it makes enough for 3 pizzas and you can freeze the extra dough for use at a later time.

Servings: Makes enough dough for three thin crust 12-inch pizzas. (serving size = 1/8 pizza, or 1 slice)

Ingredients:
1 ¾ cup warm water
1 packet active dry yeast
1 tablespoon unsulfured molasses
1 tablespoon agave nectar
5 ½ cups whole spelt flour
½ teaspoon garlic powder
1 tablespoon Italian seasoning
1 tablespoon sea salt
¼ cup extra virgin olive oil
coconut oil, for greasing bowl
cornmeal for sprinkling the pizza pan

Instructions:
To make the dough, you can use an electric mixer with a dough hook, such as a Kitchen-Aid, or just mix by hand.

Pour the warm water into a large mixing bowl. Add the agave nectar, molasses, and the yeast. When the yeast is active, mix in the first cup of flour. Once combined, mix in the olive oil, salt, Italian seasoning, and garlic powder.

Add 4 more cups of flour, ½ cup at a time, while continuing to mix the dough. After adding each ½ cup of flour and mixing, you will notice the dough becoming more formed and less sticky.

To knead the dough, sprinkle the last half a cup of flour out onto your kneading surface, turn out the dough and knead for about 6 minutes. Let it rest while you clean and grease your bowl with coconut oil. Continue kneading your dough till it feels smooth and springy. (Note: if you are using a Kitchen Aid, you do not need to knead the dough, the Kitchen Aid is doing that for you while mixing).

Form the dough into a ball and place it in the greased bowl. Turn the dough so it is evenly coated with the oil. Cover it with a towel and place it in a warm place away from drafts. Let the dough rise until it has doubled in size, about 1 hour.

Preheat oven to 400°F. Turn the dough out on a floured surface. Punch it down and break up the large bubbles. Divide it into 2 even balls for thick crust or 3 even balls for thin crust. (At this point you may place your extra dough into a freezer bag and place in the freezer for future use. When you want to use it, take it out of the freezer, let thaw and come to room temperature, and then follow the remaining steps.)

Roll each ball of dough out to the desired size and thickness. Poke the dough with a fork (known as docking) about every inch so that the crust does not inflate while prebaking.

To pre-bake your crust, sprinkle a pizza pan or pizza stone with some corn meal and place your crust on it. Bake for about 10 minutes.

Remove the pre-baked crust from the oven and then put all of your desired toppings on it.

Place the pizza back in the oven and bake until the toppings are cooked to the desired state. By pre-baking the crust, you ensure that the crust is fully cooked. Remove from the oven and slice into 8 equal pieces.

Nutrition per serving:
113 calories; 4 g Total Fat; <1 gram saturated fat; <1 g protein; 16 g carbohydrates; 3 grams dietary fiber; 0 mg cholesterol; 280 mg sodium.

Did you know?
The addition of herbs and spices to the dough gives it wonderful flavor on its own, so you aren't depending as much on the toppings to bring out the flavor of the pizza.

Southwestern Sweet Potato Wraps

The combination of sweet potatoes and kidney beans pack a high fiber punch and a delicious flavor. These burritos are absolutely fabulous and a staple at the McCaffrey household!

Servings: 6 (serving size = 1 burrito)

Ingredients:
½ tablespoon unrefined coconut oil
½ onion, chopped
2 cloves garlic, minced
2 cans (15 ounce) red kidney beans (preferably organic), drained and rinsed
1 cup water
1 ½ tablespoon chili powder
1 teaspoon ground cumin
2 teaspoons yellow mustard
1 pinch cayenne pepper, or to taste
1 ½ tablespoons reduced sodium soy sauce or reduced-sodium wheat-free tamari sauce
1 ½ pounds sweet potatoes, baked and then peeled and mashed
6 (10-inch) whole-wheat tortillas or whole spelt tortillas, warmed
4 ounces cheddar cheese (preferably organic), shredded, about 1 cup

Instructions:
Preheat oven to 350°F. Place whole sweet potatoes on a baking sheet and bake in the oven for 30 minutes or until soft through the center. Remove from the oven but leave the oven on for warming the burritos.

Allow sweet potatoes to cool, then cut open and scrape out all of the inside part of the potatoes and place them in a bowl. Mash the potatoes with a potato masher. They can still be slightly lumpy. Set aside.

Heat coconut oil in a skillet over medium heat. Add onion and garlic and sauté until soft. Stir in the beans, and mash them with a masher. Gradually stir in the water, and heat until warm. Remove from heat, and stir in the chili powder, cumin, mustard, cayenne pepper, and soy sauce or tamari sauce.

Warm tortillas by placing them in a dry skillet over medium heat. When the tortilla is warm to the touch, remove from the skillet and lay the tortilla on a flat surface, such as a cutting board or a plate. Add equal amounts of the bean mixture and the mashed sweet potatoes down the center of each tortilla. Top with cheese. Roll up the tortilla burrito style, and place burrito on a baking sheet. Repeat with remaining tortillas.

Bake the burritos for 10 to 12 minutes in the preheated oven, just enough to lightly brown the tops of the tortillas. Serve immediately.

This recipe can be doubled to make 12 burritos, and the extras can be individually wrapped and frozen for reheating later.

Nutrition per serving:
357 calories; 6.92 g Total Fat; 3.96 grams saturated fat; 18 g protein; 55 g carbohydrates; 4.5 grams dietary fiber; 0 mg cholesterol; 491 mg sodium.

Did you know?
Sweet potatoes contain high amounts of the antioxidants vitamin A (in the form of beta-carotene) and vitamin C. Both beta-carotene and vitamin C are very powerful antioxidants that work in the body to eliminate free radicals. Free radicals are chemicals that damage cells and cell membranes and are associated with the development of conditions like arteriosclerosis, diabetic heart disease, and colon cancer. This may explain why beta-carotene and vitamin C have both been shown to be helpful for preventing these conditions.

Best Ever Black Bean Burgers

These burgers can be served in a variety of ways—on top of a salad, as a taco stuffing, on a sprouted grain bun, or as an entrée with raw or cooked vegetables. The recipe makes two burgers but can easily be scaled up to make more. You can substitute different beans, veggies, or seasonings to suit your taste.

Servings: 2 (serving size = 1 burger)

Ingredients:
1 can (15 ounce) black beans, rinsed and drained
1/3 cup red onion, diced
1/3 cup red or green bell pepper, or a mixture of both, diced
1 small carrot, grated
2 cloves garlic, minced
¼ cup oat bran
2 tablespoons fresh salsa
1 can (4 ounce) mild diced green chilies
1 teaspoon cumin
2 teaspoons taco seasoning, see page 240
1 tablespoon coconut oil, plus more for frying the burgers

Instructions:
Sauté the onions, peppers, and garlic in a skillet with 1 tablespoon of coconut oil over medium heat until onions are translucent and peppers are soft. Set aside.

In a large mixing bowl, mash the beans with a fork or masher, but don't puree. Add the sautéed veggies (but don't clean the skillet) and remaining ingredients into the mixing bowl. Using moistened hands, knead ingredients to mix well. Divide the bean mixture in half and form into two balls, then press each ball into a patty.

Add a small amount of coconut oil to the same skillet that was used to sauté the vegetables. Heat over low to medium heat, add the burgers, cover, and cook for 4 to 5 minutes. Flip and cook uncovered for another 4 to 5 minutes. These burgers can also be grilled.

The burgers should be somewhat crispy on the outside and soft on the inside. Let cool slightly before serving.

Nutrition per serving:
300 calories; 8 g Total Fat; 6 grams saturated fat; 11 g protein; 45 g carbohydrates; 11 grams dietary fiber; 0 mg cholesterol; 270 mg sodium.

Did you know?
Black beans are an excellent source of dietary fiber, with a whopping 15 grams in

one cup. Additionally, research published in the Journal of Agriculture and Food Chemistry indicates that black beans are as rich in antioxidant compounds called anthocyanins as grapes and cranberries, two fruits long considered antioxidant superstars.

Black Bean Burger and Avocado Quesadillas

I grew up making quesadillas, which is traditionally a toasted white-flour tortilla with melted cheese inside. To make this healthy version, I traded the cheese for avocado and use corn tortillas instead of flour.

Servings: 1 (serving size = 1 quesadillas)

Ingredients:
1 Best Ever Black Bean Burger (see recipe page 227)
½ avocado, sliced lengthwise into about 6 pieces
2 large tomato slices
2 (6-inch) stone ground corn tortillas

Instructions:
Cut the black bean burger in half.

Heat a large skillet over medium heat. Take one of the tortillas and place it in the pan to warm it. Flip the tortilla over a few times, 10 seconds between flips.

Place one half of the burger on the tortilla, with the round edge outward and the straight edge toward the center of the tortilla. Top with tomato slices and then avocado slices. Fold over the tortilla to that the fillings are covered.

Cook for about 3 to 4 minutes, and then flip onto the other side for an additional 3 minutes.

Repeat to make the other quesadilla. Serve with a generous portion of Mexican No-Cabbage Coleslaw (page 232)

Nutrition per serving:
322 calories; 9 g Total Fat; 4 grams saturated fat; 8 g protein; 52 g carbohydrates; 10 grams dietary fiber; 0 mg cholesterol; 149 mg sodium.

Did you know?
You can put practically anything in a quesadilla. My favorites are avocado, olives, tomatoes, and beans.

Tantalizing Taco Salad

This is my absolute favorite salad. The avocado, cheese, and salsa add so many flavors that there's no need for any other dressing!

Servings: 1

Ingredients:
1 ½ cups Romaine lettuce, chopped
¼ cup diced tomatoes
2 tablespoons green bell pepper, diced
2 tablespoons red bell pepper, diced
2 tablespoons celery, diced
2 tablespoons red onion, diced
1 tablespoon black olives, sliced
1 tablespoon green onions, sliced
½ cup black beans, warmed
½ avocado, sliced
1 ounce reduced fat Monterey Jack cheese, preferably organic
1 tablespoon toasted pepitas
½ cup fresh chunky salsa

Instructions:
Place Romaine lettuce on the bottom of a large plate or bowl. Top with veggies, warm beans, cheese, avocado and salsa. Sprinkle with pepitas. Enjoy!

Nutrition per serving:
394 calories; 14 g Total Fat; 5 grams saturated fat; 22 g protein; 46 g carbohydrates; 16 grams dietary fiber; 20 mg cholesterol; 457 mg sodium.

Hardy Barley Salad

Barley is a wonderfully versatile whole grain with a rich nutlike flavor and an appealing chewy, pasta-like consistency.

Servings: 6 (serving size = ½ cup barley mixture over 1 cup greens)

Ingredients:
¾ cup pearl barley
½ cup frozen petite peas, thawed
½ cup celery, diced
½ cup zucchini, diced
½ cup carrot, diced
12 small cherry tomatoes, halved
½ cup frozen corn, thawed
2 green onion tops, sliced
6 tablespoons fresh dill, minced
6 tablespoons Sweet Herb Vinaigrette (see page 236)
2 ounces feta cheese, crumbled
6 cups Spring Mix, or other leafy green salad mix

Instructions:
In a medium saucepan, bring 4 cups water to a boil. Add barley, reduce heat and simmer, until barley is tender and chewy, about 40 to 50 minutes. Drain barley in a colander and rinse with cold water. Allow barley to cool to room temperature or cool it faster by refrigerating it.

While barley is cooking, dice the celery, carrots, and zucchini. Cut cherry tomatoes in half and slice green onion tops. Place them all in a large bowl with the corn and peas.

When barley is cooled, add it to the bowl. Add in the minced fresh dill and the vinaigrette, then toss to mix thoroughly.

To serve, line individual salad plates with 1 cup Spring Mix. Spoon ½ cup barley mixture into center. Sprinkle with feta cheese. Serve immediately.

Nutrition per serving:
244 calories; 12 g Total Fat; 3 grams saturated fat; 7 g protein; 30 g carbohydrates; 5 grams dietary fiber; 8 mg cholesterol; 171 mg sodium.

Did you know?
If you suffer from irregular bowel action, let barley give your intestinal health a boost. In addition to providing bulk and improving the transit time of fecal matter, thus decreasing the risk of colon cancer and hemorrhoids, barley's dietary fiber also

provides food for the "friendly" bacteria in the large intestine. When these helpful bacteria ferment barley's insoluble fiber, they produce a short-chain fatty acid called butyric acid, which serves as the primary fuel for the cells of the large intestine and helps maintain a healthy colon. Like oats, barley is high in the soluble fiber beta glucan, which helps to lower cholesterol.

No Mayo Coleslaw

Servings: 4 (serving size = 1 ¼ cup)

Ingredients:
2 ½ cups green cabbage
½ cup red cabbage
1 cup carrot, shredded
2 medium celery stalks, sliced thin
2 tablespoons fresh parsley, chopped
¼ cup unrefined toasted sesame oil
2 tablespoons raw apple cider vinegar
½ teaspoon garlic powder
dash sea salt
dash pepper

Instructions:
Slice cabbage and carrots by hand or use a shredding blade on a food processor.

Toss all ingredients in a bowl and marinate for at least one hour, tossing often to allow flavors to blend uniformly. Serve chilled.

Nutrition per serving:
155 calories; 14 g Total Fat; 2 grams saturated fat; 7 g protein; 7 g carbohydrates; 1 grams dietary fiber; 0 mg cholesterol; 316 mg sodium.

Mexican No-Cabbage Slaw

Enjoy this crunchy, refreshing slaw on a taco or on the side.

Servings: 8 (serving size = 1 cup)

Ingredients:
2 cups jicama, peeled and sliced into thin strips
2 cups zucchini, sliced into thin strips
1 cup red bell pepper, sliced into thin strips
1 cup green bell pepper, sliced into thin strips
2 cups carrots, grated
1/3-cup cilantro, chopped
½ cup brown rice vinegar
2 tablespoons extra virgin olive oil
1 teaspoon cumin
½ teaspoon coriander seeds, ground
¼ teaspoon sea salt

Instructions:
Slice cabbage and carrots by hand or use a shredding blade on a food processor or Mandoline slicer.

Toss all ingredients in a bowl and marinate for at least one hour, tossing often to allow flavors to blend uniformly. Serve chilled.

Nutrition per serving:
75 calories; 3 g Total Fat; 0 grams saturated fat; 1 g protein; 7 g carbohydrates; 1 grams dietary fiber; 0 mg cholesterol; 82 mg sodium.

Black Bean Soup with Fresh Cilantro

Canned beans make preparing this soup quick and easy. Pureeing a portion of the soup gives it a nice creamy consistency.

Servings: 8 (serving size = 1 cup)

Ingredients:
2 tablespoons coconut oil
1 medium yellow onion, finely chopped
4 medium carrots, sliced
¼ cups red bell pepper, diced
4 medium garlic cloves, minced
2 teaspoons cumin
2 teaspoons Mexican oregano
1 ½ teaspoons chili powder
3 cans (15 ounce) black beans, rinsed and drained
5 cups low sodium chicken broth or vegetable broth
1 cup low sodium tomato sauce
dash sea salt
dash pepper
½ cup fresh cilantro leaves, chopped

Instructions:
Heat the oil in a 6-quart saucepan over medium heat. Add the onion and sauté for 3 minutes. Add the carrots, bell pepper, garlic, cumin, oregano, and chili powder and sauté for 3 more minutes.

Add the beans, broth, and tomato sauce and bring to a boil, then reduce heat and simmer, uncovered, for 20 minutes, or until the carrots are tender.

Allow the soup to cool slightly, then puree 3 cups of it in a blender or food processor. Return the pureed portion to the saucepan, stir, and adjust the seasoning. Add the cilantro and serve immediately.

Nutrition per serving:
267 calories; 4 g Total Fat; 3 grams saturated fat; 15 g protein; 38 g carbohydrates; 13 grams dietary fiber; 0 mg cholesterol; 425 mg sodium.

Red Lentil Soup with Mint

Lentils are very low in fat, high in fiber and are frequently referred to as a wonder food for their health promoting qualities.

Servings: Makes about 9 cups (serving size = 1 cup)

Ingredients:
1 onion, finely chopped
2 garlic cloves, minced
3 large carrots, sliced thin
1 ½ cups red lentils
dash paprika
7 cups reduced sodium vegetable broth
dash salt
dash pepper
1 teaspoon dried mint leaves
2 tablespoons coconut oil

Instructions:
Heat the oil in a 6-quart saucepan over medium heat. Add the onion and sauté for 3 minutes. Add the garlic, mint, paprika, carrots, red lentils, and broth and bring to a boil.

Reduce the heat and simmer, uncovered, for 30 minutes, or until the carrots are soft and the lentils are mushy. Thin the soup with additional broth or water if it gets too thick. For a finer, creamier consistency, puree all of the soup, or portion, of it. Serve immediately.

This soup keeps refrigerated for about 1 week, and can be frozen for up to 1 month.

Nutrition per serving:
195 calories; 5 g Total Fat; 3 grams saturated fat; 10 g protein; 28 g carbohydrates; 5 grams dietary fiber; 0 mg cholesterol; 460 mg sodium

Did you know?
The red lentils, also called pink lentils (which really are orange) will lose their color during cooking and the finished soup will be a golden yellow color!

Roasted Garlic Hummus

Hummus is an excellent dip for raw veggies, a great sandwich spread, or for dipping baked tortilla chips.

Servings: 4 (serving size = 1/2 cup)

Ingredients:
1 can (15 ounce) garbanzo beans
6 medium garlic cloves, skins left on
½ teaspoon cumin
Juice of 1 large lemon, about 2 tablespoons
1 tablespoon extra virgin olive oil
1 tablespoon sesame Tahini
¼ cup water (add more or less for the desired consistency)
dash of sea salt

Instructions:
Preheat oven to 425°F.

To roast the garlic, wrap the garlic in parchment paper and bake for about 30 minutes, or until the inside of the garlic is soft and oozing. Let cool. Remove garlic from skins.

Combine all ingredients in the bowl of a food processor or in a blender and process until smooth, stopping to scrape down the sides as needed. Adjust the seasoning and serve.

Top with chopped fresh parsley, a dash of cayenne pepper, or toasted pine nuts.

Refrigerate any leftovers for up to 5 days.

Nutrition per serving:
193 calories; 6 g Total Fat; <1 grams saturated fat; 6 g protein; 27 g carbohydrates; 8 grams dietary fiber; 0 mg cholesterol; 155 mg sodium.

Sweet Herb Vinaigrette

This sweet and tangy vinaigrette can be used on any salad or as a marinade.

Servings: Makes about 1 ½ cups (serving size = 1 tablespoon)

Ingredients:
1 cup extra virgin olive oil
½ cup raw apple cider vinegar
3 teaspoons Italian seasoning
2 garlic cloves, fresh
1 tablespoon fresh lemon juice
¼ teaspoon liquid stevia extract
¼ teaspoon Herbamare or sea salt

Instructions:
Place all ingredients in a blender and blend to combine thoroughly. Let the blender run for about 2 minutes for a creamy type Italian vinaigrette. Place any leftover dressing in a glass jar or cruet. Keeps for up to 3 weeks in the refrigerator.

For an omega-3 variation, replace half the olive oil with flaxseed oil or hempseed oil.

Nutrition per serving:
82 calories; 9 g Total Fat; 1 grams saturated fat; 0 g protein; 0 g carbohydrates; 0 grams dietary fiber; 0 mg cholesterol; 27 mg sodium.

Agave Cilantro Lime Dressing

Great on top of any salad!

Servings: Makes about 1 ½ cups (serving size = 1 tablespoon)

Ingredients:
1 cup extra virgin olive oil
½ cup lime juice
½ cup cilantro leaves
2 tablespoons agave nectar

Instructions:
Place all ingredients in a blender and blend to combine thoroughly. Let the blender run for about 2 minutes for a creamy sweet dressing. Place any leftover dressing in a glass jar or cruet. Keeps for up to 1 week in the refrigerator.

For an omega-3 variation, replace half the olive oil with flaxseed oil or hempseed oil.

Nutrition per serving:
83 calories; 9 g Total Fat; 1 grams saturated fat; 0 g protein; 0 g carbohydrates; 0 grams dietary fiber; 0 mg cholesterol; 0 mg sodium.

Fresh Basil Pesto

Use this pesto as a dip for raw veggies or mix it with shredded raw zucchini, carrots, and cabbage for a yummy quick salad.

Servings: 8 (serving size = 1 tablespoon)

Ingredients:
2 cups fresh basil leaves
¼ cup extra virgin olive oil
1 garlic clove, minced
¼ cup pine nuts

Instructions:
Place basil, oil, garlic, and salt into the bowl of a food processor and blend until basil is chopped. Add the pine nuts and blend until smooth. Stop occasionally to scrape down the sides of the bowl with a rubber spatula. This pesto will keep for 5 days in the refrigerator.

For an omega-3 version, replace half or all of the olive oil with flaxseed oil or hemp oil.

Nutrition per serving:
93 calories; 9 g Total Fat; 1 grams saturated fat; 1 g protein; 2 g carbohydrates; 1 grams dietary fiber; 0 mg cholesterol; 3 mg sodium.

Green Enchilada Sauce

I created this sauce because I could not find a commercially prepared enchilada sauce that didn't have hydrogenated oils or preservatives in it. It's great for enchiladas, but can also be used as a taco sauce, in burritos, or on top of eggs.

Servings: Makes 1 quart (serving size = ½ cup)

Ingredients:
1 pound tomatillos
2 onions, chopped
¼ cup extra virgin olive oil
8 garlic cloves
1 ½ teaspoons cumin
1 tablespoon chili powder
1 can (4 ounce) mild diced green chilies
3 cups reduced sodium chicken broth

Instructions:
Heat oil in a skillet over medium heat. Add onions and garlic and cook until soft and translucent. Add the broth, tomatillos, cumin, chili powder and green chilies and bring to a boil.

Reduce heat to a simmer and cover, continue cooking until the tomatillos are soft. Remove from heat and allow to cool. When cool enough to handle, transfer the sauce to a food processor or blender and blend until smooth. Use immediately or store the leftover sauce in the refrigerator or freezer to use another time.

Nutrition per serving:
120 calories; 7 g Total Fat; 1 grams saturated fat; 2 g protein; 11 g carbohydrates; 1 grams dietary fiber; 0 mg cholesterol; 398 mg sodium.

Make Your Own Taco Seasoning Mix

The taco seasoning mixes that come in packets usually contain monosodium glutamate (MSG) and other undesirable additives. This one tastes identical to the commercial variety, without the chemical ingredients. Try it on ground beef, ground turkey, chicken, and beans.

Servings: Makes ½ cup (serving size = 1 teaspoon)

Ingredients:
4 tablespoons chili powder
1 teaspoon garlic powder
1 teaspoon onion powder
¼ teaspoon cayenne pepper
1 teaspoon Mexican oregano
2 teaspoons paprika
2 tablespoons cumin
2 teaspoons sea salt
4 teaspoons coriander

Instructions:
In a small bowl, mix all ingredients. Store in an airtight container or spice jar.

Nutrition per serving:
9 calories; 0 g Total Fat; 0 grams saturated fat; 0 g protein; 1 g carbohydrates; 0 grams dietary fiber; 0 mg cholesterol; 199 mg sodium.

VEGGIES AND SIDES

Patapar Steamed Vegetables

Using Patapar Paper for steaming vegetables is the best way to retain the valuable nutrients that are typically lost during steaming. See Chapter 10 for a complete description of how to use and where to purchase Patapar Paper.

Servings: 4 (serving size = 1 cup)

Ingredients:
2 cups broccoli, florets and stems
1 cup carrots, sliced
1 cup cauliflower florets
1 sheet Patapar Paper (vegetable parchment paper)

Instructions:
Place vegetables in moistened Patapar Paper (see chapter 10). Tie the paper up in a bundle using a twist tie or string. Place the bundle in a steamer basket over boiling water.

Steam vegetables for approximately 15 minutes, or until tender. Remove bundle from steam, open carefully, and transfer vegetables to a serving plate. Season if desired.

Rinse paper thoroughly and let dry. It can be reused up to 50 times if kept in good condition.

Nutrition per serving:
49 calories; 0 g Total Fat; 0 grams saturated fat; 3 g protein; 8 g carbohydrates; 1 grams dietary fiber; 0 mg cholesterol; 31 mg sodium.

Did you know?
For maximum nutrition it is, of course, important to consume the vegetable juices that collect inside the parchment bundle. The juice can be poured off and drunk as a "vitamin cocktail," mashed in with root vegetables or squash, added to soups and stews, or used in making homemade baby food.

Garlic Mashed Cauliflower

Servings: 4 (serving size = ½ cup)

Ingredients:
1 large head cauliflower
1 tablespoon organic butter
4 to 6 garlic cloves, roasted
¼ cup coconut milk
½ teaspoon Herbamare or sea salt
1 tablespoon fresh chives, chopped
dash paprika

Instructions:
Preheat oven to 425°F.

To roast the garlic, wrap the garlic in parchment paper and bake for about 30 minutes, or until the inside of the garlic is soft and oozing. Let cool. Remove garlic from skins.

Wash cauliflower and remove the florets from stems. Steam the cauliflower florets in Patapar paper (see chapter 10) until tender, about 20-25 minutes. Remove from paper and drain.

In a food processor, add drained cauliflower, 4 cloves of peeled roasted garlic, butter, Herbamare or salt, and half of the coconut milk. Puree until smooth but stiff, adjusting consistency with a bit of extra coconut milk as needed. Do not over process or the mashed cauliflower will be too runny. Add more garlic and Herbamare if needed, to taste.

Transfer to a bowl, and mix in most of the chopped chives.

Garnish with remaining chopped chives, parsley, or a dash of paprika.

Nutrition per serving:
68 calories; 4 g Total Fat; 2 grams saturated fat; 2 g protein; 6 g carbohydrates; <1 grams dietary fiber; 7 mg cholesterol; 375 mg sodium.

Mixed Vegetable Curry

Servings: 4 (serving size = 1 cup)

Ingredients:
2 cups onions, chopped
2 tablespoons brown rice flour
½ cup coconut milk
½ cup water
2 cups reduced sodium vegetable broth
2 tablespoons curry powder
1 cup carrots, sliced thick
1 cup red bell pepper, sliced thin or cut into chunks
1 cup sweet potato, peeled and cut into cubes
1 cup cauliflower florets
1 cup broccoli florets
2 tablespoons fresh mint leaves
1 tablespoon coconut oil

Instructions:
In a large saucepan, heat oil over medium heat. Add onions and cook, stirring often, until soft and translucent, about 4 to 5 minutes. Stir in brown rice flour and cook, stirring, for 1 minute.

Slowly stir in coconut milk, water, broth, carrots, sweet potato, mint leaves and curry. Cook mixture until thick and bubbly, about 2 to 3 minutes.

Add cauliflower, and broccoli. Reduce heat to medium low, cover and cook 5 minutes more. Serve hot over brown rice or quinoa.

Nutrition per serving:
210calories; 8 g Total Fat; 6 grams saturated fat; 5 g protein; 30 g carbohydrates; 3 grams dietary fiber; 0 mg cholesterol; 125 mg sodium.

Gingered Beets and Fennel

Servings: 6 (serving size = 1/2 cup)

Ingredients:
4 medium sized red beets, peeled and cut into cubes
1 fennel (stalks only), sliced
½ inch piece of ginger, diced
water

Instructions:
Preheat oven to 350°F.

Place all ingredients in a 2-quart casserole dish. Fill with about 1 inch of water.

Cover and bake about 30 minutes, or until beets are tender. Serve hot or chilled.

Nutrition per serving:
33 calories; 0 g Total Fat; 0 grams saturated fat; 1 g protein; 7 g carbohydrates; 1 grams dietary fiber; 0 mg cholesterol; 56 mg sodium.

Sesame Broccoli

Servings: 4 (serving size = 1 ½ cups broccoli with sauce)

Ingredients:
6 cups broccoli florets
1 tablespoon unrefined toasted sesame oil
2 tablespoons reduced sodium soy sauce or wheat-free tamari sauce
1 tablespoon hoisin sauce
1 tablespoon natural peanut butter
1 teaspoon minced garlic
1 tablespoon toasted sesame seeds (see recipe for toasted sesame seeds on page 246)
6 tablespoons water, adding more if necessary

Instructions:
In a small bowl, combine the soy sauce or tamari sauce, peanut butter, and hoisin sauce. Whisk together with a wire whisk until smooth. Set aside.

Add the 3 tablespoons water and sesame oil to a large skillet or wok and heat over medium high heat. Add the broccoli florets and sauté for 2 minutes. Add the garlic and sauté for 30 seconds, then add 3 more tablespoons water and cook, stirring, for 2 minutes. (Note: the broccoli florets should still be slightly crisp; do not overcook). Add the reserved soy sauce or tamari sauce mixture and cook for 1 minute more. Adjust the seasoning to your taste.

Transfer the broccoli and sauce to a serving dish, garnish with the toasted sesame seeds.

Nutrition per serving:
117 calories; 6 g Total Fat; 1 grams saturated fat; 6 g protein; 9 g carbohydrates; 2 grams dietary fiber; 0 mg cholesterol; 440 mg sodium.

Did you know?
Broccoli is very perishable and should be stored in an open plastic bag in the refrigerator crisper where it will keep for a week. Since water on the surface will encourage its degradation, do not wash the broccoli before refrigerating. Leftover cooked broccoli should be placed in a tightly covered container and stored in the refrigerator where it will keep for a few days.

Toasted Sesame Seeds

You may buy sesame seeds already toasted, but they taste better and are more fragrant when you toast them yourself. Buy raw sesame seeds and toast them on the stove or in the oven.

Servings: 1 (serving size = 1 Tablespoon toasted sesame seeds)

Ingredients:
1 tablespoon or more of raw sesame seeds

Instructions:
For stovetop toasting, add raw sesame seeds to a dry skillet and heat over medium heat, shaking the pan occasionally or stirring with a flat spatula. Remove the seeds when they darken and become fragrant. Be careful not to burn them. It takes between 3 and 5 minutes to toast sesame seeds on the stovetop.

To toast sesame seeds in the oven, preheat the oven to 325°F. Spread the seeds out on a dry baking sheet. Bake until the seeds are brown and become fragrant. It takes about 15 minutes to toast sesame seeds in the oven.

For both methods, allow the toasted seeds to cool, then store at room temperature in a tightly covered jar with little air space.

Nutrition per serving:
10 calories; <1 g Total Fat; 0 grams saturated fat; 0 g protein; 0 g carbohydrates; 0 grams dietary fiber; 0 mg cholesterol; 0 mg sodium.

Did you know?
Not only are sesame seeds a very good source of manganese and copper, but they are also a good source of calcium, magnesium, iron, phosphorus, vitamin B1, zinc and dietary fiber. In addition to these important nutrients, sesame seeds contain two unique substances: sesamin and sesamolin. Both of these substances belong to a group of special beneficial fibers called lignans, and have been shown to have a cholesterol-lowering effect in humans, and to prevent high blood pressure and increase vitamin E supplies in animals. Sesamin has also been found to protect the liver from oxidative damage.

Mashed Sweet Potatoes with Coconut Milk

Sweet potatoes are high in vitamin A, lower in starch than white potatoes, and absolutely delicious.

Servings: 4 (serving size = ¼ pound, or approximately ½ cup)

Ingredients:
1 ½ pound sweet potatoes
2 tablespoons coconut milk
dash of cinnamon (optional)

Instructions:
Preheat oven to 450°F.

Scrub potatoes. Arrange potatoes on oven rack and bake for 35 to 40 minutes, until tender. Remove from the oven and prick with a fork to let steam out. Cut in half, scoop out flesh, and place it in the bowl of a food processor. Discard peels.

Add coconut milk to the potatoes and a dash of cinnamon if desired, and process until smooth and creamy. Serve immediately.

Nutrition per serving:
125 calories; <1 g Total Fat; <0.5 grams saturated fat; 2 g protein; 28 g carbohydrates; 1 grams dietary fiber; 0 mg cholesterol; 18 mg sodium.

Minty Quinoa

Servings: 4 (serving size = ½ cup)

Ingredients:
2/3 cup quinoa, washed and drained
1 ¼ cup water
2 teaspoons wheat-free reduced sodium Tamari Sauce
1/3-cup pine nuts
3-½ tablespoons scallion top, finely chopped
2 ½ tablespoons fresh mint leaves, chopped
½ cup frozen peas, thawed

Instructions:
Place the quinoa and water in a saucepan, cover and bring to a boil. Reduce heat to medium-low and simmer for 20 minutes.

Remove from heat, transfer to a bowl and allow to cool for a few minutes. Sprinkle with tamari sauce, pine nuts, scallions, mint, and peas. Mix and serve.

Nutrition per serving:
200 calories; 8 g Total Fat; 1 grams saturated fat; 6 g protein; 25 g carbohydrates; 3 grams dietary fiber; 0 mg cholesterol; 128 mg sodium.

MAIN DISHES

Pan Grilled Chicken Fajitas

Servings: 4 (serving size = 4 oz. cooked chicken with veggies and 2 tortillas)

Ingredients:
1 ½ pounds boneless skinless chicken breasts, fat removed and cut into strips
1 tablespoon extra virgin olive oil
1 tablespoon coconut oil
3 tablespoons lime juice
2 garlic cloves, minced
1 cup cilantro leaf, chopped
1 onion, peeled and sliced into thin strips
1 green bell pepper, seeded and sliced into thin strips
1 red bell pepper, seeded and sliced into thin strips
2 tablespoons taco seasoning (see page 240), divided use
dash of salt
dash of pepper
8 (6-inch) stone ground corn tortillas, warmed
¼ cup reduced sodium chicken broth

Instructions:
Place chicken strips in a glass baking dish.

In a blender combine olive oil, lime juice, garlic, cilantro, 1 tablespoon taco seasoning, salt and pepper. Blend until smooth and pour over the chicken strips. Cover with plastic wrap and let chicken marinate in the refrigerator for 30 minutes or longer.

Heat chicken broth and coconut oil in a large skillet over medium heat. Add onions and peppers. Sprinkle with the remaining taco seasoning and cook, stirring frequently, until they are tender and begin to brown. Transfer onions and pepper to another dish or bowl. Keep the skillet nearby but off the heat.

Remove chicken from marinade and add it to the skillet. Discard marinade. Return the skillet to the heat and cook the chicken for 5 to 7 minutes, stirring frequently, or until no longer pink in center. Serve hot with onions and peppers, and warm tortillas.

Nutrition per serving:
433 calories; 14 g Total Fat; 5 grams saturated fat; 40 g protein; 37 g carbohydrates; 3 grams dietary fiber; 96 mg cholesterol; 406 mg sodium.

Roasted Lemon Herb Chicken

Servings: 8 (serving size = 4 oz. cooked chicken, skin removed)

Ingredients:
2 teaspoons Italian seasoning
½ teaspoon Herbamare
½ teaspoon dry mustard
2 garlic cloves, minced
½ teaspoon ground black pepper
1 (3 pound) whole chicken
2 lemons
2 tablespoons extra virgin olive oil

Instructions:
Preheat oven to 350°F.

Combine the Italian seasoning, Herbamare, dry mustard, garlic powder and black pepper; set aside.

Rinse the chicken thoroughly, and remove the giblets. Place the chicken in a 9x13 inch baking dish. Sprinkle 1 ½ teaspoons of the spice mixture inside the chicken. Rub the remaining mixture under the skin of the chicken and also on the outside of the chicken.

Squeeze the juice of the 2 lemons into a small bowl or cup, and mix with the olive oil. Drizzle this oil/juice mixture over the chicken. Place one of the squeezed lemons inside the cavity of the chicken.

Bake in the preheated oven for 1 ½ hours, or until juices run clear, basting several times with the remaining oil mixture.

Nutrition per serving:
244 calories; 12 g Total Fat; 3 grams saturated fat; 32 g protein; 2 g carbohydrates; 0 grams dietary fiber; 96 mg cholesterol; 260 mg sodium.

Sensational Sweet and Sour Turkey Meatballs

It's hard to find a bottled sweet and sour sauce without a skyrocketing amount of sugar in it. This lovely version is the best ever. Try it on chicken and tofu as well.

Servings: 6 (serving size = ½ cup sauce plus 4 ounces cooked turkey meatballs)

Ingredients:

Sauce
¼ cup unrefined peanut oil, divided
¼ cup brown rice vinegar
¾ cup 100% fruit apricot jam
1 cup ketchup (unsweetened or naturally sweetened)
¼ cup onion, diced
1 teaspoon dried oregano

Meatballs
1 pound ground turkey
3 garlic cloves, minced
1 teaspoon dried basil
1 teaspoon dried parsley
1 teaspoon dried oregano
¼ teaspoon pepper
2 scallions, white and green parts, chopped
1 egg
½ cup oat bran

Instructions:
Preheat oven to 350°F.

To make meatballs, combine all meatball ingredients a large bowl and mix together. Form into small meatballs and place them in a baking dish. Bake in oven for 20 minutes. Remove from oven and transfer to a clean baking dish.

While meatballs are baking, make the sauce. In a large bowl, whisk together vinegar, apricot jam, ketchup, oregano, and all but 1 tablespoon of the peanut oil. Set aside.

Heat the remaining 1 tablespoon peanut oil in a skillet over medium heat. Add the onion and sauté until it is translucent. Add in the remaining whisked ingredients. Cook until bubbling, then reduce heat and allow to simmer until thick, stirring occasionally, about 5 minutes. Remove from heat and pour over top of meatballs in the baking dish.

Return meatballs and sauce to the oven and bake an addition 10 minutes. Serve immediately. Goes great with sesame broccoli (page 245).

Nutrition per serving:
337 calories; 15 g Total Fat; 2 grams saturated fat; 18 g protein; 30 g carbohydrates; 2 grams dietary fiber; 79 mg cholesterol; 466 mg sodium.

Quinoa Pasta Fagioli

Fagioli means "beans" in Italian. This is a vegetarian gluten-free version of a traditional Italian soup. Serve with a crisp salad and you have a complete meal!

Servings: 4 (serving size = 1 ½ cups)

Ingredients:
2 stalks celery, chopped
1 carrot, sliced
1 onion, chopped
3 garlic cloves, minced
2 tablespoons fresh parsley, chopped
1 teaspoon Italian seasoning
2 tablespoons fresh basil, chopped
½ green bell pepper, chopped
½ red bell pepper, chopped
1 cup broccoli florets
1 bunch dark green leafy vegetable, such as chard or spinach, chopped
1 cup frozen green peas
dash sea salt
1 can (8 ounce) tomato sauce
2 cups reduced sodium chicken broth
2 tomatoes, peeled and chopped
1 package (8 ounce) uncooked quinoa pasta (spirals or shells)
1 can (15 ounce) cannellini beans (also called white kidney beans), rinsed and drained
1 tablespoon coconut oil

Instructions:
In a large stockpot over medium heat, sauté celery, carrots, onion, garlic, parsley, basil, and Italian seasoning in coconut oil until onion is translucent. Stir in chicken broth, tomatoes and tomato sauce, and bring to a boil.

Add broccoli, peppers and pasta and simmer on medium heat for 15 to 20 minutes, or until pasta is tender. Reduce heat to low. Add beans, peas, and greens and mix well. Cook for 5 minutes. Turn off heat. Serve immediately.

Nutrition per serving:
452 calories; 6 g Total Fat; 3 grams saturated fat; 18 g protein; 30 g carbohydrates; 7 grams dietary fiber; 0 mg cholesterol; 471 mg sodium.

Turkey Meatloaf Florentine

Having trouble fitting in those dark leafy greens? Try putting them in your meatloaf!

Servings: 6 (serving size = 4 ounces cooked meatloaf)

Ingredients:
1 can (8 ounce) tomato sauce
1 teaspoon dried oregano
1 teaspoon dried basil
¼ teaspoon garlic powder
1 ½ pounds ground turkey
¼ cup oat bran
1 egg
½ teaspoon sea salt
¼ teaspoon pepper
1 package (10 ounces) frozen spinach, thawed

Instructions:
Preheat oven to 350°F.

Drain the frozen spinach in a colander and press out most of the water. You may have to squeeze it between your hands to get most of the water out. It should be damp but not dripping wet. Set aside.

In a small bowl, combine tomato sauce, oregano, basil and garlic powder.

Combine ground turkey, oat bran, egg, salt, pepper and half of the tomato sauce mixture in a large bowl; mix well and form into a ball.

Place ball of meat mixture on a sheet of wax paper. Press down and spread out the meat, forming a rectangle about 8x10-inches.

Spread the spinach over half of the meat. Fold meat over so that the spinach is inside. Pinch edges of meat to seal.

Place meatloaf in a shallow baking pan, or into a loaf pan. Top with remaining tomato sauce.

Bake, uncovered, 1 hour. Let stand 5 to 10 minutes before slicing. Serve hot or cold.

Nutrition per serving:
200 calories; 8 g Total Fat; 0 grams saturated fat; 26 g protein; 30 g carbohydrates; 2 grams dietary fiber; 66 mg cholesterol; 555 mg sodium.

Simply Baked Sesame Halibut

This simple recipe can be made with salmon or tilapia as well.

Servings: 4 (serving size = 4 ounces cooked fish)

Ingredients:
1 ½ pounds halibut fillets
dash sea salt
dash pepper
2 tablespoons unrefined toasted sesame oil
water for filling the pan

Instructions:
Preheat oven to 350°F.

Brush both sides of halibut filets with sesame oil. Season with salt and pepper. Place filets in a baking dish, add a small amount of water to the bottom of the baking dish to keep the fish moist.

Bake uncovered for about 20 minutes, or until fish flakes easily.

Nutrition per serving:
240 calories; 11 g Total Fat; 1 grams saturated fat; 26 g protein; 0 g carbohydrates; 0 grams dietary fiber; 56 mg cholesterol; 373 mg sodium.

Herb Crusted Salmon on Greens

Servings: 2 (serving size = 4 ounces cooked fish on greens with dressing)

Ingredients:
Ginger Dressing for Greens
2 tablespoons lime juice
1 teaspoon fresh ginger root, minced
2 teaspoons Dijon mustard
2 tablespoons toasted sesame oil, divided
salt and pepper to taste

Salmon
2 (6 ounce) salmon fillets
2 ½ tablespoons fresh dill weed, divided
2 ½ tablespoons fresh basil, divided
1 bag (5 ounce) mixed baby greens

Instructions:
Whisk together the lime juice, ginger, and mustard in a small bowl. Slowly whisk in 1 tablespoon sesame oil. Sprinkle in salt and pepper.

Brush salmon on both sides with 1 tablespoon oil, then 1 tablespoon dill and 1 tablespoon basil. Press herbs to adhere.

Heat 1 tablespoon oil in large nonstick skillet over medium-high heat. Add the salmon to the skillet, herb side down and sauté for 4 minutes. Gently turn each fillet over and sauté until the salmon is just opaque in the center, about 5 minutes.

Toss the greens in a bowl with the remaining herbs and some dressing. Divide between 2 plates. Top with warm salmon and remaining dressing.

Nutrition per serving:
339 calories; 23 g Total Fat; 4 grams saturated fat; 27 g protein; 6 g carbohydrates; 0 grams dietary fiber; 74 mg cholesterol; 266 mg sodium

Pecan Crusted Dijon Tilapia

Most crusted fish recipes call for mayonnaise and bread crumbs. This recipe omits both and yields the same wonderful flavor!

Servings: 4 (serving size = 4 ounces of cooked fish)

Ingredients:
4 (4-6 ounce) Tilapia filets, skinless, preferably wild caught
1 cup plain non-fat Greek style yogurt, preferably organic
1/3 cup Dijon mustard
½ cup pecans, finely chopped

Instructions:
Preheat oven to 375°F. Line a baking sheet with parchment paper or coat it with coconut oil to prevent the fish from sticking.

Chop the pecans until they are very finely chopped but still have some small pieces intact. Set aside.

Combine the yogurt and Dijon mustard in a small shallow bowl and mix thoroughly to combine. Dip each Tilapia filet in the yogurt/Dijon mixture and place on a plate. Sprinkle both sides of the coated filet with the chopped pecans. Place pecan crusted filets on the prepared baking sheet.

Bake in preheated oven for about 10 to 12 minutes unless filets are extra large, then add about 2 minutes.

Nutritional facts per serving:
240 calories; 11 g Total Fat; 1 grams saturated fat; 27 g protein; 4 g carbohydrates; 1 grams dietary fiber; 50 mg cholesterol; 270 mg sodium.

Rainbow Veggie Pizza

Servings: 8 (serving size = 1 slice)

Ingredients:
1 Herbed Spelt Pizza Crust (12-inch) (see recipe page **223**) or ready to bake natural whole wheat pizza dough
1 ½ cups marinara sauce or pizza sauce
2 cups fresh spinach leaves, chopped
1 cup red onion, thinly sliced
1 cup fresh mushrooms, stems removed, thinly sliced
1 cup fresh basil leaves, chopped
1 can (4 ounce) sliced black olives
½ green bell pepper, thinly sliced
½ red bell pepper, thinly sliced
½ cup pine nuts
1 cup low moisture mozzarella cheese, shredded (preferably organic)
corn meal for sprinkling the pizza pan

Instructions:
Preheat oven to 400°F.

Roll dough out to the desired size and thickness. Poke the dough with a fork (known as docking) about every inch so that the crust does not inflate while prebaking.

To pre-bake your crust, sprinkle a pizza pan or pizza stone with some corn meal and place your crust on it. Bake for about 10 minutes.

Remove the pre-baked crust from the oven. Spread the marinara or pizza sauce over the top of the crust, leaving a ½ inch border. Top sauce with spinach, basil, mushrooms, onions, bell peppers, olives and pine nuts. Sprinkle the cheese over the top.

Place the pizza back in the oven and bake until the toppings are cooked to the desired state. By pre-baking the crust, you ensure that the crust is fully cooked. Remove from the oven and slice into 8 equal pieces.

Nutrition per serving:
272 calories; 14 g Total Fat; 3 gram saturated fat; 6 g protein; 26 g carbohydrates; 5 grams dietary fiber; 8 mg cholesterol; 693 mg sodium.

Spinach Enchiladas

These enchiladas are an absolute favorite. Another way to eat your dark green leafys!

Servings: 5 (serving size = 2 enchiladas)

Ingredients:
1 tablespoon coconut oil
1 cup onion, chopped
4 garlic cloves, minced
1 package (10 ounce) frozen spinach, thawed and drained
½ cup fat free ricotta cheese, preferably organic
½ cup nonfat plain Greek style yogurt, preferably organic
1 cup reduced fat Monterey Jack cheese, preferably organic
10 stone ground corn tortillas
2 ½ cups Green Enchilada Sauce (see recipe page 239)

Instructions:
Preheat oven to 375°F.

Warm enchilada sauce in a saucepan over medium heat until it bubbles, reduce heat to low. Cover the bottom of a 9 x 13-inch baking dish with a thin layer of the enchilada sauce. Set aside.

Meanwhile, heat oil in a skillet over medium heat. Add garlic and onion; cook for a few minutes until fragrant, but not brown. Stir in spinach, and cook for about 5 more minutes. Remove from the heat, and mix in ricotta cheese, yogurt, and ½ cup of Monterey Jack cheese. Set aside.

Dip one tortilla into the hot enchilada sauce, making sure they get fully coated and flexible, about 15 seconds. Place the sauce-covered tortilla on a plate.

Spoon about ¼ cup of the spinach mixture onto the center of the tortilla. Roll up, and place seam side down in the baking dish. Repeat with remaining tortillas.

When all enchiladas are in the baking dish, pour enchilada sauce over the top, and sprinkle with the remaining Monterey Jack cheese.

Bake for 15 to 20 minutes in the preheated oven, until sauce is bubbling and cheese is lightly browned at the edges.

Nutrition per serving:
499 calories; 15 g Total Fat; 5 gram saturated fat; 21 g protein; 67 g carbohydrates; 6 grams dietary fiber; 19 mg cholesterol; 526 mg sodium.

Three Sisters Casserole

A Native American expression, "three sisters" refers to the practice of growing beans, corn and squash together.

Servings: Makes one 8 x 11-inch baking dish, about 6 servings (serving size = 1/6 of pan)

Ingredients:

Polenta Topping
1 ½ cup course grind whole grain cornmeal
2 tablespoons chili powder
¼ teaspoon sea salt
4 ½ cups water

Three Sisters Filling
3 tablespoons coconut oil, divided use
1 cups onion, chopped
1 red bell pepper, chopped
2 cups butternut squash, peeled and cubed into 1" cubes
1 can (15 ounce) diced tomatoes
1 can (4 ounce) mild diced green chilies
2 garlic cloves, minced
1 teaspoon coriander
1 teaspoon cumin
½ teaspoon sea salt
1 can (15 ounce) kidney beans, drained and rinsed
1cup frozen corn kernels, thawed

Instructions:
Preheat oven to 375°F.

To make polenta topping, whisk together the cornmeal, chili powder, salt and 4 ½ cups water in a double boiler, or place in a large metal bowl over barely simmering water. Cook for 40 minutes, or until the polenta is thick and stiff, stirring 3 or 4 times. Remove from heat.

To make Three Sisters Filling, heat 2 tablespoons oil in large saucepan over medium heat. Add onion, and cook 7 minutes, or until softened, stirring often. Add bell pepper, and cook 5 minutes more, stirring often.

Stir in squash, tomatoes, chilies, garlic, coriander and cumin. Cook 5 minutes, stirring occasionally. Stir in ½ cup water and salt. Bring mixture to a boil. Reduce heat to medium low, and simmer, partially covered, 10 to 15 minutes, or until squash is tender. Stir in beans and corn, and cook 5 minutes, or until slightly thickened, stirring occasionally.

Coat an 8x11-inch baking dish with coconut oil. Spread 2 cups polenta over bottom of prepared dish. Spoon squash mixture over polenta. Smooth remaining polenta (about 2 ½ cups) over top.

Score casserole into 6 squares with knife. Brush top with remaining 1 tablespoon oil. Bake 30 minutes, or until heated through and top is lightly browned.

Nutrition per serving:
335 calories; 9 g Total Fat; 6 gram saturated fat; 9 g protein; 55 g carbohydrates; 8 grams dietary fiber; 0 mg cholesterol; 466 mg sodium.

HIGH QUALITY SNACK FOODS AND DESSERTS

Flourless Chocolate "Cake"

This cake is always a hit in my classes. Its texture is amazingly like that of a traditional cake—very rich, sweet and chewy.

Servings: 18 (serving size = 1/18 of the cake, very thin slice)

Ingredients:
1 cup chopped or crushed dates, pits removed and soaked for 1-2 hours
3 cups finely ground almonds (also called almond meal or almond flour)
1 tablespoon coconut oil
½ teaspoon sea salt
½ cup shredded coconut, or more if needed
1 teaspoon pure vanilla extract
½ cup carob powder or unsweetened cacao powder
Peel from 4 tangerines or 2 oranges, finely chopped in a food chopper or food processor (use the oranges or tangerines for snacking or for topping the cake)
¼ cup fresh raspberries
¼ cup fresh blueberries
1 kiwi fruit, sliced

Instructions:
Make a date paste by placing the soaked dates in the bowl of a food processor and pulsing until the dates are mushy and form a sticky paste.

Transfer the date paste to a large bowl. Add ground almonds, coconut oil, salt, shredded coconut, vanilla, carob or cocoa powder, and finely chopped orange or tangerine peel to the bowl and mix with a wooden spoon or with your hands, until it forms a ball of "dough". If mixture is not firm enough, add more shredded coconut.

Place the ball of "dough" onto a flat plate. Using your hands, form it into a round cake shape.

Top with raspberries, blueberries, kiwi slices, and the sections from your peeled orange or tangerine. Refrigerate until chilled. Slice into18 thin pieces and serve.

Nutrition per serving:
221 calories; 14 g Total Fat; 3 gram saturated fat; 5 g protein; 17 g carbohydrates; 2 grams dietary fiber; 0 mg cholesterol; 66 mg sodium.

Did you know?
Every ingredient in this recipe is alkaline forming. You can enjoy this sweet treat on a regular basis!

Agave Granola Bars

These bars are chewy and sweet.

Servings: 24 (serving size = 1 bar)

Ingredients:
2 cups rolled oats
½ cup toasted pepitas
¼ cup sesame seeds
½ cup pecans, chopped
½ cup almonds, chopped or sliced
2 tablespoons ground flaxseeds
2/3 cup unsweetened coconut flakes
2/3 cup coconut oil (warm enough to be in a liquid state)
1 teaspoon liquid stevia
½ cup agave nectar

Instructions:
In a large bowl combine all dry ingredients. Mix well. Add in coconut oil, stevia, and agave nectar and mix well.

Transfer mixture to a 9 ½ x 11-inch baking dish. Spread evenly and pat down. Cover the pan and refrigerate several hours or overnight, or place in the freezer for 30 minutes. To serve, slice into 24 bars.

Due to the coconut oil becoming soft when warm the bars may lose their shape if left out in a warm place. They are best kept in the refrigerator until ready to be eaten.

Nutrition per serving:
156 calories; 13 g Total Fat; 7 gram saturated fat; 3 g protein; 7 g carbohydrates; 1 grams dietary fiber; 0 mg cholesterol; 20 mg sodium.

Did you know?
Instead of forming this mixture into bars, you can just put it in a container and eat it like granola.

Tamari Seasoned Nut Mix

This is a great on-the-go snack.

Servings: 16 (serving size = 1 ounce)

Ingredients:
½ pound raw almonds
½ pound raw cashews
2 tablespoons wheat free reduced sodium Tamari Sauce

Instructions:
Preheat oven to 250°F.

Place nuts and tamari sauce in a bowl. Mix together thoroughly.

Transfer to baking sheet and place in the oven for 20 minutes. Remove from oven. Let cool. Keep in an airtight container.

Nutrition per serving:
178 calories; 14 g Total Fat; 2 gram saturated fat; 5 g protein; 7 g carbohydrates; 1 grams dietary fiber; 0 mg cholesterol; 88 mg sodium.

Flourless Oatmeal Raisin Cookies

This recipe makes large cookies and has NO flour. Due to the natural sweeteners, nuts, and peanut butter, they're very satisfying and won't set you up for craving more.

Servings: 24 (serving size = 1 cookie)

Ingredients:
1/3 cup organic butter, unsalted
½ cup Rapadura unrefined whole cane organic sugar
1 teaspoon liquid stevia
1 cup natural chunky peanut butter
2 eggs
1 teaspoon pure vanilla extract
1 ¼ teaspoons baking soda
1 tablespoon agave nectar
3 cups rolled oats
1 cup raisins

Instructions:
Preheat oven to 350°F.

In a large bowl, cream together the butter, Rapadura, and peanut butter until smooth. Beat in the eggs, one at a time, then stir in the agave nectar, stevia and vanilla. Mix in baking soda and oats until well blended. Stir in the raisins.

Roll dough into 2-inch balls, and place 3 inches apart on baking sheet lined with parchment paper. Flatten slightly with a fork.

Bake for 12 to 15 minutes in the preheated oven. Cool on cookie sheets for a few minutes, then transfer to wire racks to cool completely.

Nutrition per serving:
175 calories; 9 g Total Fat; 3 gram saturated fat; 5 g protein; 18 g carbohydrates; 1 grams dietary fiber; 25 mg cholesterol; 64 mg sodium.

Spelt Chocolate Chip Cookies

The cookies are wheat-free and dairy-free. You will not believe how good they are!

Servings: 12 (serving size = 1 cookie)

Ingredients:
1 ¼ cups whole spelt flour
¼ teaspoon sea salt
1 teaspoon non-aluminum baking powder
½ teaspoon baking soda
¼ cup Rapadura unrefined whole cane organic sugar
1/3 cup pure maple syrup
1/3 cup coconut oil (warm enough to be in a liquid state)
1 ½ teaspoon pure vanilla extract
½ cup grain-sweetened chocolate chips

Instructions:
Preheat oven to 350°F.

In a large bowl, use a wire whisk to thoroughly mix together the spelt flour, salt, baking powder, baking soda, and Rapadura.

In a second large bowl, whisk together maple syrup, coconut oil, and vanilla extract. Whisk until the entire mixture is thick and syrupy.

Add half of the flour mixture to the syrup mixture. Using a rubber spatula, stir to combine. The mixture will be very wet. Add in the chocolate chips and stir.

Add in the rest of the flour mixture and stir to combine, making sure to scrape the sides of the bowl with the rubber spatula to get all of the flour mixed in. At this point the dough should be soft but not overly oily or wet.

Break off tablespoon-size pieces of the dough and place them 1 inch apart on a baking sheet lined with parchment paper. You do not need to roll the dough into balls, however the sizes of the dough pieces should be somewhat round.

Bake for 11 to 15 minutes. Cookies should be a slightly puffy when removed from the oven, but will flatten out a little during cooling. Let cool on the cookie sheet for 5 minutes and then transfer to a wire rack to cool completely. Cookies will be chewy when completely cooled.

Nutrition per serving:
155 calories; 8 g Total Fat; 6 gram saturated fat; 2 g protein; 21 g carbohydrates; 2 grams dietary fiber; 0 mg cholesterol; 108 mg sodium.

Minty Chocolate Chocolate-Chip Cookies

This is a minty twist on my spelt chocolate chip cookies. So awesome!

Servings: 12 (serving size = 1 cookie)

Ingredients:
1 ¼ cups whole spelt flour
¼ teaspoon sea salt
1 1/8 teaspoon non-aluminum baking powder plus
½ teaspoon plus 1/8 teaspoon baking soda
2 tablespoons unsweetened cocoa powder
¼ cup Rapadura unrefined whole cane organic sugar
1/3 cup pure maple syrup
1/3 cup coconut oil (warm enough to be in a liquid state)
1 teaspoon pure vanilla extract
1 teaspoon mint extract
½ teaspoon liquid stevia
½ cup grain-sweetened chocolate chips

Instructions:
Preheat oven to 350°F.

In a large bowl, use a wire whisk to thoroughly mix together the spelt flour, salt, baking powder, baking soda, cocoa powder and Rapadura.

In a second large bowl, whisk together maple syrup, coconut oil, vanilla extract, mint extract, and stevia. Whisk until the entire mixture is thick and syrupy.

Add half of the flour mixture to the syrup mixture. Using a rubber spatula, stir to combine. The mixture will be very wet. Add in the chocolate chips and stir.

Add in the rest of the flour mixture and stir to combine, making sure to scrape the sides of the bowl with the rubber spatula to get all of the flour mixed in. At this point the dough should be soft but not overly oily or wet.

Break off tablespoon-size pieces of the dough and place them 1 inch apart on a baking sheet lined with parchment paper. You do not need to roll the dough into balls, however the sizes of the dough pieces should be somewhat round.

Bake for 11 to 15 minutes. Cookies should be a slightly puffy when removed from the oven, but will flatten out a little during cooling. Let cool on the cookie sheet for 5 minutes and then transfer to a wire rack to cool completely. Cookies will be chewy when completely cooled.

Nutrition per serving:
159 calories; 8 g Total Fat; 6 gram saturated fat; 2 g protein; 21 g carbohydrates; 2 grams dietary fiber; 0 mg cholesterol; 161 mg sodium.

Allowable Sin™

These are my famous sugar-free chocolate truffles. These treats are loaded with protein, good fat, and fiber. Beware, these treats are addicting!

Servings: 32 (serving size = 1 piece)

Ingredients:
¼ cup coconut oil
2 ounces unsweetened baking chocolate
¼ cup vanilla flavored whey protein powder
2 tablespoons carob powder or unsweetened cocoa powder
¼ cup unsweetened shredded coconut
¼ cup raw cashews, chopped
¼ cup raw almonds, chopped
¼ cup raisins or chopped dates
½ cup chunky natural peanut butter
1 teaspoon vanilla extract
1 teaspoon liquid stevia
32 mini size paper baking cups (cupcake liners), about the size of truffles

Instructions:
Chop the baker's chocolate into small pieces.

Place the coconut oil in a small saucepan and add the chopped chocolate. Place the pan over a low heat and allow the chocolate to melt into the coconut oil. Stir frequently with a rubber spatula. When the chocolate is completely melted, remove from heat and set aside.

In a large bowl, combine the protein powder, carob or cocoa powder, coconut, chopped almonds, chopped cashews, chopped dates or raisins, and shredded coconut. Mix together well with a spoon. Add in the peanut butter and mix thoroughly. At this point the mixture should be somewhat crumbly.

Add the vanilla extract and the stevia to the melted chocolate mixture in the saucepan and stir to mix thoroughly. Transfer the melted chocolate mixture to the bowl, using the rubber spatula to scrape out the saucepan.

Stir the mixture thoroughly to combine. Use a small measuring spoon, such as a teaspoon, to scoop and fill the baking cups with the chocolate mixture. Put them in a baking dish or other large flat container and place in the freezer until the truffles harden, about 30 minutes. Store in the freezer until ready to eat.

Note: when frozen, the paper cup peels off easily and you will have a chocolate delight that resembles a mini Reese's Peanut Butter Cup (without the sugar and trans-fats)!

Nutrition per serving:
80 calories; 6 g Total Fat; 3 gram saturated fat; 3 g protein; 3 g carbohydrates; 1 grams dietary fiber; 0 mg cholesterol; 8 mg sodium.

CHAPTER 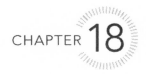 18

Frequently
Asked Questions

Q: *On a sugarless/flourless diet are these products allowed: Baked Brown Rice Snaps, Gluten Free pastas made from organic rice, spelt, potato and soy flours?*

A: On a sugarless/flourless diet, we should be very careful not to fall into the trap of replacing white flour foods with a bunch of foods made from alternative flours. The idea of a flourless lifestyle is to eat foods in their more whole form--closest to natural form as possible. Occasionally we can enjoy crackers, muffins, and pastas made from brown rice flour, amaranth flour, spelt flour, quinoa flour, buckwheat, and oat flours. However, for the most part, it is best to eat these grains in their more whole forms, such as the brown rice, steel cut oats, buckwheat, and quinoa. Whenever a grain is ground into flour so that it can be used to make pastas cookies, muffins, or cakes—usually other ingredients have to be added to "hold" the flour together into a muffin, bread, or cracker. When we eat the whole grain, all that is required is some water and heat to cook it, along with some natural herbs and spices for seasoning.

Additionally, all flours, including whole grain flours, are considered potentially troublesome because research has shown that they all create a brain chemical response in the form of increased serotonin levels. This serotonin "high" may lead to cravings for more carbohydrates, which in turn may lead to overconsumption of carbohydrates in general. Also, although whole wheat flour and other whole grain flours are absorbed more slowly than white flour, whole grain flours can still destabilize blood glucose levels by triggering the pancreas into an insulin release. Too much insulin creates an upsetting imbalance and many of our bodily functions and organs are affected.

My best recommendations are to eat whole grains in their closest to natural state, and save the alternative flour foods for special occasions, not everyday consumption. For instance, I eat brown rice and oat bran regularly, and only on special occasions (like a once every so often camping trip or special homemade brunch) will eat whole-wheat pancakes for breakfast. On a day when I eat something like that, I am careful not to eat any other type of flour foods. For instance, if I have the whole-wheat pancakes, on that day I will not eat any other food with wheat in it, and I also will not eat any other flour foods, such as a brown rice cracker. For those who are interested, I do not eat any pasta at all for good scientific and personal reasons. First, pastas are made with flours that are finely ground, which contribute to that serotonin "high" much more quickly. Second, probably due to that serotonin high, pasta was a food I used to eat in mass quantities, therefore I have eliminated it from my life entirely.

Q: *My diabetic daughter wonders why eating sugar is any worse than eating natural sugar in fruit, for instance, since our bodies convert most foods into glucose anyway?*

A: I get this question frequently, so I am glad that you asked. Sugar content in foods and how sugar is processed in the body is often oversimplified. It is very important that we all realize the detrimental effects of eating sugar in its refined forms. Sugar from fruit IS NOT the same as refined white sugar from a cookie or a candy bar. Eating refined sugar is like putting rocket fuel into your body. The sugar is absorbed very quickly leading to a sharp rise in blood sugar (referred to as a "sugar high") followed by a quick drop in blood sugar (the crash). This plays serious havoc with the entire digestive system, which puts stress on the pancreas and liver as they must work extra hard to metabolize such a large sugar rush. In fact, when the pancreas is stressed to continually provide insulin to convert sugar to energy it can literally be worn out and will not work any more (that is the cause of diabetes).

When natural occurring sugars are eaten as part of a whole food like a fruit or a vegetable, this type of stress on the digestive organs does not occur. When the fruit is intact and whole, its fiber will moderate the release of fructose and subsequently insulin into your bloodstream. This happens slowly so that there is no huge onslaught of sugar for your body to metabolize.

Yes, the end result of carbohydrate metabolism is glucose, but the source of the glucose and the rate at which the glucose enters the body is what we should keep in mind. It's time we realize that we cannot keep abusing our bodies with refined sugars. We are killing ourselves with this sweet poison and it's time that we stop lying to ourselves and rationalizing our addiction to sugars.

Q: *My husband insists that if I ate 5 lbs. of fudge I wouldn't gain any more weight than if I ate 5 lbs. of lettuce. He said I couldn't gain any more weight than the weight of the food eaten?*

A: Although we might be tempted to think in simplistic terms that we gain as much weight as the weight of the food we eat, our bodies are not that simplistic. Metabolism of food, assimilation of nutrients, burning of calories, and storage of fat is a complex process based on several scientific laws of physics, chemistry, and thermodynamics (energy). In fact, to illustrate this, we can look at the human body's consumption of water. If a person drinks a gallon of water a day, and if the water is at room temperature, that water will weigh 8.3 pounds. Drinking 8.3 pounds of water does not make us gain 8.3 pounds of body weight. First, all substances change in weight depending upon the temperature and pressure. This is called density. When water is heated it becomes heavier, and when it is cooled or frozen, it becomes lighter (this is why ice floats in water). Second, water is metabolized and utilized in various ways by the body. Some of it is absorbed, some of it is used to transport nutrients to bones and tissues, and some of it flushes out wastes. We do not necessarily flush out all of the water we drink, nor do we absorb all of it and hold on to it in the body. If we eat five pounds of lettuce, we will not gain five pounds. In fact, if we eat five pounds of lettuce, we will most likely lose some weight. That is because lettuce is a form of insoluble fiber that requires more calories to be expended just to digest it than the calories it provides the body. Five pounds of lettuce contains 260 calories, but it takes more than 260 calories to digest it. Additionally, most of that lettuce will leave our bodies undigested because it is insoluble and used in the body as roughage (helpful for maintaining healthy bowel function).

As for the five pounds of fudge, we will most likely gain some weight, although we will not gain the weight of the fudge itself. Fudge is pure sugar and carbohydrates that contains no fiber; therefore it takes little energy to digest the fudge. Also, most of the carbohydrates will break down easily into simple sugars that, if not converted to energy will be stored as fat.

Q: *What is "fractionated palm oil" and "fractionated coconut oil"? Are they the same as hydrogenated oils?*

A: Fractionation is a further phase of coconut oil or palm oil processing, designed to extract and concentrate specific fatty acid fractions. Fractionated coconut or palm oil is used for the convenience of manufacturers who like its stability and melting characteristics. The healthful aspects of natural coconut or palm oil are largely lost in the process. I've noticed that fractionated palm oil is a common ingredient in many power bars sold in health-food stores.

You should only eat organic, expeller pressed or extra virgin coconut or palm oil. It is difficult to know how the oils are processed when they appear on an ingredient label. Fractionated coconut or palm oil is NOT good for you. It isn't known if this processed oil is any better than hydrogenated fats, and it is my educated opinion that it should be avoided. Remember to eat foods in their closest to natural form. Fractionating oils is not natural.

Q: *What is your opinion on Smart Balance buttery spread? Is it healthy or something we should avoid, perhaps use real butter instead?*

A: Smart Balance is a patented mixture of olive, soy, palm and canola oils along with chemical emulsifiers, synthetic antioxidants, and artificial flavors. It's unfortunate that soybean oil and canola oil are part of this proprietary blend. They are both unhealthy oils. The regular SMART BALANCE also contains vegetable diglycerides, sorbitan esters, calcium disodium EDTA and something called TBHQ.

Foods that contain mono-diglycerides should be avoided. They are merely hydrogenated oils in disguise. Very bad for you!

Sorbitan esters are chemicals used to emulsify foods; that means it holds them together and prevents separation.

EDTA stands for ethylenediaminetetraacetic acid. EDTA can perform the following specific functions in food: sequestering metals, preventing discoloration of potato products, stabilizing vitamins, preventing discoloration of fish and shellfish, preventing flavor changes in milk, inhibiting the thickening of stored condensed milk, enhancing the foaming properties of reconstituted skim milk, preventing color changes of scrambled eggs prepared from egg powder, preserving canned legume, preventing gushing in beer, promoting flavor retention and delaying loss of carbonation in soft drinks, preventing oxidation of meat products, and preventing discoloration of canned fruits and vegetables. EDTA is also often added to detergents, liquid soaps, shampoos, agricultural chemical sprays, pharmaceutical products, oil emulsions and to textiles to improve dyeing, scouring and detergent operations. Wow, with so many uses, one must wonder how safe it really is for human consumption.

Tert-butylhydroquinone (TBHQ) is a white, crystalline solid having a characteristic odor. It is practically insoluble in water but soluble in alcohol and in ether. TBHQ is a general-purpose antioxidant used to preserve various oils, fats and food items by retarding their oxidative deterioration. It is used in formulating varnish, lacquer, resins and oil field additives. It is used a fixative in perfumery to reduce the evaporation rate and improve stability. I repeat, wow, with so many uses, one must wonder how safe it really is for human consumption.

I personally use real butter or coconut oil, two naturally occurring whole foods that have been consumed for generations without chemicals added to them to make them taste better or make them stable for longer.

Q: *Is Earth Balance Natural Buttery Spread OK to eat? The ingredient list is as follows: Expeller-Pressed Natural Oil Blend (soybean, palm fruit, canola and olive), filtered water, pure salt, natural flavor (derived from corn, no MSG, no alcohol, no gluten), soy protein, soy lecithin, lactic acid (non-dairy, derived from sugar beets), and beta-carotene color (from natural source). If not, what do you recommend as a butter replacement?*

A: Earth Balance, or any other new fangled tub spreads are not healthy. Even though they don't contain hydrogenated oils, they contain soy protein isolates, which are not healthy.

I actually don't recommend replacing butter in the diet. What I do recommend is that the butter you eat be organic so that you don't also eat hormones and pesticides that get absorbed into cow's milk fat and subsequently into the butter made from that milk fat.

My question to you would be why don't you want to eat butter? Have you (along with the rest of America) been a victim of the disinformation campaign that butter and tropical saturated fats are the root cause of heart disease and cancer? If so, then read on.

For millennia, butter has been a staple of the diets of supremely healthy peoples, and valued for its life-sustaining properties. Butter does not cause diseases, but rather protects against them. Heart disease was rare in America a hundred years ago. At that time the average amount of butter people ate was 18 pounds per year. Imagine, eating 18 pounds of organic butter per year and still being healthy!

Unfortunately, between 1920 and 1960 the amount of butter people were eating dropped to only 4 pounds per year. During that same time, heart disease rose to become the number one killer in America. How can it happen that when people eat less butter they develop heart disease at alarmingly higher rates than at any other time in human history?

Because butter (and it has to be organic butter these days) actually contains many nutrients that protect us from heart disease. First among these is vitamin A, which is needed for the health of the thyroid and adrenal glands, both of which play a role in maintaining the proper functioning of the heart and cardiovascular system.

Butter also contains lecithin, a substance that assists in the proper assimilation and metabolism of cholesterol and other fat constituents.

Butter contains a number of anti-oxidants, especially Vitamin A, Vitamin E and the mineral Selenium, that protect us against the kind of free radical damage that weakens the arteries.

Butter also helps strengthen the immune system. The vitamin A in butter is essential in this role as well. The short and medium chain fatty acids (also found in coconut oil) have immune strengthening properties. But hydrogenated fats and excess of long chain polyunsaturated oils and many butter substitutes both have a deleterious effect on the immune system.

If you want to replace butter in your diet with oil that is even more supremely effective, use extra virgin coconut oil. I recommend a combination of the two.

Q: *I was wondering your thoughts on spirulina and chlorella? Could you please tell me more about them? Do they each have something that I cannot get through my normal healthy diet?*

A: Before I talk about chlorella and spirulina, I talk about chlorophyll. Chlorophyll is the element in plants that gives the leaves their green color. The plants are able to "make" chlorophyll from their exposure to sunlight through photosynthesis. Chlorophyll not only supplies the green color to the plants but also supplies a form of vitality or energy that enables the plant to live independently and separately from other plants. Fungi, for instance, and many similar forms of vegetation or living matter which do not have chlorophyll, become parasites and have to attach themselves to something else that does have chlorophyll in order to derive the vitality and essence necessary to life.

Having said that, we humans also need to attach ourselves to, or rather ingest, chlorophyll to give us the vitality and essence necessary to life. If we do not eat enough green foods, we have low energy and degenerate into poor health.

Chlorella and spirulina both contain chlorophyll, as does wheat grass, alfalfa grass and barley grass, and of course all green vegetables and plant foods. Chlorella and spirulina have extremely high amounts of chlorophyll and enzymes, which aid in digestion and help to proliferate the growth of good bacteria in the intestine.

Chlorella is a green single-celled algae cultivated in fresh water ponds. It has a grass-like smell because of the high amounts of chlorophyll in it, the highest concentration of any plant in the world. It has existed on the planet for billions of years and was one of the first foods to appear. Chlorella is one of the healthiest, most potent foods in existence.

Chlorella is a potent detoxifier; it actually binds with heavy metals in the blood to pull them out of the tissues and bloodstream. Chlorella is also a fibrous material that greatly augments healthy digestion and overall digestive tract health.

Spirulina (Spirulina Pacifica) is a microscopic freshwater plant, an aquatic micro-vegetable/organism composed of transparent bubble-thin cells stacked end-to-end forming a helical spiral filament, hence the name.

Spirulina will not bind to heavy metals the way chlorella will. Spirulina has other properties that compliment the properties of chlorella. Spirulina is the richest source of natural antioxidants of any whole-food source. It contains every natural known antioxidant including zinc, manganese, selenium, and copper, vitamin E, vitamins B1 and B6, Methionine, and beta-carotene.

Spirulina contains more beta-carotene than any other whole food. Beta-carotene allows the body to signal cancerous cells to stop dividing. Foods rich in beta-carotene may not only be able to prevent but also reverse cancers. Research has demonstrated that beta-carotene reduces the size of tumors.

Spirulina and chlorella are both excellent sources of protein. Earthwise or Jarrow are good brands for chlorella and spirulina.

Q: *Is carrageenan from seaweed OK? Many prepared foods contain this ingredient.*

A: My thoughts on carrageenan are that it should be avoided.

Carrageenan is a common food additive that comes from red seaweed also known as Irish Moss or *Chondrus Crispus*. Carrageen has long been used as a thickener and emulsifier in ice cream, yogurt, cottage cheese and other processed food products, including soy milk. Carrageenan is extracted from red seaweed by using powerful alkali solvents. These solvents would remove the tissues and skin from your hands as readily as would any acid

Results of a study published in October 2001 suggest that carrageenan may not be as safe as once thought. Findings from animal studies and a review of the scientific literature showed that degraded forms of carrageenan can cause ulcerations and cancers of the gastrointestinal tract. Carrageenan is a gel. It coats the insides of a stomach, like gooey honey or massage oil. Digestive problems often ensue, especially in those with intestinal problems such as Chron's, IBS and colitis. People with those condition should avoid it.

Concerns about carrageenan have centered on the "degraded" type which is distinguished from the "undegraded" type by its lower molecular weight. Most of the studies linking carrageenan to cancer and other gastrointestinal disorders have focused on degraded carrageenan. But Dr. Joanne Tobacman, a leading carageenan researcher, thinks that undegraded carrageenan - the kind most widely used as a food additive - might also be associated with malignancies and other stomach problems. She suggests that such factors as bacterial action, stomach acid and food preparation may transform undegraded carageenan into the more dangerous degraded type.

Given this new information on carrageenan, I would recommend avoiding regular consumption of products containing it. Product labels do not distinguish between degraded and undegraded carrageenan.

Q: *I have a question concerning grinding my own flax seeds. I heard that if you grind them yourself, there is a harmful chemical produced. Could you please elaborate on this?*

A: Raw flaxseeds are safe in the proper amounts. However, they do contain a substance called cyanogenic glycosides, as do lima beans, sweet potatoes, yams, and bamboo shoots. Once ingested, these glycosides are metabolized into another compound called thiocyanate, which is what I talked about in the class. Thiocyanate has the potential, over time, to suppress the thyroid's ability to take up enough iodine. This biochemical occurrence raises the risk of developing goiter.

In order to avoid this problem, you should limit the amount of RAW ground flaxseeds to 3-4 tablespoons per day. Another way is to lightly bake the flaxseeds before grinding them. Toasting them at a very low temperature of 250 degrees Fahrenheit for 15-20 minutes will deactivate and decompose the cyanogenic glycosides but will not destroy the beneficial omega-3 oil contained in the seeds. DO NOT bake at temperatures above 300 because you will destroy the oil and turn it into a free radical).

When you purchase flaxseeds already ground, they have already been toasted at a low temperature.

Notes

PREFACE

Razden, Anjula. "The Shopping Cart Cure." *Experience Life Magazine.* January/
February 2007:38-40.

Schatz, Hale Sofia. *If The Buddha Came to Dinner* (New York: Hyperion, 2004), 12.

INTRODUCTION

1. Rubin, Jordan S., N.M.D., PhD. *The Makers Diet* (Florida: Siloam, 2004), 2.
2. Associated Press, "Study: Childhood Obesity Expected to Soar Worldwide,"
   msnbc.msn.com, March 7, 2006, http://www.msnbc.msn.com/id/11694799/.
3. Gardner, Amanda. "Obese Kids Have Old Arteries," *US News and World
   Report,* usnews.com, November 11, 2008, http://health.usnews.com/articles/
   health/healthday/2008/11/11/obese-kids-have-old-arteries.html.
4. Edward Bauman, M.Ed., Ph.D. "Eating For Health: A New System, Not
   Another Diet" baumancollege.org, 2007, http://www.baumancollege.org/
   newsite/index.php?option=com_content&task=view&id=93&Itemid=55
5. Schmid, Ronald F., N.D., *Traditional Foods are Your Best Medicine* (Vermont:
   Healing Arts Press, 1997), xiv.
6. Ibid, xv.
7. Ibid, xiv.
8. Schatz, Hale Sofia. *If The Buddha Came to Dinner* (New York: Hyperion, 2004),
   3.

CHAPTER 1:
FROM OBESE JUNK FOOD JUNKIE TO SLIM TRIM NUTRITION SAVVY EXPERT: SEVENTEEN YEARS OF SUSTAINED WEIGHT LOSS

1. Overeaters Anonymous. "Fifteen Questions." oa.org, 1998-2008, www.oa.org.
2. Wikipedia. "Cognitive Dissonance." Wikipedia.org, January 4, 2009, http://en.wikipedia.org/wiki/Cognitive_dissonance.
3. Rubin, Jordan S., N.M.D., Ph.D. *The Maker's Diet* (Florida: Siloam, 2004), 29.
4. Schmid, Ronald F., N.D., *Traditional Foods are Your Best Medicine* (Vermont: Healing Arts Press, 1997), xiv.

CHAPTER 2:
GLOBESITY AND THE FATALLY FLAWED FOOD GUIDE

1. Associated Press, "Obesity an 'International Scourge,'" cbsnews.com, September 3, 2006, http://www.cbsnews.com/stories/2006/09/03/health/main1962961.shtml.
2. Associated Press, "Globesity Gains Ground as Leading Killer," msnbc.msn.com, May 10, 2004, http://www.msnbc.msn.com/id/4900095/.
3. Johns Hopkins Bloomberg School of Public Health, Public Health Newsletter, "Study Suggests 86 Percent of Americans Could be Overweight or Obese by 2030," July 28, 2008, http://www.jhsph.edu/publichealthnews/press_releases/2008/wang_obesity_projections.
4. Associated Press, "Study: Childhood Obesity Expected to Soar Worldwide," msnbc.msn.com, March 7, 2006, http://www.msnbc.msn.com/id/11694799/.
5. Associated Press, "Globesity Gains Ground as Leading Killer," msnbc.msn.com, May 10, 2004, http://www.msnbc.msn.com/id/4900095/.
6. Ibid.
7. Associated Press, "European Nations Sign Anti-Obesity Charter," cbsnews.com, November 15, 2006, http://www.cbsnews.com/stories/11/16/world/main2188875.shtml.
8. Associated Press, "Study: Childhood Obesity Expected to Soar Worldwide," msnbc.msn.com, March 7, 2006, http://www.msnbc.msn.com/id/11694799/.
9. Light, Luise, Ed.D. "A Fatally Flawed Food Guide." *Evergreen Monthly.* November, 2004, 37-38.
10. Ibid.
11. United States Department of Agriculture. "Inside the Pyramid: Discretionary Calories." MyPyramid.gov, October 8, 2008, http://www.mypyramid.gov/pyramid/discretionary_calories.html
12. Willett, Walter C., M.D. *Eat, Drink, and Be Healthy.* New York: Simon & Schuster, 2001, 16.
13. Ibid, 12.
14. Ibid, 16.
15. Ibid, 22-24.

CHAPTER 3:
A DOCTOR, A DENTIST AND A PSYCHIC

1. Price Pottenger Nutrition Foundation, "What is the Price-Pottenger Foundation?" 1997-2008, http://www.ppnf.org/catalog/ppnf/whois.htm.
2. Pottenger, Francis M., M.D., *Pottenger's Cats* (La Mesa: Price-Pottenger Nutritional Foundation, 2nd Edition, 2005), 113.
3. Ibid, 114.
4. Ibid, 116.
5. The Master Cleanse/Raw Food Site, "Pottenger's Cats-A Study in Nutrition," 2003-2008, http://therawfoodsite.com/cats.htm.
6. Ibid.
7. Ibid.
8. Pottenger, Francis M., M.D., *Pottenger's Cats* (La Mesa: Price-Pottenger Nutritional Foundation, 2nd Edition, 2005), 2.
9. Ibid, 5-6.
10. Nutrition Really Works, "The Pottenger Cat Experiments Illustrate the Genetic Tendency Principle." 2005, http://nutritionreallyworks.com/Pottengers-cats. html.
11. Wikipedia, "Francis M. Pottenger, Jr.," October 13, 2008, http://en.wikipedia. org/wiki/Pottenger.
12. Pottenger, Francis M., M.D., *Pottenger's Cats* (La Mesa: Price-Pottenger Nutritional Foundation, 2nd Edition, 2005), 42.
13. Ibid, 3.
14. Schmid, Ronald F., N.D., *Traditional Foods are Your Best Medicine* (Vermont: Healing Arts Press, 1997), 7.
15. Byrnes, Stephens, Dr. "The Neglected Nutritional Research of Dr. Weston Price, DDS," http://www.mercola.com/2001/jan/21/weston_price.htm.
16. Schmid, Ronald F., N.D., *Traditional Foods are Your Best Medicine* (Vermont: Healing Arts Press, 1997), 7.
17. Rubin, Jordan S., N.M.D., Ph.D. *The Maker's Diet* (Florida: Siloam, 2004), 43.
18. Byrnes, Stephens, Dr. "The Neglected Nutritional Research of Dr. Weston Price, DDS," http://www.mercola.com/2001/jan/21/weston_price.htm.
19. Schmid, Ronald F., N.D., *Traditional Foods are Your Best Medicine* (Vermont: Healing Arts Press, 1997), 8.
20. Byrnes, Stephens, Dr. "The Neglected Nutritional Research of Dr. Weston Price, DDS," http://www.mercola.com/2001/jan/21/weston_price.htm.
21. Schmid, Ronald F., N.D., *Traditional Foods are Your Best Medicine* (Vermont: Healing Arts Press, 1997), 8.
22. Ibid.,31.
23. The Weston A. Price Foundation, "Principles of Healthy Diets," 1999, http:// www.westonaprice.org/brochures/wapfbrochure.html.
24. Byrnes, Stephens, Dr. "The Neglected Nutritional Research of Dr. Weston Price, DDS," http://www.mercola.com/2001/jan/21/weston_price.htm.
25. Ibid.

26. Schmid, Ronald F., N.D., *Traditional Foods are Your Best Medicine* (Vermont: Healing Arts Press, 1997), 20-21.
27. Byrnes, Stephens, Dr. "The Neglected Nutritional Research of Dr. Weston Price, DDS," http://www.mercola.com/2001/jan/21/weston_price.htm.
28. Ibid.
29. Schmid, Ronald F., N.D., *Traditional Foods are Your Best Medicine* (Vermont: Healing Arts Press, 1997), 9.
30. Byrnes, Stephens, Dr. "The Neglected Nutritional Research of Dr. Weston Price, DDS," http://www.mercola.com/2001/jan/21/weston_price.htm.
31. Ibid.
32. Ibid.
33. Schmid, Ronald F., N.D., *Traditional Foods are Your Best Medicine* (Vermont: Healing Arts Press, 1997), 39.
34. Pottenger, Francis M., M.D., *Pottenger's Cats* (La Mesa: Price-Pottenger Nutritional Foundation, 2nd Edition, 2005), 118.
35. Kirkpatrick, Sydney D. and Thurlbeck, Nancy, "Edgar Cayce's View of Health and Healing," 2004-2008, http://www.healingcancernaturally.com/edgar-cayce-health-healing.html.

CHAPTER 4:
THE PERFECTION OF WHOLE FOODS

1. Rubin, Jordan S., N.M.D., Ph.D. *The Maker's Diet* (Florida: Siloam, 2004), 31
2. Egan, Hope. *Holy Cow!* (Colorado: First Fruits of Zion, 2005), 12.
3. Ibid., 13.
4. Rose, Natalia. "Raw Food Life Force Energy," ereader.com, Excerpt from Raw Food Life Force Energy (Harper Collins, January 2, 2007), http://www.ereader.com/servlet/mw?t=book_excerpt&bookid=42987&si=59.
5. Hunt, Charles J., *The Christ Diet: Connect Your Cells to Your Soul* (California: Heartquake Publishing, 1992), 69.
6. Ibid.
7. Rose, Natalia. "Raw Food Life Force Energy," ereader.com, Excerpt from Raw Food Life Force Energy (Harper Collins, January 2, 2007), http://www.ereader.com/servlet/mw?t=book_excerpt&bookid=42987&si=59.
8. Hunt, Charles J., *The Christ Diet: Connect Your Cells to Your Soul* (California: Heartquake Publishing, 1992), 107-111.
9. Murray, Michael, N.D., *The Encyclopedia of Healing Foods* (New York: Atria Books, 2005), xi.
10. Balch, Phyllis, CNC., *Prescription for Nutritional Healing, 4th Edition* (New York: Avery Publishing Group, 2006), 12.

CHAPTER 5:
THE TRUTH AND NOTHING BUT THE
TRUTH ABOUT SUGAR AND FLOUR

1. Murray, Michael, N.D., and Pizzorno, Joseph N.D., and Pizzorno, Lara, M.A., L.M.T., *The Encyclopedia of Healing Foods* (New York: Atria Books, 2005), 69.
2. Ibid., 70
3. Appleton, Nancy, Ph.D., *Lick the Sugar Habit* (New York: Avery Penguin Putnam, 1996), 10-11.
4. Ibid., 17-18.
5. Ibid., 11.
6. Ibid., 22.
7. Warner, Melanie. "A Sweetener With a Bad Rap – New York Times," www.nytimes.com, July 2, 2006, http://www.nytimes.com/2006/07/02/business/yourmoney/02syrup.html?pagewanted=1.
8. Ibid.
9. Ibid.
10. Ibid.
11. Cohen, Mark Francis. "What's Worse Than Sugar." *AARP Bulletin*. April 2004, p. 24.
12. Starr Hull, Janet, Dr., *Splenda: Is It Safe Or Not?* (Texas: The Pickle Press, 2004), 5.
13. Wilson, Lawrence. "Food Additives." *Arizona Networking News*, December/January 2005, 1-2.
14. Starr Hull, Janet, Dr., *Splenda: Is It Safe Or Not?* (Texas: The Pickle Press, 2004), 10-11.
15. Gabbay, Simone, *Nourishing the Body Temple* (Virginia: ARE Press, 1999), 96-97.
16. Ibid., 98.
17. Ibid.
18. Ibid.
19. Higgins, Mary Meck, Ph.D, R.D., L.D., CDE. "Healthful Whole Grains!" Kansas State University, September 2002, 4.

CHAPTER 6:
THE BIG "FAT" LIE

1. McCullough, Fran, *The Good Fat Cookbook*, (New York: Scribner, 2003), 13.
2. Byrnes, Stephens, Dr. "The Neglected Nutritional Research of Dr. Weston Price, DDS," http://www.mercola.com/2001/jan/21/weston_price.htm.
3. Fallon, Sally W., M.A. and Enig, Mary, Ph.D. "The Truth About Saturated Fats." mercola.com, August 17, 2002, excerpt taken from *Nourishing Traditions: The Cookbook That Challenges Politically Correct Nutrition and the Diet Dictocrats*, second ed., (New Trends Publishing, 2000), http://www.mercola.com/2002/aug/17/saturated_fat1.htm#
4. Ibid.

5. Ibid.
6. Ibid.
7. Ibid.
8. Fallon, Sally W., M.A. and Enig, Mary, Ph.D. "The Great Con-ola." westonaprice.org, July 28, 2002, http://www.westonaprice.org/knowyourfats/conola.html
9. Ibid.
10. Ibid.
11. Ibid.
12. Ibid.
13. Ibid.
14. McCullough, Fran, *The Good Fat Cookbook*, (New York: Scribner, 2003), 25
15. Ibid.
16. Fallon, Sally W., M.A. and Enig, Mary, Ph.D. "The Truth About Saturated Fats." mercola.com, August 17, 2002, excerpt taken from *Nourishing Traditions: The Cookbook That Challenges Politically Correct Nutrition and the Diet Dictocrats*, second ed., (New Trends Publishing, 2000), http://www.mercola.com/2002/aug/17/saturated_fat1.htm#
17. Ibid.
18. BBC News World Edition. "Fish Oil Keeps Arteries Clear," February 7, 2003, http://news.bbc.co.uk/2/hi/health/2732647.stm
19. Fallon, Sally W., M.A. and Enig, Mary, Ph.D. "The Truth About Saturated Fats." mercola.com, August 17, 2002, excerpt taken from *Nourishing Traditions: The Cookbook That Challenges Politically Correct Nutrition and the Diet Dictocrats*, second ed., (New Trends Publishing, 2000), http://www.mercola.com/2002/aug/17/saturated_fat1.htm#

CHAPTER 7:
TRANS FATS: THE WORST NUTRITIONAL DISASTER IN HISTORY

1. Fallon, Sally W., M.A. and Enig, Mary, Ph.D. "The Truth About Saturated
2. Fats." mercola.com, August 17, 2002, excerpt taken from *Nourishing Traditions: The Cookbook That Challenges Politically Correct Nutrition and the Diet Dictocrats*, second ed., (New Trends Publishing, 2000), http://www.mercola.com/2002/aug/17/saturated_fat1.htm#
3. McCullough, Fran, *The Good Fat Cookbook*, (New York: Scribner, 2003), 35.
4. Ibid., 36.
5. Ibid., 34-35
6. Ibid., 37.

CHAPTER 8:
LIVING PROCESSED-FREE IN A PROCESSED FOOD WORLD

1. The Popcorn Agri-Chemical Handbook 2008 Edition, www.popcorn.org, The Popcorn Board, http://www.popcorn.org/handbook/handbook.cfm.

2. USFDA website, http://www.cfsan.fda.gov/~comm/tds-toc.html, accessed 12-6-08
3. Schecter, A., et el., "Congener-Specific Levels of Dioxins and Dibenzofurans in U.S. Food and Estimated Daily Dioxin Toxic Equivalent Intake." *Environmental Health Perspectives,* 1994, 102: 962-966.

CHAPTER 9:
FOOD ADDITIVES: WHAT'S SAFE AND WHAT'S NOT

1. Hoza Farlow, Christine, D.C., *Food Additives, A Shopper's Guide to What's Safe & What's Not* (KISS For Health Publishing: California, 2004), 12-13.
2. Ibid.
3. Balch, James, M.D, and Phyllis A. Balch, C.N.C., and. *Prescription for Nutritional Healing, 3rd Edition* (Garden City Park, NJ: Avery Publishing Group, 1997), 8.
4. Tuormaa, Tuula, E. "The Adverse Effects of Food Additives on Health." 1994, http://www.foresightpreconception.org/booklet_foodadditives.htm
5. Wilson, Lawrence. "Food Additives." *Arizona Networking News*, December/January 2005, 1-2.
6. Hickman, Martin. "Expert Links Additive to Cell Damage." http://news.indepent.co.uk/health/article2586652.ece.
7. Hoza Farlow, Christine, D.C., *Food Additives, A Shopper's Guide to What's Safe & What's Not* (KISS For Health Publishing: California, 2004), 18-70.
8. Dunham, Will. "Study Ties Cured Meats to Higher Lung Disease Risk", April 17, 2007, http://www.reuters.com.
9. Geis, Sonya. "Flavoring Suspected in Illness: California Considers Banning Chemical Used in Microwave Popcorn", May 7, 2007, p. A03, http://www.washingtonpost.com.
10. Harris, Gardiner. "Doctor Links a Man's Illness to Microwave Popcorn Habit," www.nytimes.com, September 5, 2007, http://www.nytimes.com/2007/09/05/us/05popcorn.html

CHAPTER 10:
ALKALINITY AND THE MOST IMPORTANT
FOODS FOR GOOD HEALTH

1. Lipsky, Elizabeth, M.S., C.C.N., *Digestive Wellness* (California: Keats Publishing, 1996), 4.

CHAPTER 11: PLAN-D SUPERFOODS

1. Holzapfel, Cynthia. *Apple Cider Vinegar for Weight Loss and Good Health* (Tennesee: Healthy Living Publications, 2002), 13.
2. McCullough, Fran, *The Good Fat Cookbook*, (New York: Scribner, 2003), 58.
3. Chappell, Mary Margaret. "South American Super Foods." *Vegetarian Times.*_

April 2008, p.76.

4. Ibid.
5. Murray, Michael, N.D., *The Encyclopedia of Healing Foods* (New York: Atria Books, 2005), 422.
6. Ibid.
7. McCullough, Fran, *The Good Fat Cookbook*, (New York: Scribner, 2003), 46.
8. Fallon, Sally W., M.A. and Enig, Mary, Ph.D. "Butter is Better." *Health Freedom News*. December 1995, 58.
9. Ibid., 59.
10. All-About-Lowering-Cholesterol.com, "Lowering Cholesterol With Avocado Fat," http://www.all-about-lowering-cholesterol.com/avocado-cholesterol-and-avocado-fat.html.
11. Ibid.
12. Gabbay, Simone. *Nourishing the Body Temple, Edgar Cayce's Approach to Nutrition* (ARE Press: Virginia, 1999), 82-83.
13. Murray, Michael, N.D., *The Encyclopedia of Healing Foods* (New York: Atria Books, 2005), 589-590.

CHAPTER 12:
PROCESSED-FREE VITAMINS

1. Obikoya, George, M.D. "Why take a Vitamin?" http://vitamins-nutrition.org/vitamins/why-take-vitamin.html
2. Shayne, Vic, Ph.D. "Symptoms of Vitamin B Deficiency: Why Vitamin Pills are Not Enough." chetday.com, 2005, http://www.chetday.com/vitaminbdeficiencies.html.

CHAPTER 13:
SWING YOUR ARMS AND BOUNCE

1. Rubin, Jordan S., N.M.D., PhD. *The Makers Diet* (Florida: Siloam, 2004), 174.
2. Health World Online, "Exercise Better Than Drugs to Lower Cholesterol – What Doctors Don't Tell You," 2002, http://www.healthy.net/scr/article.asp?Id=2893
3. Prosch, Gus J, Jr., M.D., "Twelve Vital Nutritional and Health Topics,"hbci.com, http://www.hbci.com/~wenonah/riddick/prosch12.htm, accessed December 21, 2008.
4. Gittleman, Ann Louise, M.S., C.N.S. *The Fat Flush Plan* (New York: McGraw-Hill, 2002), 93.
5. Prosch, Gus J, Jr., M.D., "Twelve Vital Nutritional and Health Topics,"hbci.com, http://www.hbci.com/~wenonah/riddick/prosch12.htm, accessed December 21, 2008.
6. Duggan, Sandra, R.N. *Edgar Cayce's Guide to Colon Care* (Virginia: Inner Vision Publishing Company), 21.

CHAPTER 14:
PLAN-D: A PLAN FOR BALANCED EATING AND LIVING

1. Ford, Debbie. *The Right Questions* (California: HarperSanFrancisco, 2003), 7-8.

Appendix A
GLOSSARY

FOOD ITEMS UTILIZED ON PLAN-D

Throughout this book there are a number of ingredients that may be new to you which are either referenced in chapter narratives or included in recipes. I have included a brief explanation of them for your clarification. Most of these items are available at regular grocery stores although some are more commonly sold at natural food stores.

- **Agave Nectar:** Agave nectar, (also referred to as agave juice), is extracted from agave cactus, and is suitable for any sweetening use. It is not as thick as honey and will not solidify. It pours quickly even when cold, and blends and dissolves easily in or on all foods. It is unrefined with a mild flavor and exceeds the sweetening power of white sugar thus requiring less of it when used as a substitute for sugar in recipes.
- **Carob:** Carob powder is obtained from the processing of pods from the carob tree. The powder which has a flour like consistency is used as a substitute for cocoa. It is caffeine and theobromine free, and thus does not have the stimulative effect of chocolate. It can be used in drinks, in baking, or boiled to create a honey-like syrup.
- **Flaxseed:** Flaxseeds are harvested from the flax plant, and are available as whole flaxseeds, ground flaxseed meal, or as flaxseed oil. Flaxseeds are rich in *alpha linolenic acid* (ALA), an omega-3 fat which can help reduce inflammation in the body which affects conditions such as asthma, osteoarthritis, rheumatoid arthritis, migraine headaches, and osteoporosis.
- **Quinoa:** Quinoa is a grain grown in the Andes Mountains of South America. It is light, tasty, and easy to digest, and contains more protein than any other grain - an average of 16.2% per serving. It is a complete protein which is also

high in essential linoleic acid, fiber, minerals, and vitamins.
- **Rapadura Sugar:** Rapadura sugar is a sweetener which is unbleached and unrefined and can be used in place of refined sugars. It is whole, pure, and organic dried sugar cane juice with a mild, caramel-like flavor. Its unique flavor and nutrient qualities are due to its method of processing which does not separate the sugar from its molasses content.
- **Sucanat:** Sucanat is similar to Rapadura sugar in taste and use. It is a close cousin to Rapadura, but contains less nutrients.
- **Tahini:** Tahini is a paste or nut butter that is made from ground sesame seeds. It has a strong flavor and high fat content and is typically used in hummus recipes.
- **Tamari Sauce (Wheat-Free, reduced sodium):** Tamari sauce is a soy sauce made from whole soybeans, sea salt, water, and koji (Aspergillus hacho). It is thicker and a darker brown than regular soy sauce, and has a smooth, rich flavor to it. Some tamari sauces contain wheat, however I recommend using the wheat-free variety.
- **Tempeh:** Tempeh is similar to tofu as it is made from soybeans that are cultured and fermented into a cake form. However, tempeh is a whole soybean product that gives it a firmer texture and stronger flavor. Tempeh is also higher in protein, fiber, and vitamin content than tofu.
- **Tofu:** Tofu, also known as bean curd, is made typically made from coagulated soy milk, although some tofu is made from almonds or black beans. The resulting curds are then pressed into blocks of tofu. Tofu, besides being low in calories and having no cholesterol, contains many nutrients including iron, protein, magnesium, and calcium. Tofu on its own does not have a particular taste but instead absorbs and reflects the other ingredients with which it is cooked.

Appendix B
RESOURCES

RESOURCE LIST

Below is a list of resources you may be interested in checking out. While not endorsing specific manufacturers or products, the following websites are good sources of general health and nutrition information.

1. **Plan-D Website: www.plandee.org**
   - I invite you to visit our Plan-D website. There you can find new recipes, great articles and up-to-date nutrition information. We also have a forum, audio programs, video clips, and a link to receive The Center for Processed-Free Living's monthly Nutrition e-Newsletter.
   - We also have a calendar listing of free events and upcoming Plan-D workshops. There is also a special place for you to submit your own Plan-D success story and your own recipes.

2. **The Center for Processed-Free Living: www.processedfreeliving.org**
   - The Center for Processed-Free Living is the non-profit organization that owns the Plan-D program, which includes the book you are holding, its accompanying cookbook, and the Plan-D DVD. The Center's mission is to eliminate childhood and adult obesity through nutrition education. At the time of this writing, the Center has conducted over a dozen nutrition education classes at Boys and Girls Clubs throughout the Phoenix, Arizona metropolitan area. It is my desire to have these classes be offered all over the United States and beyond.
   - If you'd like to help me with my wish, please visit our website. There you can sign up to help and receive the Center's very popular Nutrition e-Newsletter.

3. Overeaters Anonymous (OA): www.oa.org
- Overeaters Anonymous (OA) is a support-based program that helps people who want to stop eating compulsively, and those who suffer from bulimia and anorexia. OA is not a diet club and does not endorse any particular plan of eating. It deals instead with underlying causes and recommends using a plan of eating that best suits each individual. Patterned after the 12-Step program of Alcoholics Anonymous, the basis of the OA program addresses physical, emotional and spiritual well-being.
- There are OA meetings in every part of the world, and in nearly every city in the United States. Many on-line and telephone meetings are also available. There are no dues or fees for membership, no weighing in at meetings, and no one is too fat or too thin to be welcome. OA provides valuable support from other members and has helped thousands to recover from compulsive eating.

4. Braggs Health Products and Books: www.bragg.com
- Dr. Paul C. Bragg, Life Extension Specialist, was the founder of the American Health Movement. His daughter, Patricia Bragg, N.D., Ph.D, continues to carry on her father's work taking the Bragg Healthy Lifestyle message worldwide. The Bragg website is a great resource to locate all of the Bragg products, books, and current health related information.

5. Environmental Working Group (EWG): www.ewg.org
- EWG is a non-profit organization whose mission is to help protect our environment and public health by the distribution of public information. The EWG staff investigates data which relates to potential health and environmental threats and shares this information with the general public. As explained on their website, EWG provides practical information that will assist your efforts to protect the health and well-being your family and community.
- You can download a printable wallet guide of the EWG's *Dirty Dozen* and *Clean 15* at **www.foodnews.org**. Carry the list in your purse or pocket when you go shopping.

6. Weston A. Price Foundation: www.westonaprice.org
- The Weston A. Price Foundation supports the use of modern technology to promote the use of science and traditional farming methods as a force to help improve our environment and human health. Per this website, information is provided about "accurate nutrition instruction, organic and biodynamic farming, pasture-feeding of livestock, community-supported farms, honest and informative labeling, prepared parenting and nurturing therapies."

7. Price-Pottenger Nutrition Foundation: www.ppnf.org
- The Price-Pottenger Foundation, a public, non-profit educational resource

organization, is the guardian of the archival materials from Dr. Weston A. Price and Dr. Francis M. Pottenger, Jr.'s research. The Foundation also maintains a library of over 10,000 historical and contemporary references. Additionally, as stated on their website, the foundation "provides accurate information about whole foods and proper preparation techniques, soil improvement, natural farming and pure water, preventing disease and birth defects, avoiding personality disturbances and delinquency, enhancing the environment, and enabling all people to achieve long life and excellent health."

8. **Tropical Traditions: www.tropicaltraditions.com**
   - This is the ideal source for the purchase of coconut oil at bulk discount prices. They also produce a wide range of organic food products, skin care products, home care items, supplements, and healthy oils.

9. **Vitacost.com: www.vitacost.com**
   - This site offers top brand vitamins at significantly lower prices than retail. The site is a source of nutrition- and body care-related products, from name-brand manufacturers including Garden of Life, New Chapter, and Natural Factors in addition to other brands.

10. **Patapar Paper Source: www.baar.com**
    - Baar Products is the official supplier of Edgar Cayce health care products. You can order Patapar paper at a reasonable price from this site. Just type in the name of the item in the search box on the top left side of the site for the link to the product. The site also offers nutritional supplements, books, and natural beauty products.
    - Baar Products is the only source of CayceCare products—unique products and remedies drawn from the work of Edgar Cayce. Cayce, considered by many to be the Father of Modern Holistic Medicine, produced a tremendous legacy of information about the human body.

11. **Association for Research and Enlightenment (A.R.E.): www.are.org**
    - Edgar Cayce's Association for Research and Enlightenment (A.R.E.), the nonprofit founded by Cayce in 1931, houses the entire set of 14,306 readings in a database available through the association's website. The readings can also be found in their entirety in their onsite library, located at the headquarters in Virginia Beach, Virginia, which is open to the public daily.

12. **A.R.E. Integrative Medical and Wellness Center (formerly The A.R.E. Clinic): www.arecenter.org**
    - The A.R.E. Integrative Medical and Wellness Center, located in Scottsdale, Arizona, is a nonprofit medical clinic with a focus on Conventional and Alternative Medicine, as well as related Education and Outreach. The clinic offers a wide range of medical services and bodywork. Integrative Medicine advocates a blend of both conventional and alternative treatments. These

include what you would expect to find at your every day doctor's office, and those that you might not. The idea is to treat more than just the body, but also the mind and spirit.

- The A.R.E. Center derives much of its information on Holistic Medicine from the prominent 20th Century American Psychic, Edgar Cayce, who through clairvoyant diagnosis found alternative treatments for many diseases and ailments. His 14,000 readings have been compiled and analyzed to build a branch of medicine far more comprehensive than conventional medicine alone, by treating the person as a whole, rather than just the body. At the A.R.E. Integrative Medical & Wellness Center, doctors and practitioners work along side clients to promote healing, and greater wellness of body, mind, and spirit.

Appendix C
HOLISTIC NUTRITION EDUCATION RESOURCES

I have received many e-mails and phone calls from people asking me about the type of training I received and how to become a holistic nutrition professional. For their benefit, I wrote a synopsis of the curriculum I took to become certified.

If you have a passion for healthy eating, cooking, or teaching and want to channel that passion into a career, or if you simply want to expand your own personal knowledge of nutrition to improve your health and the health of your family, this information may help you decide if formal training is for you.

BAUMAN COLLEGE

In 2001 I attended a satellite campus of Bauman College (formerly called The Institute for Educational Therapy) in Sacramento, California. The main campus is located in Penngrove, California, just north of San Francisco near the wine country. The college now has three satellite campuses located in Berkeley and Santa Cruz (both in California), and Boulder, Colorado, as well as a self-paced distance learning program for those who cannot attend one of the campuses. The satellite campus in Sacramento no longer exists.

Bauman College is a holistic nutrition school that offers nutrition education programs that train individuals to become Nutrition Educators, Nutrition Consultants, and Natural Chefs. The curriculum will quickly expand your basic knowledge of nutrition and dispel the nutrition myths that keep many people from experiencing optimal health. You will learn how your body operates and how its functions are affected by the foods you eat.

The programs offered at Bauman College have been revamped in recent years. At the time I attended there were three programs offered in nutrition—Diet Counselor (200 hours), Nutrition Educator (200 hours), and Nutrition Consultant (400 hours). I attended the Diet Counselor program and the Nutrition Educator program. The 200-hour Diet Counselor program is no longer offered separately; instead its coursework has been combined with the coursework for what used to be the 200-hour Nutrition Educator program into a new 400-hour program called Nutrition Educator.

SYNOPSIS OF MY BAUMAN COLLEGE EDUCATION
Diet Counselor
The Diet Counselor training involved courses in learning about different types of diets. We had quizzes for every course, wrote papers, and had homework activities that involved working with real clients. We also did presentations in front of the class and had a written final exam at the end of the program. Here's a synopsis of the classes:

- **Changing Trends in Nutrition** – This was a study of an emerging shift in American dietary patterns toward the use of whole foods, nutritive condiments and food supplements to provide essential micronutrients lacking in the Standard American Diet (SAD). I also learned about the government-endorsed dietary guidelines for heart disease and cancer prevention espoused by the Surgeon General.
- **Personal Diet Planning** – In this course I learned the specific keys to working with one's relationship to food and to methods of formulating personal diet plans. I was challenged to critique many of the current dietary philosophies. I also learned the properties of various foods and culinary herbs, as well as how to substitute healthy foods for poor quality non-foods. I learned how to design eating plans for health conditions using food and supplements. For homework I had to experiment with different food plans to ascertain personally which foods and lifestyle habits provide optimal support for my own body, mind and spirit.
- **Keys to Successful Weight Management** - I actually had a thing or two to teach them about this area, but in this course I learned about how to address the issues of eating disorders, obesity, overweight, and weight loss. Bauman College is of the philosophy that *diets do not work*, and that learning to practice responsible eating and lifestyle habits empower clients to feel better as they shape up. In addition to the physical aspects of weight management, I also studied the factors of emotional and social problems associated with being overweight or underweight.
- **Cross Cultural Health Systems** - In this course I explored several key aspects that contribute to wellness or illness, such as one's constitution, ancestral heritage, blood typing, metabolism, and cultural influences. Oriental healing systems were studied to demonstrate the similarities and differences between Eastern and Western approaches to healing. I learned about the cultural as well as the medicinal foods and herbs that contribute to balance and recovery from illness and injury.
- **Cooking for Health** - This was one of my favorite classes because we learned how to do cooking demonstrations while teaching others how to eat healthy. Each person in the class had to demo a recipe and tell all of the health aspects of

the ingredients being used. Of all the classes I have taken, this is the one that I am using on the most regular basis, as I teach cooking and food prep classes to my clients and students to help them understand how to shop and prepare food to satisfy their need for flavor, zest, and ethnic and emotional appeal.

- **Allergy and Immune Support** - I studied the Model of the Allergy Cycle as it demonstrates the relationship between stress, toxins, trauma, mal-nutrition and chronic allergy patterns.
- **Herbal Preparation** - This was a great hands-on class where I learned about plant biochemistry and energetic action. I learned the therapeutic use of herbs for regeneration and each person in the class made their own herbal first aid kit. I learned how to make salves, tinctures, tea blends and custom herbal formulas.
- **Interview and Research Skills** – This was a most valuable course on how to conduct a client intake to assess their nutritional needs. I also learned skills for investigating nutritional research and health conditions.

Nutrition Educator

The Nutrition Educator courses were more rigorous and scientific in nature. We did several research papers for every course and we had to do a final thesis research paper on a particular topic of interest. I did mine on colon disorders as they relate to diet (everything relates to diet!) As in the Diet Counselor program, we presented all of our research papers as formal lectures in front of the class.

- **Digestive Physiology** - I learned all about the digestive system—the anatomy of the digestive tract and the major functions of each organ. This was the world of digestive enzymes and hormones, bacterial action, and metabolism of proteins, fats, and carbohydrates.
- **Macronutrients** - Macronutrients are carbohydrates, fats, and proteins. I learned about the chemical nature and classification of the macronutrients and also the types and functions of fiber in the diet. In this course I also learned the basic chemical classifications, structures, reactions, and functions of fats and oils. Everything I always wanted to know about saturated vs. unsaturated, cholesterol, triglycerides and essential fatty acids. I also learned about amino acids, and the challenges and opportunities of a vegetarian diet. A homework assignment was to experimentally vary my choices of proteins, fats, and carbohydrates and observe any changes in mood, energy, and productivity. I learned that I don't need very much animal protein at all and that I can thrive on a diet consisting mainly of plant-based protein sources.
- **MicroNutrients** – Micronutrients are the vitamins and minerals that are embedded in the macronutrients. Each person in the class had to write several reports on the vitamins and minerals, stating their history and discovery, features, physiologic functions, route of absorption, transport, and storage, significant food sources, signs of excess and deficiency, RDA, and optimal and toxic levels of particular nutrients. We also devised menu plans featuring foods rich in micronutrients for our classmates and clients.
- **Nutritional Assessment and Therapy** - This is another class that I use in my daily practice for one-on-one nutrition counseling. In this course I learned how

to evaluate a client's diet using research methods, computerized diet evaluations, hair analysis, and urine pH analysis.

- **Nutrition and the Life Cycle** – In this course I learned specific nutritional demands for different times of life such as pregnancy, menopause, aging, childhood, etc.
- **Business Practices** - I learned how to write a business and marketing plan, mission statement, vision statement, etc.
- **Final Paper** – Instead of having a written final exam, each person in the class had to write and present a final research paper at the end of the program.

My time at Bauman College was one of the most valuable and memorable experiences of my life. I learned so much about food, the body, and how to help others change their diets, and in essence their lives. Some of the most valuable aspects of the training for me were the presentations that I had to give in front of the class, the eclectic variety of reading material, and the guidelines for successful diet counseling. I looked forward to my classes every week—just being with the instructors and my classmates in the environment of learning a healthful approach to life was so affirming. It nurtured my spirit and filled me in ways that have continued to keep my passion burning.

To Contact Bauman College:
Bauman College
10151 Main Street Ste. 128, Penngrove, CA 94951
800-987-7530
www.baumancollege.org

CLAYTON COLLEGE OF NATURAL HEALTH

Clayton College of Natural Health (CCNH) offers bachelor's degrees, master's degrees, and Ph.D.'s in holistic nutrition. Some of my classmates from Bauman College have obtained advanced degrees in holistic nutrition from Clayton College, and have highly recommended it.

CCNH is a self-paced distance learning institution offering certification and degree programs in a variety of natural health disciplines. The self-paced distance learning programs allow students all over the world to pursue an innovative high quality education in natural health. From their website:

"People from all walks of life, from health and fitness professionals to stay-at-home parents, have discovered this convenient and revolutionary way to attend an established natural health school. If you have ever dreamed of starting a career as a natural health consultant, this is your opportunity to make that dream come true by attending a respected holistic health school."

Clayton College of Natural Health
2140 11th Avenue South, Suite 305, Birmingham, AL 35205
Admissions: 1-800-995-4590
www.ccnh.edu

Index

Breinigsville, PA USA
23 June 2010
240465BV00001B/28/P